Psychiatry in Context
EXPERIENCE, MEANING & COMMUNITIES

Philip Thomas

PCCS Books

Books

First published 2014

PCCS BOOKS
The Wyastone Business Park
Wyastone Leys
Monmouth
NP25 3SR
contact@pccs-books.co.uk
www.pccs-books.co.uk

Psychiatry in Context: Experience, Meaning and Communities

British Library Cataloguing in Publication data: a catalogue record for this book
is available from the British Library.

ISBN 978 1 906254 72 8

Cover photographs of fabrics by Philip Thomas
Cover designed in the UK by Old Dog Graphics
Typeset in the UK by Old Dog Graphics
Printed by Lightning Source

Contents

Preface

The design on the front of this book incorporates illustrations of textiles from around the world, from places that I have been fortunate to visit during my career. Kente cloth (top left) was the textile of the Ashanti kings of West Africa. Woven of cotton and silk, it was worn at times of high ceremony; its patterns and figures have symbolic meanings. The Sindhi mirror textile (top centre) is richly embroidered with gold thread and hundreds of tiny glass mirrors on a black background. It was bought in a wonderfully chaotic market full of heat, dust and voices in Karachi. The Guinea brocade (top right) also comes from West Africa, in this case The Gambia. It is a sophisticated cotton textile incorporating spiral patterns woven into the fabric, which is then dyed using the process of batik. This example is known as kingfisher. The woollen kirking shawl (second row, centre) was made in Edinburgh in the mid-nineteenth century. It was traditionally worn by a mother on her first attendance at church following the birth of a child. Finally there is a piece of woven cotton fabric from the beautiful Spanish colonial town of Flores in Guatemala, situated on an island in the middle of the Lago Petén Itzá, close to the border with Belize. It was bought in a small shop run as a collective by a group of women of Mayan heritage, and shows a man playing a marimba.

These beautiful textiles symbolise two issues that are at the heart of this book. The first is that of human difference, the fact that we live in an increasingly diverse world. Despite the increasing 'homogenisation' of culture, its reduction to a set of 'rational' universals that within neoliberalism serve primarily the commercial interests of the large multinationals, our societies are paradoxically becoming more diverse. Other tensions in globalisation are resulting in national boundaries becoming porous. Britain along with other European countries is becoming increasingly culturally diverse. Over 300 different languages are spoken by London schoolchildren (Baker & Eversley, 2000), and a recent briefing paper using Labour Force Survey data collected in London found that 18 per cent of the capital's population spoke a first language other than English at home (Greater London Authority, 2006). Many of these people were forced to flee their countries of origin to escape war, destruction and persecution. Their stories are told through a heterogeneity of languages, of faith traditions, of folklore, myth and meaning, and this leads to the second issue; the central position of stories and narratives in our lives. Narrative is at the heart of how we make sense of our experiences, and one of the main purposes of this book is to show how this is true of states of psychosis and distress. This is why the word 'context' is so important.

We use the word every day without pausing to think about what it means, but it is important that I am clear about the meaning I have in mind when I use the word in this book. *The Shorter Oxford English Dictionary* (*SOED*, 2007) gives the origin of the word from the Latin contexere, meaning to weave together. The word's origin is tied to the metaphor of weaving. The Latin word texere, meaning to weave, is also the root of our word 'text'. We weave fabrics, and in a similar manner we weave stories. It gives a linguistic sense to the modern usage of the word 'context' as 'the part or parts immediately preceding or following a passage or word as determining, or helping to reveal its meaning ...' (*SOED*, 2007: 504). It is the sense of weaving and meaning that lie at the heart of the way I use the word in this book. Contexts are indispensable if we are to understand human experience. It is by examining contexts, what preceded an activity, what followed on from it, that we begin to grasp the meaning and significance of human acts as we grapple with the meaning of the stories we encounter in clinical practice.

Stories are deeply embedded in our cultural traditions, and psychiatry, as Lewis (2011) points out, is full of them, from stories about the dopamine theory of schizophrenia, to stories of adversity and trauma. Stories about weaving abound in myth and folklore: Penelope weaving a shroud to keep her suitors at bay when her husband Odysseus was on his travels; Tennyson's Lady of Shalott who weaved images at her loom of a world she could only see reflected in her mirror; or the Grimm brothers' tale of the six swans. But the story that resonates most powerfully with the moral purpose of this book is that of Philomela in Ovid's *Metamorphoses*. It (Ovid, 1986) describes how Procne, wife of the warrior king Tereus of Thrace, asked her husband to travel to Greece to bring back her sister, Philomela, whom she longed to see. Tereus sailed to Athens where he presented his wife's request to King Pandion, the father of the two sisters. Pandion had misgivings about letting his only other daughter out of his protection. He told Tereus that Philomela could go on condition that he protected her as he would his own daughter. However, from the first moment that Tereus set eyes upon Philomela he was seized with passion for her, and when they arrived back in Thrace he imprisoned her in a remote cabin where he raped her. He warned her not to tell anyone what had happened, but she refused to promise this, so in his rage, Tereus cut out Philomela's tongue, rendering her speechless.

Determined to let the world know of the terrible thing that had been inflicted upon her, she wove a tapestry in which she told the full story, and sent it to Procne. Upon discovering what had happened to her sister, Procne was so incensed that she murdered her son by Tereus, boiled his body, and served it as a meal to her husband. When he finished the meal, she then presented him with their son's severed head. Tereus was intent on revenge and pursued the two sisters. Just as he was about to catch them, the Gods interceded, turning Procne into a swallow, and Philomela, a nightingale.

The stories of many people who use mental health services in the twenty-first century are not unlike Philomela's story. They are accounts of struggles for justice, for narratives of adversity, suffering and trauma to be heard and witnessed by others. This book, I hope, creates a space and a clearing for listening to and hearing these stories, and thus for healing.

This book is dedicated to the memory of Terry McLaughlin and Ian Murray.

Acknowledgements

Over the years many voices have shaped my ideas about psychiatry, especially those of people who were my patients, starting when I did my training at the Royal Edinburgh Hospital. Some of the most influential of these encounters occurred early in my career as a consultant at Manchester Royal Infirmary. Every Tuesday afternoon I had what was euphemistically called a 'continuing care clinic' in the long-demolished Hulme Clinic. Two or three memorable individuals taught me the importance of listening carefully to their stories, especially their experiences of medication. It was there that I took the first faltering steps in learning how to work with service users over months and years to help them reduce or discontinue their long-term neuroleptic medication. And outside the walls of the clinic and the hospital, people in the Black communities of Moss Side and Alexandra Park told me about the role that psychiatry played in their lives, and especially the lives of their young people, and of their fears about mental health services. The stories and experiences of dozens of patients it has been my privilege to try to help formed the matrix out of which the stories in Chapters 8, 9 and 10 came into being.

As I was exposed to all these influences I began to discover that many other psychiatrists had had similar experiences, shared the same concerns, and were starting to work in similar ways. Over the last fifteen years, especially since I wrote my tyro's book, *The Dialectics of Schizophrenia*, agreements and disagreements with friends and colleagues closely associated with the Critical Psychiatry Network (CPN) have played a vital role in the development of my ideas. In my view CPN is the single most important professional development in British psychiatry to have occurred since 1971 (the year the Royal College of Psychiatrists came into being), and it is gratifying to see its ideas influencing thought across the Atlantic, in Europe and Australia and New Zealand. That said, what you will read in these pages represents my own views, and there will no doubt be many in the Critical Psychiatry Network who will disagree with some of what I have to say.

As far as individuals are concerned, Pat Bracken in particular continues to be a great source of encouragement and constructive criticism. I have learnt a great deal from Pat over the last twenty years, and his wise hand has guided my reading and understanding of what little philosophy I have grappled with. Since he moved back to Ireland in 2003, I have really missed our long evening discussions in the New Beehive pub in Bradford about Foucault, Heidegger, Wittgenstein and Merleau-Ponty! I am particularly grateful to him for his helpful and constructive criticism about Chapter 6.

Several other people have been kind enough to comment and offer constructive criticism on various chapters. Joanna Moncrieff, whose painstaking academic investigations of the role of drug treatments in psychiatry is in my view the single most important outcome of critical psychiatry thus far, offered helpful critical comments on Chapter 3. I am especially grateful to Eleanor Longden who, busy though she was writing up her PhD thesis, managed to find time to offer valuable comments on Chapter 4. Suman Fernando, whose writing over the last thirty years in my opinion represents the first flourishing of Critical Psychiatry in Britain, was kind enough to offer critical comments about Chapter 5. I am also grateful to Jayasree Kalathil and Mohammad Shabbir, both of whom made helpful comments about Chapter 8.

I am particularly grateful to Andy Smith and Eleanor Dace for their forthright and helpful comments on Chapter 11, and the ideas contained within this chapter benefited from discussion with Louise Pembroke over many years. Chapter 12 benefited from the unique insights and experience of Marius Romme and Sandra Escher, as well as that of Jacqui Dillon whose work nationally and internationally has inspired many service users and professionals. Marius and Sandra's work has had a great influence on my thinking over the years, and along with Joanna Moncrieff's work will prove to be of historic significance. Salma Yasmeen and Mohammad Shabbir, whose work at the community development project Sharing Voices Bradford has inspired me since 2002, offered constructive comments on Chapter 13.

Heather Allan and Pete Sanders at PCCS Books provided tremendous help and support over the two years it took to write this book. Pete gave me incredible latitude as my editor (although I'm not sure if that is how he sees his role). He let me get on with it, didn't interfere, but was always on hand to offer advice that invariably glittered with gentle wit and wisdom. His impeccable sense of style and tone really helped to smooth off many rough edges in this work. The final manuscript benefited enormously from Sandy Green's close scrutiny. I am also very grateful to Alastair Thomas and Chris Wrench at Creative Graphics for assisting with some of the figures. Finally, one person alone witnessed the frustration, passion, despair, elation, defeat, obstinacy and day-to-day tedium that it is to live through a project like this: my wife, Stella. Without her love, belief and support I would never have managed it.

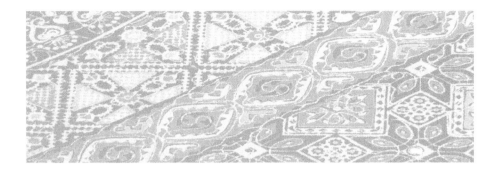

Section 1

The Problems of the Technological Paradigm

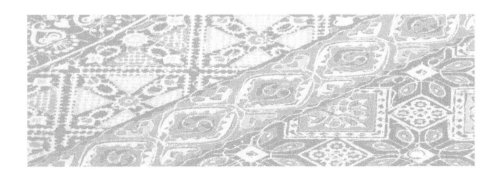

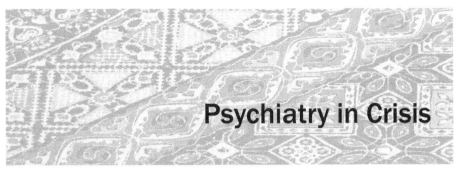

Psychiatry in Crisis 1

Of all tyrannies, a tyranny sincerely exercised for the good
of its victims may be the most oppressive.

C.S. Lewis, *God in the Dock*

These are deeply unsettling times for the profession of psychiatry. It is in the midst of a crisis. Or perhaps it is more accurate to say that it is in the midst of a number of crises, some closer to home than others. Evidence of turmoil is to be found in many places. Much of it originates within the profession, in the writings of British psychiatrists in the pages of the *British Journal of Psychiatry*. But the fissures that are opening up are deep, and extend beyond these shores. This is no local difficulty. They are apparent in the furore that greeted the publication of the fifth edition of the American Psychiatric Association's *Diagnostic and Statistical Manual* (*DSM*) in May 2013, and across the globe in the pharmaceutical industry's retreat from funding research in new drugs for psychiatry. There are even signs that the profession is reconsidering the status of drug therapies in psychiatry. Peter Tyrer, the editor of the *British Journal of Psychiatry*, recently wrote of 'the end of the psychopharmacological revolution' (Tyrer, 2012: 168). For fifty years the pharmaceutical industry and profession have maintained a liaison that both would prefer to have kept hidden beneath the sheets. Now there is talk of a split, and evidence that the pharmaceutical industry too is in 'crisis' (Sanders, 2013). The industry has significantly reduced new investment into the identification and development of new drugs for depression, bipolar disorder and schizophrenia (Hyman, 2013).

Some of the reasons for this emerged in a recent editorial in the journal *Schizophrenia Bulletin* which started as follows:

> The data are in, and it is clear that a massive experiment has failed: despite decades of research and billions of dollars invested, not a single mechanistically novel drug has reached the psychiatric market in more than 30 years. (Fibiger, 2012: 649)

The author, Christian Fibiger, is a psychopharmacologist whose life has been spent in the search for new drugs for psychiatric disorders. He has held academic appointments at the University of British Columbia, and more recently in the pharmaceutical industry with companies such as Lilly Research Laboratories and Amgen. His editorial confirms that most major pharmacological companies are abandoning the search for new drugs in psychiatry. One of the tasks of this book is to examine why it is that this 'experiment' has failed, and what opportunities this presents for new directions for psychiatry.

As well as psychiatry, mental health services in England are in crisis, with a desperate shortage of beds in acute psychiatric units across the country. An investigation by *Community Care* magazine found that across the country over 1,700 acute psychiatric beds have been cut over the last two years (McNicoll, 2013). Consequently many patients are admitted to units hundreds of miles from their families and communities. The government claims that bed losses have been necessary to fund more community resources, but it is difficult not to believe that the real reason for bed losses has to do with the recession following the cataclysmic economic crisis of 2008.

The recession has had far-reaching consequences across the globe. In the UK it has resulted in savage cuts in public spending on social security, health and education. The effect of these cuts is felt most acutely through changes to the benefit system for people who use mental health services, those who have the most profound experiences of marginalisation, alienation and exclusion; people whose lives are lived against a backdrop of poverty, fear and adversity. The effects of stigma on the lives of people who use mental health services have been well known for many years. But the recession has brought with it a malediction from the government and the 'popular' media. Political leaders have kindled a debate, the rhetoric of which is redolent of the 'worthy' and 'unworthy' poor of the Elizabethan Act for the Relief of the Poor of 1601. This rhetoric is echoed on the front pages of the tabloid press – '4M scrounging families in Britain' declared the headline in the *Express* on 2nd September 2011.[1] According to the Association of Chief Police Officers, disability hate crime in England and Wales has almost doubled in three years, from just over 1,000 reported incidents in 2009, to just under 2,000 in 2011 (*The Guardian*, 2012a). Many of those affected are people who are long-term users of mental health services.

At the same time income inequality has grown faster in the UK than in any other rich country (Ramesh, 2011). A report from the Organisation for Economic Co-operation and Development (OECD) found that the ratio between the average annual income of the richest 10 per cent of the population and the poorest 10 per cent in the UK had increased from 8 to 1 in 1985 to 12 to 1 in 2008 (OECD, 2011). And while the economic crisis ratchets up income inequality, health inequalities linked to

1. http://www.express.co.uk/news/uk/268681/4m-scrounging-families-in-Britain. Accessed on 8th November 2013.

income inequality continue to grow unchecked (Pickett & Wilkinson, 2013).

In the first chapter of *Anatomy of an Epidemic*, Bob Whitaker (2010) draws attention to the extraordinary increase in people in the USA struggling with disability. He points out that since the 1990s increasing numbers of people suffering from depression and bipolar disorders feature in government disability figures. By 2010 there was an estimated 1.4 million such people of working age receiving federal payments for affective disorder. This increase occurred over the same period of time that prescriptions for psychiatric drugs exploded. Broadly similar figures are to be found in the UK. There is evidence that between 2000 and 2013 there has been a 41 per cent increase in the number of people claiming benefits of one sort or another (up from 725,000 to 1,021,000) who have a mental health problem (James Davies, personal communication, January, 2014). This suggests that psychiatric drugs are having little impact on the number of people claiming benefits. It points to the ineffectiveness of psychiatric interventions.

Although these crises appear to be unrelated, they act as threads that draw together and bind several themes that run through this book. But for the moment I want to return to the crisis in psychiatry by examining recent papers published in the *British Journal of Psychiatry* that set out contrasting views on the matter. It is important that I acknowledge that I was a co-author of one of these so what I have to say about the crisis represents my own position.

The Crisis in Psychiatry

The last five years have been remarkable on account of four special articles or editorials published in Britain's leading academic journal of psychiatry, the British Journal of Psychiatry. The first of these (Craddock *et al*, 2008) was co-authored by thirty-seven people, evidence of the strength of feeling and agreement about the issues raised, and their appeal at least in some sections of the profession. It argued that psychiatry faces an identity crisis brought about by a 'downgrading' of core elements of medical care in psychiatry, such as the belief that the profession offers specific treatments based in diagnosis. This is seen in the '… uneasiness in colleagues in defending the medical model of care …' (Craddock *et al*, 2008: 6) and subtle shifts in language exemplified by a move away from the use of the word 'patient' to 'service user'. They identify a number of factors they consider to be important in understanding how this happened. These include a broadening of the concept of 'mental illness', especially the trend to include more people with relatively 'mild symptoms' in the concept. This has diverted attention away from those with 'severe mental disorders' for whom demedicalisation of their problems is 'damaging' or even 'life threatening'. One consequence of this is that it undermines the priority of serious mental illness for those responsible for commissioning and purchasing mental health services.

Other factors that threaten the medical identity and status of the profession include scepticism within the profession towards the value of biomedical studies of mental illness. They also refer to interprofessional rivalries between psychiatrists and other professional groups in mental health, as well as the provision of services that assume that severe mental illness signifies chronicity and poor outcome. They continue:

> The net effect of these influences, however, is the same: to obstruct our primary medical duty towards patients with severe psychiatric disorders. Hence, it is imperative that we take action to ensure that patients with mental illness are not disadvantaged compared with others within the National Health Service (NHS). (*ibid*: 7)

They claim that patients have a right to expect more than what they describe as 'non-specific psychosocial support'.

They regard the changing interprofessional relationships between psychiatrists and other staff working in mental health services as a particular threat to the profession of psychiatry. They are referring here to New Ways of Working, a programme of work undertaken jointly by the Royal College of Psychiatrists and the Department of Health (Department of Health, 2005a), which they see as an attack on medical leadership in multidisciplinary teamwork in psychiatry. The traditional relationship between general practitioner (GP) and hospital specialist was based historically in the right of the GP to refer patients to hospital specialists of her or his choice. This specialist then assumed responsibility for the patient's care. The distributed model of care supported by *New Ways of Working* means that not all people referred to an 'anonymous team' for specialist mental health care would be assessed by a consultant psychiatrist.

The paper then goes on to propose a view of psychiatry as a 'medicine of the brain', in which psychiatric patients should expect '… prompt and accurate diagnosis followed by implementation of appropriate evidence-based treatment – much as is expected by the cardiology patients of today' (Craddock *et al*, 2008: 8). They promise that, in future, major advances in molecular biology and neuroscience will provide psychiatry with '… powerful tools that help to delineate the biological systems involved in psychopathology and impairments suffered by patients' (*ibid*: 8). In the future they claim these developments will yield diagnostic approaches with improved biological validity that will be useful in predicting treatment response, and they hold out the promise of '… completely novel treatments … based on detailed understanding of pathogenesis' (*ibid*: 8).

The second paper to appear was that written by Bullmore and colleagues (2009). They agree with many of the points raised by Craddock *et al*, but their paper focuses more specifically on what they see as the central role of neuroscience in psychiatry. It is a call for psychiatry as a modern and progressive medical speciality '… fully engaged with the science of the brain.' (Bullmore *et al*, 2009: 293). They assert that neuroscience is central to the use of drugs in psychiatry, which is one of the profession's '... defining operational characteristic[s] ...' (*ibid*: 293). They are, however, concerned about the profession's reluctance to embrace the theoretical and therapeutic potential of neuroscience. They set out a model of scientific analysis that they consider to be helpful in formulating '... integrated mind–brain models that incorporate both the genotype and its expression in hierarchical and complex phenotypes of the brain ...' (*ibid*: 293), as well as interactions between the physical and social environments. I will return to this shortly. They do, however, admit that it may take several decades of effort for the therapeutic benefits of the new neuroscience to be realised. And this is despite their acknowledgement that current physical models of mental function are, to use their words, 'scientifically primitive'. Nevertheless they believe that such is the pace of theoretical and technological developments in neuroscience that this will change. In support of this assertion they give as an example the acceptance within the profession that ventricular enlargement (or brain shrinkage) is a cardinal feature of schizophrenia. Although many in the profession were initially reluctant to accept this view, they claim that the evidence for cortical atrophy in schizophrenia has been established beyond doubt by the latest generation of brain imaging technologies.

They also reject the accusation that neuroscientific accounts of psychosis are reductionist, arguing that systems biology and 'modern complexity theory' will provide non-reductionist explanations of the interactions between genes, molecules and cells in understanding the '... integrated hierarchical phenotype ...' of psychiatric disorders (*ibid*: 294). Complexity here refers not to aspects of behaviour, but to its biological correlates. They reject the fear that neuroscience gives rise to a form of reductionism that results in what they call 'soulless' psychiatric practice. They see this as an objection raised by those possessed by the 'admirable determination' to respect the uniquely personal aspects of psychosis but they claim that this is no argument against a neuroscientific psychiatry.

The third paper by Oyebode and Humphreys (2011) sees the crisis in terms of a threat to the existence of psychiatry. Like apothecaries, psychiatrists may become extinct, a professional blind alley, an evolutionary dead-end. They restate many of the concerns expressed by Craddock *et al* (Femi Oyebode was a co-author of that paper), identifying the 'challenges' to psychiatry as the demedicalisation of health care in mental health services, and the marginalisation of psychiatrists in service development. They also see internal disputes within the profession about the nature of mental disorders, and claims made about the ineffectiveness of neuroleptics and antidepressants as contributing to the crisis. Other threats include the growth of clinical psychology and professional groups such as graduate mental health workers. In other areas of psychiatry neurologists are increasingly becoming involved in the care of people suffering from dementias. They argue that if psychiatry is to have a future it must focus more on how '... advances in scientific knowledge and basic understanding of mental illnesses will influence how psychiatric conditions are assessed and managed' (Oyebode & Humphreys,

2011: 440). They argue that training and education in psychiatry has failed to keep up with developments in other branches of medicine, especially neurology. As a result the profession has become distanced from the rest of the medical profession. This separation anxiety (my expression) should be rectified by giving junior psychiatrists greater exposure to other branches of clinical medicine in their training.

The fourth paper proposed a completely different analysis of the crisis. It (Bracken *et al*, 2012), was co-authored by twenty-nine British psychiatrists, whose input was coordinated through the Critical Psychiatry Network. Although the paper was not published formally as coming from the Network, it may be seen as representing a significant body of opinion within the group, and indeed more generally in the profession.

In sharp contrast to the assertions made by the others on the 'specific' nature of psychiatric treatments, the core argument in this paper was that good psychiatric practice primarily involves engagement in the non-technical, or non-specific, aspects of clinical care, particularly human relationships, meanings and values. In this view the crisis of psychiatry has arisen because technical aspects of care, or the 'technological paradigm' (diagnostic systems, causal models of mental distress, evidence-based medicine), has obscured the significance of the non-specific aspects of care. This technological paradigm has three features:

(a) Mental health problems arise from faulty mechanisms or processes of some sort, involving abnormal physiological or psychological events occurring within the individual.

(b) These mechanisms or processes can be modelled in causal terms. They are not context-dependent.

(c) Technological interventions are instrumental and can be designed and studied independently of relationships and values.
(Bracken *et al*, 2012: 430)

These assumptions set the priorities for the education, training and continuing professional development of psychiatrists. This can be seen in the content of academic journals, conferences, training courses, and exam syllabuses. The problem with this is that they place non-technical aspects of care in a secondary position.

The paper draws attention to a serious flaw in the technical paradigm. Craddock *et al* (2008) claimed that psychiatry offers 'specific' treatments based in diagnosis. The difficulty with this, as Bracken *et al* point out, is that empirical evidence from within evidence-based medicine indicates that the benefits people gain from psychiatric drugs and psychotherapy have less to do with the 'specific' properties that these drugs and therapies are supposed to possess than they have to do with non-specific elements of care. The effectiveness of the specific elements of psychiatric care, argues the paper, has been grossly inflated.

The arguments put forward in this paper have implications for the relationship between people who use mental health services and psychiatrists. In contrast to what one might be led to believe by Craddock *et al*, only a relatively small proportion of people who use mental health services find psychiatrists helpful (as low as 12 per cent in one study, Rogers *et al*, 1993). Superficially it might be reasonable to assume that this group is happy with the view that their experiences are mental disorders arising from brain dysfunction, and the drug treatment that follows from this. However, many people who use mental health services are either opposed to such a view of their experiences, or have much more complex, subtle and shifting understandings of them (Furnham & Bower, 1992).

The service user/survivor movement consists of many different shades of opinion, but a common theme, shared by many, challenges the right of psychiatry to interpret and respond to their experiences. Increasingly, service users cope with psychosis and distress without recourse to psychiatry. In other words, to use the title of a recent book that presented many examples of this, they rely on alternatives beyond psychiatry (Stastny & Lehmann, 2007). In addition, organisations like the Hearing Voices Network offer voice hearers a wide range of different understandings of psychosis through peer support. These understandings do not preclude biomedical and cognitive explanations, but technological accounts are not allowed to dominate, and must take their place alongside alternatives based in cultural and spiritual beliefs, personal narrative and experiences of adversity and trauma, and political and social contexts. Bracken *et al* continue:

> Thus, large sections of the service user movement seek to reframe experiences of mental illness, distress and alienation by turning them into human, rather than technical, challenges. (Bracken *et al*, 2012: 432)

And the paper concludes by setting out the challenge this poses for the future of the profession of psychiatry:

> The evidence base is telling us that we need a radical shift in our understanding of what is at the heart (and perhaps soul) of mental health practice. If we are to operate in an evidence-based manner, and work collaboratively with all sections of the service user movement, we need a psychiatry that is intellectually and ethically adequate to deal with the sort of problems that present to it. As well as the addition of more social science and humanities to the curriculum of our trainees we need to develop a different sensibility towards mental illness itself and a different understanding of our role as doctors. We are not seeking to replace one paradigm with another. A post-technological psychiatry will not abandon the tools of empirical science or reject medical and psychotherapeutic techniques but will start to position the ethical and hermeneutic aspects of our work as primary, thereby highlighting the importance of examining values, relationships, politics and the ethical basis of care and caring. (Bracken *et al*, 2012: 432)

What Is the 'Crisis' Really About?

Psychiatry has always been in the grip of a tension between different schools of thought about the nature of psychosis and distress. Until recently this tension was regarded by many in the profession as something of value, an indicator that psychiatry is an 'eclectic' discipline. But many psychiatrists feel that this is no longer the case. Something has changed. Over the last thirty years, as psychiatric knowledge and practice has fallen under the influence of the technological paradigm, there is a feeling of growing intolerance to approaches to psychosis that are not grounded in neuroscience and genetics. Although the first three papers appear not to be overtly hostile to non-neuroscientific or genetic approaches to psychosis, they barely receive a mention. There are three issues arising from these papers that I want to draw attention to before I move on to outline the contents of this book. These are the issue of psychiatry and harm, the scientific basis of psychiatry, and the relationship between the profession of psychiatry and service users.

Psychiatry and harm

Craddock *et al* claim that changes in service organisation have threatened the leadership role of the psychiatrist in mental health care: '... this creeping devaluation of medicine is damaging our ability to deliver excellent psychiatric care' (Craddock *et al*, 2008: 6), and 'for those with severe mental illness, to avoid medicalisation is at worst damaging or even life-threatening' (*ibid*: 6). The problem here is that they do not specify how and in what way demedicalisation is harmful or life-threatening. They present no evidence in support of this. We are entitled to ask the question: on what basis is this assertion made?

This is an important question, because Chapter 3 of this book casts doubt on the effectiveness and safety of psychiatric drugs. There is good scientific evidence that psychiatric drugs and ECT used in depression are much less effective than we have been led to believe. This applies, albeit for slightly different reasons, to neuroleptics. As far as antidepressants are concerned the evidence indicates that they confer little extra benefit over placebo. In psychosis, some people may gain short-term benefit from neuroleptics, but this probably arises from non-specific effects related to tranquillisation and the induction of a state of indifference. In contrast to the assertion made by Craddock *et al* that the demedicalisation of people suffering from serious mental illness leads to harm, there is scientific evidence that casts doubt on the effectiveness and safety of neuroleptics in the long-term management of psychoses.

Chapter 3 examines the growing body of research evidence that the diagnosis of schizophrenia and treatment with neuroleptics are associated with significant health risks. These health problems include obesity, type-2 diabetes and heart disease. Indeed, there is evidence that people who receive a diagnosis of schizophrenia have a much reduced life expectancy compared to people who do not have the diagnosis. It is of course difficult to interpret these relationships. For example, it remains unclear the extent to which reduced life expectancy in people with schizophrenia is a direct consequence of the serious physical health problems that are associated with the use of neuroleptics, or whether they are mediated by a third factor associated with the diagnosis and medication, such as 'life-style' (lack of exercise, smoking, poor diet). In addition, the effects of chronic poverty and stress may be equally as important.

A related issue here is Bullmore *et al*'s claim that brain-imaging studies have established that cortical atrophy is a central feature of some forms of schizophrenia. It is indisputable that some people with the diagnosis of schizophrenia show evidence of loss of brain tissue on brain scans, but at issue here is the interpretation of this evidence. Does it indicate the existence of a distinct sub-type of schizophrenia, or is it an artefact associated with long-term treatment with neuroleptic drugs? In summary, when Craddock *et al* raise the issue of the harmfulness of demedicalisation, it is important to point out that the medicalisation of distress and psychosis brings many risks to health. In the absence of any supporting evidence it is difficult to avoid the conclusion that Craddock et al's assertion that demedicalisation is harmful or life-threatening is based in an ideological view of the centrality of biomedical science in the practice of psychiatry. This leads to the second issue.

The scientific basis of psychiatry

The first three papers make strong claims for psychiatry as a discipline grounded in scientific theory and methods. The first question this raises is in what sort of science should psychiatry be based? All three are quite clear about this: neuroscience and molecular genetics. This is hardly surprising. Craddock is a psychiatric geneticist; Bullmore a psychiatrist trained in neuroscience who uses neuro-imaging to investigate brain activity in psychoses. Craddock *et al* claim that psychiatrists are '... trained in diagnosing physical and mental illness ... [and are] ... competent to formulate diagnoses that incorporate *physical, mental and social factors* and, where appropriate, recommend initiation of one or more of a range of possible medical treatments' (*ibid*: 7, emphasis added). This raises a number of questions. The first is the claim that psychiatrists are competent to formulate diagnosis based in physical, mental and social factors. It is not clear precisely which 'physical' factors they are referring to here, but they are presumably referring to unsubstantiated biological theories such as the monoamine theory of depression and dopamine theory of schizophrenia. Again, they present no evidence in support of this assertion, so we must question its basis.

Fibiger's (2012) remarks at the start of this chapter are pertinent here. He indicates that there is no established physical basis for any psychiatric disorder. There are, to put it bluntly, no known physical factors that are aetiologically important in any psychiatric condition, and that possess diagnostic, prognostic or therapeutic implications, as is the case in all other branches of medicine. In the next chapter, we will see that there is simply no factual basis for the claim made by Craddock *et al* concerning the physical basis of psychiatric diagnoses. That said, there is an important caveat. It is important to be aware that the state of a person's physical health and their mental state and wellbeing are inextricably bound together. For example, some neurological disorders such as multiple sclerosis are associated with profound changes in mood, which might be misidentified as major depressive disorder, as well as cognitive changes that indicate early dementia. Drug treatments used in physical illnesses such as steroids can cause profound changes in a patient's mental state, such as acute paranoid psychosis. In other words, medical knowledge and training are an important component of mental health care as far as the complex interface between physical illness and mental health are concerned. This is particularly so given the need we all have to find meaning in our experiences of illness and suffering.

Setting aside physical factors, Craddock *et al* also claim that psychiatrists are competent to formulate diagnoses that incorporate psychological and social factors. What are we to make of this? It seems distinctly odd that when all three papers see the salvation of psychiatry in the hands of molecular genetics and neuroscience, they claim that psychiatrists are also competent in the assessment of psychological and social factors. If, as these authors imply, all that matters about us as human beings, our hopes and fears, doubts and joys, despair and alienation, is to be accounted for solely in terms of genes, molecules and networks of brain cells, on what basis can a claim for competency in the assessment of psychological and social factors rest? Indeed, Bullmore *et al* set out a hierarchy in which genetic variation drives complex brain phenotypes that ultimately culminate in behaviour. It is important to note that the words 'mind', 'mental', 'psychological' and 'social' simply don't feature in the model.

Notwithstanding this difficulty, let us for the moment assume that psychiatrists are competent to formulate diagnoses that include psychological and social factors. In Chapters 4 and 5 we will consider the extensive scientific research into psychological and social factors in psychosis. The key question here is how this evidence stands in relation to neuroscientific and molecular genetics research, and even more important, what impact does it have on clinical practice guidelines and the training and practice of psychiatrists? There is evidence that there has been a progressive marginalisation and devaluation of research into psychological and social factors in psychosis. Many psychiatrists and psychologists are increasingly concerned about the domination of scientific research into psychosis by neuroscience and genetics. John Read and colleagues (2001) have argued that the biopsychosocial model has become transformed into a stress-vulnerability model. Psychosocial factors have become incorporated into the more general concept of 'stress', which in turn has been increasingly investigated as a physiological and neuroscientific phenomenon. At the same time vulnerability is largely understood in terms of genetic vulnerability in schizophrenia research.

This makes it extremely difficult to justify the claim that psychiatrists today are competent to formulate diagnoses based in psychological and social factors. Indeed, it follows that a 'medicine of the brain' would remove our inner worlds, whether studied through psychology or philosophy, from the frame, in much the same way that behaviourism did in psychology in the 1950s and 1960s. A psychiatry informed solely by developments in molecular genetics and neuroscience (were such developments feasible in any case) is one in which the mind, our inner worlds, and the social worlds that our minds stand in relation to, are of no relevance. This is the ultimate soulless psychiatry, a sterile, decontextualised and inhuman medicine of the brain.

Furthermore, this raises the question of whether or not neuroscience and genetics are up to the task. Are they ultimately capable of telling us all we need to know about the brain to enable us to treat distress and psychosis, in much the same way as a cardiologist can treat cardiac disease through a scientific understanding of the way the heart functions? There are two issues that arise from this. The first is a moral or ethical question. What are the consequences of pursuing an approach to psychosis that fails to engage with the social contexts in which individual experiences of psychosis arise? This is a moral issue because these contexts involve great suffering, personal experiences of social adversity, trauma and abuse, including childhood trauma, loss, bullying, as well as the racism, racial harassment and abuse experienced by people from, for example, black and minority ethnic (BME) communities. Scientific evidence indicates that these social contexts are strongly implicated in the origins of psychosis. This is supported by the testimony of service users and survivors. These contexts are primarily matters of social justice, and this raises serious questions about the basis of scientific responses to psychosis and distress that fail to engage with the moral dimensions of suffering to be found in personal stories of suffering, oppression and adversity. It matters little whether the science is based in molecular genetics, neuroscience or cognitive science.

The second question that arises from a psychiatry based in molecular genetics and neuroscience is primarily a philosophical question. Is science likely to yield any information of value into the nature of these human problems that might result in new forms of treatment or therapy? This question is addressed in Chapter 6.

Whose interests does psychiatry really serve?

The first three papers make claims for the power and authority of psychiatrists in the field of mental health. These claims are ostensibly set out on behalf of people who see psychiatrists; people who, according to Craddock *et al*, prefer to be called 'patients' rather than 'service users'. The question that arises is, whom are they referring to? The authors of these papers are happy to engage with the views of the patients they encounter in their clinics, people who out of deference may be reluctant to question the judgement of hospital specialists. However, we will see that views of many people who use mental health services are much less positive about psychiatry. They are much more critical about the role it plays in their lives. However, the issue that is gnawing away at the heart of the Craddock paper is that of leadership in multidisciplinary teams. They write as follows:

> Assessment, in many cases, may lead the psychiatrist, *as a leader in the clinical team*, to conclude that the most suitable treatment is a psychological or social intervention delivered by the member of the team with the most appropriate skills. (Craddock *et al*, 2008: 7, emphasis added)

The key purpose of the paper is to assert the right of the consultant psychiatrist to lead mental health care. Over the last thirty years psychiatrists have been forced out of the Victorian asylums that spawned the speciality, first into district general hospital units, and more recently into the community. Craddock *et al* see the new patterns of working in mental health services that have emerged out of community care over the last twenty years, such as 'New Ways of Working', as a threat to medical leadership. In the asylums psychiatric leadership was unquestioned and unchallenged for over 100 years. However, once out of the asylum, and in the face of growing challenges from the service user/survivor movement (see, for example, Beeforth *et al*, 1994; Read & Reynolds, 1996; Faulkner & Layzell, 2000; Kalathil *et al*, 2011), and from other professional groups, especially clinical psychologists (Boyle, 2002; Johnstone, 2000; Bentall, 2003), the claim to leadership made by these papers is little more than an assertion completely without justification, scientific or professional.

Outline of the Book

This book is written in six sections. This first chapter has set out two perspectives on the crisis in psychiatry. One is that of psychiatrists who see the future of the profession in terms of a more intensive commitment to research in neuroscience and molecular genetics; the other broadly critical perspective is sceptical about the scientific basis of psychiatry *as it currently stands*. This caveat is important because within critical psychiatry there are different views about the future role of science. One purpose of this book is to stimulate debate more widely about the extent to which neuroscience and genetics are capable of delivering a vision of psychiatry as 'medicine of the brain'. The critical perspective, however, also draws attention to the central importance of deeply human aspects of care, the so-called non-specific factors that mobilise hope and meaning in the context of a positive therapeutic relationship. The implications of this for clinical practice of psychiatry are explored in Sections 4 and 5.

Chapter 2 continues to explore the crisis in psychiatry. It examines the failure of scientific studies to establish the validity of psychiatric diagnoses. Although modern scientific studies of psychiatric diagnoses go back nearly fifty years, it is important to recognise that this is set against a much lengthier history of failures to find the biological 'causes' of psychosis. This raises the question, 'If after 150 years of research we remain ignorant about the biological basis of psychosis, how likely are future studies to succeed where so many others have failed?' How much confidence can we place in assertions that at some unspecified future date all will be revealed?

Chapter 3 develops themes raised in Chapter 2. If there are no biological differences between the brains of people with a diagnosis of schizophrenia and those who do not have the diagnosis, then it becomes extremely difficult to provide a rational basis for biological treatments for the condition. This chapter therefore examines the evidence base for the effectiveness of drug treatments for depression and schizophrenia and for the effectiveness of electroconvulsive therapy. In contrast to what we have been led to believe, these physical treatments confer only very marginal benefits over placebo. For example, some people with the diagnosis of schizophrenia may gain limited benefits from neuroleptic drugs in the acute phase of their distress, but these benefits probably arise because these drugs have non-specific properties such as tranquillisation and the induction of a state of indifference. There is no evidence that their limited effectiveness is related to specific actions on disordered brain chemistry. Furthermore, we must offset the meagre benefits of drug treatment in psychiatry against the substantial risks associated with their use. In the case of neuroleptic drugs these include serious risks to physical health, reduced life expectancy, and the prospect that their continued long-term use may be associated with a worse outcome than in people who discontinue them. The implication of this is clear; one of the main priorities for psychiatry in the future is to lessen its dependence on the use of medication as a front-line response to psychosis and distress. Similar points emerge when we scrutinise the evidence for the effectiveness of psychotherapies, including cognitive behavioural therapy. Although safer (at least as far as physical health is concerned) we will see that much of the benefit people gain from psychotherapies is to be accounted for by non-specific factors, especially the quality of the therapeutic relationship as seen by the client. Sections 4 and 5 address the challenges these observations pose.

Although this book questions the current scientific basis of psychiatry, it should not be taken as a manifesto for those opposed to the idea that science in any form has a role to play in psychosis and distress. Scientific studies in epidemiology, social science and psychology yield important insights that are in danger of becoming submerged beneath the deluge of neuroscience. Section 2 deals with this knowledge. One of the most important themes to emerge from the writing of critical psychiatrists over the last fifteen years has been to explore the way in which scientific modes of thought decontextualise the experiences of psychosis (see, for example, Bracken & Thomas, 2005). Section 2 examines the scientific evidence that a wide range of contexts – social, economic and cultural – play a central role in the origins of psychosis. Indeed, contexts play a much more important role than simply acting as 'triggers' for psychosis in someone who is biologically predisposed. For example, there is evidence that the content of voices or unusual beliefs is related to personal experiences of trauma.

Chapter 4 deals with the links between psychosis and childhood adversity, particularly abuse (sexual, physical and emotional), emotional neglect and physical illness. It also examines the evidence that links childhood adversity to the broader socio-economic circumstances in which families struggle to bring up their children. Chapter 5 examines the unspoken assumptions that are rooted in scientific psychiatry's attempts to account for the apparently raised incidence of schizophrenia in black people. In addition to the adversity described in Chapter 4, black people in the UK must also contend with additional layers of historical adversity that places every aspect of their lives in a negative light compared to the white majority. Their lives remain haunted by the ghosts of one of the great tragedies of history – slavery. Its echoes can still be heard in twenty-first-century psychiatry. We will see how recent evidence has shown that individual experiences of racism play a key role in many black people's experiences of psychosis.

These two chapters also serve another important purpose. Personal experiences of adversity and racism are fundamentally matters of social justice. This, I shall argue, poses serious questions about the moral basis of scientific knowledge based in neuroscience and genetics, and the use of this knowledge in clinical practice. Again, these issues have featured in the work of critical psychiatrists (for example, the plea of postpsychiatry for 'ethics before technology', Bracken & Thomas, 2001). This has important implications for future practice in psychiatry. How is it possible to practise psychiatry in ways that acknowledge the importance of contexts of adversity in the lives of individual patients? Much of the rest of the book tries to respond to this question.

However, before we are in a position to consider how the practice of psychiatry must change, we need to examine two issues. The first interrogates the claim made by the first three 'crisis' papers that the future of psychiatry is secure in the hands of neuroscience and genetics. In Section 3, Chapter 6 examines this claim by considering the limits of neuroscience in psychiatry. I focus on neuroscience because other authors, most notably Mary Boyle, Lucy Johnstone and Jay Joseph, have already examined in detail the limits of genetics and molecular biology in psychiatry. We are told that although we face a long and arduous journey, ultimately a combination of neuroscience and genetics will 'crack' the problem of psychosis, yielding as-yet-undreamt-of novel treatments. Just how solid are these claims? Chapter 6 examines the limits of neuroscience research in psychiatry in three broad areas, methodological, conceptual and statistical, most of which can be traced back to a deeply problematic set of assumptions about the relationship between brain activity and consciousness. I will argue that there is no basis for the assertion that insights from neuroscience will lead to a new era of psychiatry as a medicine of the brain. Neuroscientific accounts of consciousness are deeply flawed, and there is no way around these problems.

If there is to be no neuroscientific salvation for psychiatry, how are we to find a rational and ethical basis for clinical practice? Chapter 7 tries to answer this by setting out the basis for psychiatric practice as narrative. Rather than seeing this as a new set of theories about psychosis, or indeed a new paradigm, narrative psychiatry foregrounds the relationship between patient and psychiatrist. It sees the practice of psychiatry as an ethical human and social process based in the telling and sharing of stories. At the heart of narrative psychiatry is the view that the most natural way for doctors to engage with the contexts that are important in understanding patients' experiences is by listening to and engaging respectfully with their stories. Narrative psychiatry makes it possible to work with stories told from different perspectives, the patient's, the family's, and so on. Another valuable feature of narrative psychiatry is that it has the ability to encompass a wide variety of stories, some of which may be in conflict. It is, for example, capable of engaging with 'biomedical' understandings of psychosis (using the metaphor of chemical imbalance) for those who find such narratives helpful, alongside non-medical narratives. These key aspects of narrative psychiatry, attending carefully to the stories of people's lives and the contexts in which these stories are set, through careful listening, set out the background for clinical practice that will be explored in the final parts of the book.

In Section 4 we return to the most intimate of encounters, that between a person experiencing psychosis or distress and the psychiatrist. It illustrates the use of narrative psychiatry by looking at clinical practice as stories. Each of the three chapters in this final section deal with different stories reflecting commonly encountered situations and dilemmas in the practice of psychiatry. Chapter 8 presents the stories of two women, one of South Asian heritage, the other from a white working-class background, whose sadness follows the sudden deaths of their husbands. The stories also demonstrate the value of attending to cultural understandings of and responses to sadness, and thus raise the issue of community development to be considered in Chapter 13. Chapters 9 and 10 try to show how, in practice, narrative psychiatry facilitates engagement with contexts of trauma and racism that feature so prominently in the stories of many people who experience psychosis. Chapter 9 is the story of a young woman detained on a secure unit following a violent assault on a stranger, apparently in response to voices. Chapter 10 describes how years of racial abuse and harassment drove a young African-Caribbean man mad. Both these stories also help to tease out the ethical complexities involved in the use of medication and compulsory detention. The stories in this section are not case histories in the conventional sense. They are fictional, but loosely based in the experiences of many patients I encountered during my career as a consultant psychiatrist.

The penultimate section deals with the central role of the service user/

survivor movement and communities in psychiatric practice. We (Bracken *et al*, 2012) argued that the crisis in psychiatry offers an opportunity to rethink our relationship to the wider service user and survivor movement. Chapter 11 outlines the recent history of the movement. This history antedates critical psychiatry by at least fifteen years, and we can see its influence on critical psychiatry through the writings of prominent survivors, as well as through service-user-led research, some recent examples of which are presented. Of greatest significance for the future of psychiatry is the growth of service user involvement in mental health services, and this chapter presents the evidence for this, and ends with a description of the role of the service-user development worker in services.

A key argument to be set out in the final section is that service users and survivors have a major role to play if psychiatry is to engage with the contexts that shape their lives and experiences. One way in which this is happening is through peer support. The best-known example of this is to be found in the work of the Hearing Voices Network (HVN), and Chapter 12 examines the background and development of this work, and how psychiatrists are increasingly working in alliance with these groups. The salient word here is alliance, the implication being that control ultimately rests with local voice hearers. This pioneering work offers a valuable model for psychiatrists in supporting and assisting service users/survivors to set up their own systems of support.

There are also notable examples of work by psychiatrists that foreground the potentially meaningful nature of psychosis by engaging with personal narratives, no matter how fragmented they might seem. An excellent example of this is Soteria and the work of Loren Mosher. Soteria represents a way of working in psychiatry that draws together a number of themes raised earlier in the book. Not only does it focus on the importance of meaning, but it was specifically set up to help people through psychosis with the minimal use of medication. In addition, many who had been supported through psychosis in Soteria went on to work as peer-support workers for those in acute crisis. There is also an evidence base for the effectiveness of Soteria, and Chapter 12 examines this, as well as that relating to the Scandinavian services, such as Open Dialogue and the Needs-Adapted model, that have established a broadly similar tradition.

Section 5 ends with an account of the role of community development in helping people from BME communities. If psychiatrists really are to engage with the contexts of the lives of patients from BME communities it is important that this is done in ways that reflect the cultures, traditions and histories of these communities. Chapter 13 presents community development as a set of practices that enable psychiatrists and mental health professionals to do this. Community development featured prominently in the British government's Delivering Race Equality policy, but there are, as we will see, different models of community development. The chapter ends with a description of the work of Sharing Voices Bradford, a community development project that has worked closely since 2002 with the BME communities in a town in the North of England.

Recommended Reading

Bracken, P., Thomas, P., Timimi, S., Asen, E., Behr, G. *et al* (2012) Psychiatry beyond the current paradigm. *British Journal of Psychiatry, 201*, 430–4. doi: 10.1192/bjp. bp.112.109447.

Bullmore, E., Fletcher, P. & Jones, P. (2009) Why psychiatry can't afford to be neurophobic. *British Journal of Psychiatry, 194*, 293–5. doi: 10.1192/bjp.bp.108.058479.

Craddock, N., Antebi, D., Attenburrow, M.-J., Bailey, A., Carson, A. *et al* (2008) Wake-up call for British psychiatry. *British Journal of Psychiatry, 193*, 6–9. doi: 10.1192/bjp. bp.108.053561.

Oyebode, F. & Humphreys, M. (2011) The future of psychiatry. *British Journal of Psychiatry, 199*, 439–40. doi: 10.1192/bjp.bp.111.092338.

The Problem of Diagnosis in Psychiatry

2

> There is something that causes me the greatest difficulty, and
> continues to do so without relief: unspeakably more depends
> on what things are called than on what they are ... creating new
> names and assessments and apparent truths is enough to
> create new 'things'.
>
> Friedrich Nietzsche, *The Gay Science*

On 18th May 2013, the Board of the American Psychiatric Association published the fifth edition of its *Diagnostic and Statistical Manual* (*DSM-5*). Just three weeks earlier the Director of the National Institute of Mental Health in the USA, Dr Thomas Insel, announced in his blog that the Institute would not be using *DSM-5* (Insel, 2013). Patients, he said, deserved better. Psychiatric diagnoses are based on symptoms, and by implication lack validity. In future the NIMH, the body responsible for setting the psychiatric research agenda in the US, would only fund research that used its own Research Domain Criteria (RDoC), an attempt to move to a system of psychiatric diagnosis based on findings from research in neuroscience and molecular biology.

Dr Insel wasn't the only person concerned about the problems of *DSM-5*. The Chair of the DSM-IV Task Force, Dr Allen Frances (2009) wrote in the *British Journal of Psychiatry* that *DSM-5* had failed in its grand ambition of a 'paradigm shift' in psychiatric diagnosis based on biological markers, because no such markers exist. Instead *DSM-5* turned to tinkering with the thresholds for diagnosis, and dimensional ratings, with the consequent risk of 'epidemics' of false diagnosis (or over-diagnosis) that would result in millions of people across the globe being exposed to the risk of unnecessary psychiatric treatment. The only people to benefit from this situation were those involved in the pharmaceutical industry.

The *DSM* is the authoritative voice in America on psychiatric diagnosis. Over the years it has played a major role in shaping psychiatric theory and practice. Much has been made of the publication of *DSM-III* in 1980, and its role in heralding a new scientific era in psychiatry. *DSM-III* introduced much tighter definitions of psychiatric disorders, in an attempt to improve the appallingly low levels of agreement between psychiatrists about diagnosis in individual cases. The APA carried out extensive field trials of the reliability of the twenty or so most important diagnoses in *DSM-5*, and published the results in the *American Journal of Psychiatry* in January 2013. They were far from convincing. In general the levels of kappa (the statistic used to measure levels of agreement) from the field trials were very low. The accompanying editorial (Freedman *et al*, 2013) tried to play down the significance of this. It claimed a kappa of 0.46 for schizophrenia represents an 86 per cent level of agreement between two psychiatrists in a clinic where 10 per cent of their patients have a diagnosis of schizophrenia. This editorial, however, made no reference to an influential paper published forty years earlier by the architect of *DSM-III*, Robert Spitzer, arguing that a more robust level for kappa is 0.7 (Spitzer & Fliess, 1974), a value commonly accepted in other fields of medicine. Where the rest of medicine marches on as far as diagnosis is concerned, it seems that psychiatry is moving backwards.

Diagnosis is central to the practice of medicine, and for this reason any criticism of the role of diagnosis in psychiatry is usually met with hostility from those in the profession whose identities are firmly aligned with that of the hospital specialist. This can be seen in the spate of papers in the *British Journal of Psychiatry* (Shah & Mountain, 2007; Craddock *et al*, 2008; Bullmore *et al*, 2009; Oyebode & Humphreys, 2011) that we examined in Chapter 1. That apart, others have been deeply critical of the role of diagnosis in psychiatry, including survivors and service users (Read & Reynolds, 1996; Mental Health Foundation, 1997), academics from psychology and sociology (Johnstone, 2000; Bentall, 1990, 2003; Boyle, 2002; Pilgrim, 2007), and critical psychiatrists (Fernando, 1991; Thomas, 1997; Double, 2002; Bracken & Thomas, 2005; Moncrieff, 2010; Timimi, 2011). Thomas Szasz (1960) famously refuted the idea that mental illnesses are genuine diseases, and thus diagnosis and psychiatrists have no legitimate role to play in psychosis. The position argued in this text is quite different. In Western cultures, doctors have traditionally played a role alongside the priest or minister of religion in helping people to cope with, and find meaning in, their experiences of suffering, physical or emotional. Neither is it my intention to argue that science has no role in understanding psychosis, or to imply that scientific methods have no role to play in the systematic study of psychosis and distress. However, the current scientific basis of psychiatry is deeply flawed, and we can begin to grasp the problems that stem from this by considering the problem of diagnosis. This is a necessary prelude to the examination of psychiatric treatment that follows in Chapter 3.

Over the last fifty years, scientific knowledge and methods have dominated medicine and psychiatry. However, unlike medicine, where enormous strides in diagnosis and treatment have been achieved through a firm understanding of the biological basis of disease, this is not so in psychiatry. There are, of course, marginal conditions like Alzheimer's disease, where great strides have been made in recent years in understanding the molecular pathology of the condition. But this is arguably a neurological disorder, not a psychiatric one. The present chapter explores this by setting out a common basis for approaching three aspects of the theory and practice of psychiatry that are linked, although they are not often considered together. These concern the extent to which psychiatric diagnoses have an established scientific basis, the role of evidence-based medicine (EBM) in guiding decisions about treatment in psychiatry, and in contrast, the importance of what are called non-specific factors such as trust, hope and meaning in helping people towards healing. EBM and non-specific factors will be the matter of detailed examination in the next chapter.

We start with a brief account of the role of diagnosis in general medicine. What is a diagnosis? What purposes does it serve? In psychiatry, diagnosis is commonly identified with what is called the medical model, but contemporary psychiatry is no longer limited to medical theories about psychosis. Over the second half of the twentieth century, cognitive psychology has played an increasingly important role in theories of diagnoses such as schizophrenia. Psychiatric theory and practice is no longer based exclusively in medical theories about psychiatric disorders. For this reason, we use the expression the 'technological paradigm' in preference to the medical model (Thomas *et al*, 2012). It is technological in the sense that contemporary psychiatry sees distress as a series of technical challenges to be responded to through a range of technologies, including drugs and therapies. Here we will examine the features of this paradigm through the diagnosis of schizophrenia. This is a deliberate choice. The diagnosis has been the subject of intensive investigation within the technological paradigm for well over 100 years, but it continues to defy the attempts of psychiatrists and researchers to establish its scientific basis. This failure of the technological paradigm is best understood in terms of problems associated with the validity of the diagnosis, that is to say the extent to which the diagnosis reflects fundamental biological (or psychological) differences between those who have it, and those who do not. In Chapter 6, the limitations of neuroscience in trying to account for the experiences of psychosis will be examined.

Diagnosis and the Medical Model

According to Fulford *et al* (2006), diagnosis serves four main functions in medicine. It has a descriptive function, a convenient way of summarising important information about a patient's symptoms to enable doctors to communicate with each other. It also has an aetiological function, in that medical diagnoses convey important information about the causes of diseases. Third, it has a therapeutic function, in that an understanding of what causes a disease and its associated symptoms has implications for the treatment and management of the condition.

Finally, a diagnosis is a prediction – it conveys information about what will happen to the patient if she or he is left untreated. It is also a prediction about the treatment the patient is likely to respond to. Here we are largely concerned with the aetiological (cause), therapeutic and predictive functions of diagnosis.[1]

It is impossible to grasp the significance of psychiatric diagnosis within the technological paradigm without understanding the way that scientific thought has seized medicine over the last 200 years. Scientific medicine originated in the first half of the nineteenth century. Michel Foucault (2003) and Roy Porter (1997) have described how at that time the focus of scientific progress shifted from the hospital to new sites, the clinic and the laboratory. Developments in technology such as the microscope led to the development of a new science, histology (the study of the structure and form of body tissues), which straddled anatomy and physiology. The microscope made possible the detailed examination of healthy tissues and organs, and how their structure changed as a result of morbid, or pathological, processes. Let us take cancer as an example.

Cancer was well recognised in antiquity. Practitioners of Hippocratic medicine believed that tumours were caused by an abnormal accumulation of black bile in the veins. This belief endured for centuries in various forms until the middle of the seventeenth century when the lymphatic system was first described, and implicated as a cause of cancer. Today, this system is still regarded as important in understanding how cancerous cells spread throughout the body, but no one believes that the system causes cancer. In the middle of the nineteenth century the German physician Rudolf Virchow proposed that body tissues consisted of minute units called cells, and from this the science of cellular pathology (or histopathology) developed. Virchow's proposal that cancers developed from immature cells gave rise to a great deal of descriptive work in which pathologists examined the microscopic structure of tumours. This made it possible to classify different types of cancer. This, coupled with long-term studies of the course of the disease in large numbers of patients, enabled physicians to make quite accurate predictions about the outcome of the disease, based on its histological features. Thus the diagnosis of cancer was refined in ways that enabled physicians to predict the outcome (prognosis) in individual patients.

Despite these advances, the causes of cancer remained poorly understood until the late twentieth century. In breast cancer, for example, a number of risk factors were identified (smoking, family history, diet, not having children, hormonal factors), and although this was useful in prevention, it had few implications for

---

1. It is worth noting that something important is missing from Fulford *et al*'s account. Diagnosis serves a fifth function, one that binds patient and doctor together in the process of talking about the meaning of the diagnosis for the person who is ill. This understanding, depending on the nature and severity of the diagnosis within the wider culture in which the patient and doctor are embedded, has implications for the patient's sense of self, even for his or her life and death. For these reasons I call it the 'existential function' of diagnosis. We will return to it in Chapter 7 on narrative psychiatry.

the treatment of the condition. For most women treatment meant major surgery based on a classification of the cancer through the microscopic examination of a sample of tissue removed at biopsy. Then in 1990, researchers in the University of California discovered the existence of the *BRCA1* gene, which synthesises a protein that helps to repair damaged DNA. If it isn't functioning properly then repairs cannot be made, and this increases the risk of cancerous cells developing, especially in breast and ovarian tissue. This marked a shift of emphasis in research into the treatment of breast cancer towards molecular genetics.

The outcome of this research came in 2012, when a paper published in *Nature* represented a major breakthrough in understanding breast cancer based on a 'molecular map' of the condition. The research teams (Curtis *et al*, 2012) had decoded the *BRCA* genes, and were able to classify breast cancer into ten sub-types on the basis of genetic features that predicted outcome (survival rates). This opened the way for more accurate targeting of the drugs used to treat the disease in individual cases. They also discovered several new genes that were implicated in the disease, all of which are now the subject of research that could lead to the development of new drugs. Finally, the research resulted in an understanding of the relationships between these genes, and what are known as cell-signalling pathways, the control mechanisms that are vital in regulating cell growth. This has the potential to lead to a deeper understanding of how genes cause cancer.

Advances in understanding diseases like cancer have taken place in a series of steps and plateaux. On occasions the introduction of new technology for the scientific investigation of the body, such as the microscope or chromatography (which makes it possible to identify genes and their molecular constituents) resulted in rapid progress. But there are also lengthy periods of consolidation, the plateaux, in which the implications of this technology have been extended to other diseases. The microscope, for example, led not only to an understanding of the structure and appearance of cancer tissue, but also to the identification and description of different bacteria as agents responsible for diseases like tuberculosis and cholera. At other times rapid steps in progress have had less to do with advances in technology than they have had to do with a brilliant insight that revolutionised scientific theory. The discovery of the double helix structure of DNA is such an example. Without it the recent advances in the molecular genetics of breast cancer would not have been possible.

The Technological Paradigm in Psychiatry

For well over 100 years there has been a strong belief in some quarters that psychiatric disorders can be explained in much the same way that we can explain cancer. Both Ellenberger (1970) and Marx (1970) attribute the origins of this view to Wilhelm Griesinger, the German neurologist and proto-psychiatrist. Marx described three aspects of Griesinger's work that influenced what we call the technological paradigm. First, he believed that mental disorders were brain disorders related to the presence of cerebral pathology. Thus the psychiatrist was best thought of as a physician. Second, he maintained that investigation of psychopathology must be based on an empirical, scientific psychology. Mental processes were a matter for scientific investigation not philosophical speculation. Third, he applied theoretical models developed by neurologists to psychopathology, in the belief that ultimately, mental disorders would be understood in terms of neurological processes.

The most influential figure in the history of psychiatric diagnosis and classification is the German psychiatrist Emil Kraepelin, who from 1903 to 1922 was professor of psychiatry in Munich. One of Kraepelin's main ambitions was to establish a scientific basis for psychiatry through experimental psychology. He contributed to scientific psychiatry in two ways. First, he developed a clinical method that relied on detailed clinical observation of patients' mental states, linked to their long-term follow-up. This method resulted in the second contribution, his description of the condition he called *dementia praecox*, which today we know as schizophrenia. Kraepelin's work drew on insights from neurology, experimental psychology and neuroanatomy, but of even greater significance were his detailed long-term studies of individual patients. He classified the psychoses into dementia praecox and manic-depressive insanity, based on whether or not patients recovered. In broad terms those suffering from dementia praecox did not recover; their condition deteriorated over time.

The influence of this early version of the technological paradigm waxed and waned. American psychiatry in the first half of the twentieth century was dominated by psychoanalytic schools of thought about psychosis and distress through the work of Meyer (1957), Sullivan (1956), Menninger (1963) and Fromm-Reichmann (1948). The technological paradigm was highly influential in British and European psychiatry, but over the last thirty years it swept aside the analytic tradition in America. Some (Wilson, 1993; Mayes & Horwitz, 2005) relate this to the publication of *DSM-III*. From the 1970s onwards into the 1990s, the so-called 'Decade of the Brain',[2] there was a growing preoccupation with the scientific basis of psychiatry, seen in a move away from psychoanalytic theory and a return to the accurate description and observation of clinical cases. This represented a return to the methods and values of Emil Kraepelin, hence the expression neo-Kraepelinism frequently used today. There was a strong belief that this, the use of new technologies such as CT scans, NMR scans, PET scans, and functional magnetic resonance imaging (fMRI) in tandem with the scientific methods of cognitive psychology, and the new field of molecular genetics, would reveal the biological basis of the diagnosis of schizophrenia.

---

2. On the 17th June 1990 in Presidential Proclamation 6158, George Bush Senior declared the new decade the 'Decade of the Brain' to '... enhance public awareness of the benefits to be derived from brain research through appropriate programs, ceremonies and activities' (Bush, 1990).

We are now in a position to describe the three main features of the techno-logical paradigm in psychiatry: the assumption that psychiatric diagnoses are discrete entities; that the symptoms associated with a diagnosis are caused by specific disturbances in biological or psychological function; that specific treatments for the diagnosis (whether pharmacological or psychological, such as CBT) are effective because they rectify the underlying disturbance in biological or psychological function. We will consider each of these through the example of the diagnosis of schizophrenia.

Psychiatric diagnoses are discrete entities

This view of psychiatric diagnosis bears the imprint of Kraepelin's view of clas-sification, at least in the way that neo-Kraepelinian psychiatrists have interpreted it. Kraepelin believed that dementia praecox (schizophrenia) and manic-depressive psychosis were different disorders. This view originated in his long-term follow-up studies which indicated that people who suffered from dementia praecox did not recover, and that their condition deteriorated with the passage of time (Kraepelin, 1919). His belief was that in the fullness of time biological research would reveal a discrete cause for the condition. An implicit assumption of this view is that there are fundamental differences between people with the diagnosis, and those who do not have it. This is the position taken by the late Robert Kendell (1975, see especially pp. 65–9) who argued that a diagnosis of schizophrenia should, as is the case with medical diagnoses, imply the existence of a natural boundary or discontinuity between people who have the diagnosis and those who do not. More generally in psychiatry these differences exist at two levels. First, experiences such as unusual beliefs and hearing voices do not occur in 'normal' people. There is something fundamentally different, or abnormal, about such experiences. Second, these experiences originate in, or are caused by, specific disturbances in biological function.

Specific disturbances in biological function

The assumption here is that the 'abnormal' experiences ('symptoms') that are used to establish the diagnosis of schizophrenia are caused by specific disturbances in brain function. Although the focus here is on biological disturbances, the same arguments apply to disturbances in psychological function that are thus believed to be specific to the diagnosis. These disturbances are not a feature of 'normal' people, or people with other diagnoses. This means that those diagnosed with schizophrenia are fundamentally different in a biological way from other people. One way of describing this aspect of the technological paradigm is that it 'carves nature at its joints', an expression used by Kendell (1975: 65) taken from Plato. This requires that a successful theory about the natural world should reflect some underlying distinction in that world. If schizophrenia, for example, is a valid diagnosis, this should be reflected in some underlying natural (that is to say, biological) property of people with the diagnosis, that sets them apart from those who do not have the diagnosis. In other words the diagnosis represents a natural category based on the biological (or psychological) properties of the individuals who fall into the category. There have been countless attempts to identify these 'differences' over the years, and many claims made for the discovery of the 'cause' of schizophrenia, but none has ever been confirmed. A detailed examination of these claims is beyond the scope of this text, but a summary can be found in Thomas (2011).

Specific treatments rectify the specific disturbances

We will examine the evidence for this in detail in the next chapter, but as it follows from the first two assumptions it is important to mention it here. The biological 'differences' that are assumed to be important in causing schizophrenia are widely believed to establish a rational and logical basis for the use of neuroleptic drugs in people with the diagnosis. This is important in justifying their use, for example, in making the case for forcing people to take these drugs against their wishes. In one sense it doesn't matter if there is little or no scientific evidence in support of a specific disturbance in biological function in the condition. The existence of, and belief in, the dopamine theory itself is sufficient to justify the continued use of neuroleptic drugs, through force if necessary.

Diagnosis and the Problems of the Technological Paradigm in Psychiatry

In view of the foregoing, there are two difficulties facing the use of diagnosis in psychiatry. It may be self-evident, but it is important to remember that there is a fundamental difference between physical diseases and so-called 'mental' illness. The person who has a physical disease suffers from an illness, but the illness is caused by a disease process.[3] Diseases affect bodies, and bodies are easily examined and investigated. Bodies can be inspected, palpated (felt and prodded), listened to (heart sounds, breath sounds), measured, and looked inside in various ways. This means that it is relatively straightforward for different doctors examining the same patient to agree with acceptable levels of accuracy that there is a suspicious lump in a breast. The lump can be measured and described in terms of its relationship to the surrounding breast tissue, the skin overlying it,

---

3. The *Shorter Oxford English Dictionary* (*SOED*, 2007) defines illness as '… ill health; the state of being ill'. It makes a distinction between this 'state', a property of a person, and disease (p. 1325). Interestingly, the word 'illness' originally had strong moral connotations in the sixteenth to eighteenth centuries ('Wickedness, depravity, immorality', *ibid*). The issue of illness, and the subjective experiences of disease and its meanings in personal terms, will become important later in this book. The skill and art of medicine in broad terms lies in the doctor's ability to work in the domains of disease and illness simultaneously.

and the muscle layers of the chest wall beneath. The presence of a lump in a breast is, by and large, a matter of fact that can be agreed upon by two or more doctors working independently of each other.

The problem with 'mental' illness is that in order to make a diagnosis, doctors depend on things patients tell them about their experiences, as well as observations they make about the patient's behaviour. These are not facts in the sense that the presence of a breast lump is a fact, because they are not phenomena in the physical world. The things people tell doctors about their experiences, their beliefs and so on, are aspects of their mental worlds and are thus not accessible for investigation as are bodies. They are embedded within the narratives or stories we communicate about ourselves, and as such must be interpreted by the doctor. The act of interpretation opens up the process of diagnosis in psychiatry to high levels of uncertainty and ambiguity. A consequence of this is that it is much more difficult for doctors to agree upon the presence of a 'symptom' in psychiatry, or indeed its significance, because they are drawn into making judgements about what the patient says. Of course, a doctor examining a breast lump also makes judgements about the lump, but these are of a different order. They will generally concern the significance of the physical features of the lump, its size, the speed at which it appears to be growing, and whether it is mobile or tethered to the skin or adjacent tissue. These are readily corroborated by other doctors. In contrast psychiatrists' judgements about what a patient says are based on their interpretations about what is being said, and in making these interpretations psychiatrists draw on values, for example their beliefs about what they consider to be normal or abnormal experience.

There is much evidence that both medical and psychiatric diagnoses are laden with values (Fulford, 1989, 2002; Sadler, 2005), but in contrast to medical condition, where the body stands as the irrefutable page upon which disease is inscribed, psychiatrists have nothing other than their value-laden interpretations of things their patients tell them, despite their strenuous efforts to achieve 'neutrality' and objectivity. This is the main reason why there have been poor levels of agreement between psychiatrists about diagnosis, both in regard to individual patients, and across broader groups of psychiatrists and patients. Indeed there is evidence that there have been very poor levels of agreement on whether or not a particular person is suffering from a mental disorder. This is the first problem of diagnosis in the technological paradigm, poor reliability.

The reliability of psychiatric diagnoses

A number of early studies drew attention to this problem (Beck et al, 1962; Kreitman, 1961; Blashfield, 1973; Kuriansky et al, 1974; Sandifer et al, 1964). It became a major problem when the World Health Organization (WHO) wanted to make international comparisons of the diagnostic behaviour of psychiatrists. Low reliability made it impossible to compare the frequency of different psychiatric conditions in different countries. Kramer (1961) found that the first admission rate for schizophrenia was 50 per cent higher in the USA than England and Wales, whereas manic-depressive psychosis appeared to be nine times more common in England and Wales compared with the USA.

The problem of reliability emerged even more starkly in studies that examined how smaller groups of psychiatrists made their diagnoses. Katz *et al* (1969) showed to two groups of forty-four experienced psychiatrists videos of interviews with two patients. Twelve different diagnoses were made by the first group, and fourteen by the second. Temerlin (1968) showed that social forces could manipulate the process of psychiatric diagnosis. He played a recording of an actor trained to give a convincing account of 'normality' to groups of psychiatrists and clinical psychologists. Before listening to the recording, one group was told by an influential clinician that the patient was very interesting because although he looked 'neurotic' he was 'psychotic'. A second group was told by the same figure that the patient was perfectly normal. In the first group 87 of the 95 people agreed the 'patient' was psychotic, and all twenty members of the group who were told that he was healthy made a diagnosis of healthy personality. Psychiatrists were more susceptible to social influence and suggestion than clinical psychologists.

Studies like this drew attention to an uncomfortable fact – that unlike diagnosis in other fields of medicine, psychiatric diagnosis was not an objective, scientific process. It was not based on empirical facts, but interpretations based on values and opinions, and thus amenable to influence by social factors, especially professional power and prestige. But the most devastating evidence about the lack of objectivity, and thus the poor reliability, of psychiatric diagnosis came from a famous paper published by David Rosenhan in the journal *Science* (1973). Rosenhan, a Professor of Law and Psychology at Stanford University, was interested in the lack of agreement to be found in forensic reports written by eminent psychiatrists about the sanity of the accused. He arranged for eight pseudo-patients with no psychiatric history to visit twelve hospitals across the USA, complaining of hearing voices. They were instructed to say that they were hearing a voice saying words like 'empty', 'hollow' or 'thud'. In all other respects, they were told to report the facts of their lives and early development truthfully. All were admitted and given diagnoses of schizophrenia or bipolar disorder, and offered medication. All eight were eventually discharged, but only when they said the voices had stopped. The study was recently replicated by Slater (2004), with broadly similar results.

To some extent the problem of reliability was resolved through the development of standardised interview schedules with rigorous definitions of symptoms, such as the Present State Examination (PSE), but the extent to which this successfully resolved the problem of reliability is a matter of debate. Some have argued that these improvements were not as much as one might have expected (Bentall & Jackson, 1988). Indeed the results of the reliability field trials for *DSM-5* indicate that things have barely progressed. Brockington *et al* (1978) compared ten different systems of criteria for diagnosing schizophrenia used in over 300 patients. Overall the levels of agreement between these different systems was poor. But while research focused on rigorous definitions of symptoms and countless hours of work in agreeing criteria for psychiatric diagnosis in the *DSM* and *ICD* (*International Classification of Diseases*), a silent presence lurked in the background: the problem of validity.

The validity of psychiatric diagnosis

The validity of a system of scientific classification is the extent to which it is believed to reflect the real world. A good example is the nineteenth century Russian chemist Mendeleev's classification of the chemical elements in the periodic table. He was interested in the natural order that the chemical elements appeared to obey. He noticed that if he arranged the elements according to their atomic number, a pattern, or periodicity, was observed so that every eighth member of the series shared physical characteristics. For example, the metal lithium is a light, highly reactive element with the atomic number 3. It shares these properties with the metals sodium (atomic number 11) and potassium (19). Ordering all the known elements at the time into groups based on atomic number, he noticed that there were gaps. His predictions about the properties of the missing elements were subsequently found to be very accurate when they were discovered later. Fulford *et al* (2006) suggest that such a rigorous definition of validity is beyond the ability of most sciences, especially medical sciences. For this reason they turn to what are seen to be 'lesser' validities, of which there are four types: construct validity, predictive validity, face validity, and content validity. Because the first two are the most important for the arguments I want to develop we will focus on them.

The construct validity of a diagnosis deals with the extent to which the diagnosis is related to an underlying theory about the cause of the disease. Bentall and Jackson (1988) use the term 'construct validity' to refer to the consistency with which the symptoms of a disorder cluster together. For example, if certain types of verbal auditory hallucinations are a cardinal feature of schizophrenia, then these experiences should not occur in other conditions such as depression. Likewise, if low mood is a key feature of depression, it should not occur in schizophrenia. The evidence is that this is simply not the case with psychiatric diagnoses. Throughout the course of the twentieth century psychiatrists were forced into debates about the existence of 'overlap' diagnoses such as schizoaffective disorder, because research showed that symptoms of mood disorders and schizophrenia are commonly encountered together in the same patients in clinical practice. Delusional beliefs are frequently encountered in severely depressed people (Winters & Neale, 1983), or thought disorder long considered to be pathognomonic of schizophrenia is commonly seen in patients with hypomania (Andreasen, 1979). In other words, patients simply do not conform to the idealised categories of psychiatric diagnoses.

In medicine, construct validity is important because the validity of disease categories stands or falls by the extent to which the symptoms of a disease can be tied to an underlying pathological causal mechanism. In psychiatry, this is extremely difficult for much the same reason that there are problems with reliability. This is why it has been customary to accept a weaker view of construct validity in psychiatry. For example, Robins and Guze's (1970) highly influential paper on the validity of psychiatric diagnoses refers to laboratory studies, including chemical, physiological, radiological and anatomical findings, as well as psychological tests, and family studies of the inheritance of psychiatric disorders. They assert that since most psychiatric illnesses have been shown to run in families, this implies a biological basis for a condition.

The second aspect of validity is predictive validity. This is the extent to which the subsequent course and outcome of a diagnosis in a given patient conforms to the course and outcome that one would expect for that particular diagnosis. This is a matter of vital importance in psychiatry, where the diagnosis of schizophrenia is believed to be associated with poor outcome and deterioration in social and psychological function. Kendell (1975) stresses the importance of predictive validity in psychiatry, because diagnostic concepts stand or fall by the value of their prognoses and therapeutic predictions, not because of what validity might tell us about the relationships between the symptoms of a disease and the disease process, that is to say the causes of disease. This is another instance of how the concept of validity is watered down in psychiatry.

The Fundamental Problem of Validity and Psychiatric Diagnoses

The focus now shifts to the problem of the validity of psychiatric diagnoses. Again, the issue here as we have already seen is that in the first place psychiatric diagnoses are based on reports that people make of their mental states. But there is an additional problem. Until quite recently it was not possible to study the part of the body most closely tied to mental states, the brain. Scientific studies of psychiatric diagnoses had to rely on indirect observations of brain function, through basic skull X-rays or examination of the cerebrospinal fluid that bathes the brain and spinal cord. That has changed with the introduction of new imaging technologies, so that it is now possible to examine the brain in new ways. For example, it is possible to see if there are differences in the activity of particular brain areas when people hear voices, or have strange beliefs. But this raises a third, more fundamental, problem. How can we be certain that there is a link between an 'abnormal' pattern of brain activity and a mental state like hearing the voice of God telling you that tomorrow afternoon the world will come to an end as the moon crashes into the Pacific Ocean? Such research assumes that the brain events cause the mental states, but how can we be certain that that is so? We will return to this problem in Chapter 6.

Despite these difficulties, the introduction of new brain-imaging technology, and new research techniques in molecular biology, similar to those that delivered new insights into the classification of breast cancer, have raised expectations that it would only be a matter of time before the biological basis (or validity) of the diagnosis of schizophrenia was established without any doubt (Andreasen, 1995). To what extent has this technological paradigm been successful? We will deal with this through the construct and predictive validities of the diagnosis.

Construct validity

Early attempts to establish the construct validity of the diagnosis of schizophrenia were unsuccessful (see, for example, Kendler, 1980). Bentall and Jackson (1988) point out that the problem with most of the earlier work on the construct validity of the diagnosis is that it failed to take into account the effects of years of physical treatment and institutionalisation that patients with the diagnosis experienced. In the next chapter we will see that there is a considerable body of evidence that physical treatments such as neuroleptic drugs and ECT bring about physical changes in brain structure and function. Furthermore, many of the studies were correlational in nature[4] and it is not possible to establish a causal link between the physical 'abnormality' under investigation and the diagnosis. Much the same criticism applies to the studies of structural brain changes in people with schizophrenia. Bentall and Jackson (1988) conclude that there is little reason for confidence about the validity of the diagnosis of schizophrenia.

Validity is at the heart of the claim for the scientific basis of all diagnoses in medicine. This concerns the extent to which there is evidence that people with a given diagnosis differ biologically from those who do not have the condition. The validity of a diagnosis stands or falls depending upon whether it can be tied to an underlying causal pathological mechanism. In psychiatry this has proved impossible to achieve. Since 1970, there have been four major papers in the psychiatric literature dealing with the issue: Robins and Guze (1970), Kendler (1980), Andreasen (1995) and Kendell and Jablensky (2003).[5] These papers are high on aspiration but low on evidence. My earlier comments regarding Robins

---

4. A correlation tells us that a mathematical relationship exists between two variables, A and B, in a scientific study, but it does not tell us whether A *causes* B, or B causes A. Indeed it may be possible that both A and B are caused by a third, unknown variable, C, or that A and B and C are related to a fourth variable, and so on. All that we can conclude from a correlation is that there is a relationship, but we still do not know how the relationship is brought about.

5. These papers are not the jaundiced scrivening of sceptical social constructivists or anti-psychiatrists, but from the pens of leading academic psychiatrists who dedicated their careers to the search for the biological basis of psychiatric disorders.

and Guze's (1970) highly influential paper on the validity of psychiatric diagnoses are worth repeating, wherein they refer to laboratory studies, including chemical, physiological, radiological and anatomical findings, as well as psychological tests, and family studies of the inheritance of psychiatric disorders. They assert that since psychiatric illnesses like schizophrenia run in families, they must have a biological basis, yet there is no evidence for this (see Chapter 6 of Mary Boyle's (2002) seminal *Schizophrenia: A scientific delusion?* and more recently Jay Joseph's (2003) *The Gene Illusion*, and for an equally critical view of twin studies, Goldman, 2011).

Kendler's (1980) overview confirmed that early biological studies failed to establish the construct validity of schizophrenia. Nancy Andreasen's (1995) *American Journal of Psychiatry* editorial promises future riches through molecular genetics, neurochemistry, neuroanatomy, neurophysiology and neuro-imaging, but she concedes that the long-hoped-for laboratory tests anticipated by Robins and Guze (1970) had not materialised; '... we still lack definitive diagnostic tests equivalent to the measurement of blood sugar for diabetes or the ECG for myocardial infarction' (Andreasen, 1995: 161). It is worth noting that she was writing at the mid-point of the 'Decade of the Brain', and was deeply immersed in brain studies of schizophrenia, with the latest generation of imaging technologies to map the 'broken brain'. Fifteen years on, has neuroscience delivered the promised riches?

Anckarsäter (2010) used the Robins and Guze's (1970) criteria for validity to assess meta-analyses and review papers for neurobiological markers and treatment effects in major psychiatric disorders. Apart from conditions like Huntington's disease, which has an established basis in molecular genetics (and which like Alzheimer's disease is arguably a neurological condition), no laboratory marker has been found to support the construct validity of any psychiatric diagnosis. Neither is there any evidence to support the view that they have specific outcomes and responses to treatment. He writes:

> Despite the obvious lack of empirical support for today's diagnostic models, it is not without a sense of heresy that one has to conclude that most, if not all, of the mental disorders known today, i.e., the categories that have structured both the psychiatric praxis and the research into their prevalences, patterns of distributions, 'comorbidities', and aetiologies, simply do not exist as such. (Anckarsäter, 2010: 61–2)

Although the literature is replete with studies claiming to find differences in the brains of those with a diagnosis of schizophrenia and those not so diagnosed, as Anckarsäter's study indicates, the results of replication studies have either failed to confirm initial findings, or are inconclusive. Even the most recent NICE guidelines on the treatment of schizophrenia acknowledge the lack of evidence for a biological basis for the condition:

The possible causes of schizophrenia are not well understood. Research has attempted to determine the causal role of biological, psychological and social factors. The evidence does not point to any single cause. Increasingly, it is thought that schizophrenia and related psychoses result instead from a complex interaction of multiple factors. (National Collaborating Centre for Mental Health, 2010: 22)

David Kingdon, an academic psychiatrist with expertise in the use of cognitive behaviour therapy (CBT) in psychosis, questions the extent to which 160 years' research into the physical basis of mental disorders has helped us to understand the causes of these conditions, improved their management, or contributed to destigmatising them (Kingdon & Young, 2007). He points out that there have been thousands of studies investigating the biological basis of psychosis, but the results are conflicting, inconclusive, and generally non-specific. The search for the genetic basis of specific mental disorders is a case in point. Through the early part of the twentieth century there was a shift in research away from specific genes, to 'susceptibility genes of variable effect'. Quite what the therapeutic implications of this are for individual patients is difficult to know. In terms of the diagnosis of schizophrenia, biological research has failed to reveal the point of discontinuity between people with the diagnosis and those without. Neither is there a clear biological basis to justify the use of neuroleptic drugs in schizophrenia.

Kendell and Jablensky acknowledge that since Robins and Guze's (1970) paper, the validation of the diagnosis of schizophrenia remains unresolved, either in terms of its symptom profile, or its genetic (and thus biological) basis. They note that an '… air of disenchantment …' is apparent '… in the light of the failures of the revolutionary new nosology [classification] provided by *DSM-III* and its successors to lead to major insights into the etiology of any of the main syndromes' (Kendell & Jablensky, 2003: 7). They conclude that psychiatry is 200 years behind other branches of medicine because it can only define most of its conditions in terms of syndromes (i.e., groups of symptoms that tend to occur together):

… most contemporary psychiatric disorders, even those such as schizophrenia that have a pedigree stretching back to the nineteenth century, cannot yet be described as valid disease categories. (*ibid*: 10)

Predictive validity

This refers to the extent to which a particular diagnosis predicts a specific course and outcome. Included in this is a specific response to treatment or other therapeutic interventions. In his original study, Kraepelin (1913) reported that only 13 per cent of his patients suffering from dementia praecox recovered. Table 2.1 (overleaf) summarises the results of four long-term outcome studies of people diagnosed with schizophrenia. In broad terms 50 per cent or more of people with the diagnosis make a significant recovery.[6]

Table 2.1
Summary of four recent outcome studies of schizophrenia

Author(s)	Number of Subjects	Follow-up (years)	% Improved
Bleuler (1978)	200	22	53
Huber et al (1975)	>500	21	57
Ciompi (1980)	300	37	49
Harding et al (1987)	262	32	68

Other work confirms that people who are given a diagnosis of schizophrenia have a wide range of outcomes, throwing doubt on the view that it has a poor prognosis. The work of Strauss and Carpenter (1974a, 1974b, 1977) in the USA shows that social factors such as work status and social contacts are the best predictors of outcome, along with family environment (Leff et al, 1983), not clinical, biological or psychological factors. Cultural factors are important too. Richard Warner (1985) has shown that results from the international pilot study of schizophrenia indicate that outcome in non-Western cultures, where psychiatric care and drug treatments are much harder to come by, is much better than in the Western world. Recent work confirms this. Kua et al (2003) found that two-thirds of their patients in Singapore had a good or fair outcome at twenty years. In Madras, Thara (2004) found that only 5 out of their 61 subjects followed up over twenty years had been continuously ill; more than three-quarters were in employment. Taken overall the results of these studies indicate that the predictive validity of the diagnosis of schizophrenia is very poor. This is hardly surprising, given that predictive validity and treatment response is largely determined by the the underlying pathological mechanisms (i.e. construct validity), which has not been established

---

6. There is a straightforward explanation for this. The asylums in Kraepelin's day were full of patients, many of whom were suffering from serious physical diseases that caused organic psychoses that had extremely poor outcomes leading to dementia and death. These included neurosyphillis, epilepsy, malnutrition, especially pellagra (niacin deficiency) associated with psychiatric symptoms, and chronic infections such as tuberculosis. It is quite possible that amongst his carefully documented cases there were people suffering from these conditions, whose prognosis would have been extremely poor.

Conclusions

Fulford *et al* (2006) point out that, unlike somatic medicine, psychiatric diagnoses are almost exclusively descriptive and based on symptoms rather than aetiology. A negative interpretation of this is that psychiatry is 'scientifically primitive'. Until the seventeenth century, diagnosis in somatic medicine was almost entirely descriptive, consisting of syndromes, as Kendell (1975) has shown. But as we have seen in the case of breast cancer, for example, advances in medical science have enabled somatic medicine to progress to aetiological diagnosis. An alternative interpretation of the failure to validate psychiatric diagnoses is that the nature of the scientific developments that are necessary for psychiatry to move to aetiological diagnoses are simply much more difficult and complex than those that lie behind oncology. Those involved in neuroscience research in psychiatry maintain, as did Robins and Guze nearly fifty years ago, and Andreasen twenty years ago, that it is only a matter of time before science will lift the veil that hides the biological nature of psychosis from our eyes. But how much more time must pass, and how many more aspirational pleas for more time? How much more money must be spent on more research seeking the biological substrate of psychosis? Would not this money be better spent on the scientific evaluation of alternative treatment and support options? In any case, this begs a more fundamental question: will science ever yield a full account of the human experiences of psychosis? That question will have to remain open until Chapter 6, but in the next chapter we will see that the failure to validate psychiatric diagnoses has important consequences for attempts to evaluate the effectiveness of physical and psychological therapies used in psychiatry.

Recommended Reading

Bentall, R.P. (2003) *Madness Explained: Psychosis and human nature.* London: Allen Lane.

Boyle, M. (1993) *Schizophrenia: A scientific delusion.* London: Routledge.

Kendell, R. & Jablensky, A. (2003) Distinguishing between the validity and utility of psychiatric diagnoses. *American Journal of Psychiatry, 160,* 4–12.

Pilgrim, D. (2007) The survival of psychiatric diagnosis. *Social Science and Medicine, 65,* 536–44.

Robins, E. & Guze, S. (1970) Establishment of diagnostic validity in psychiatric illness: Its application to schizophrenia. *American Journal of Psychiatry, 126,* 983–7.

Rosenhan, D. (1973) On being sane in insane places. *Science, 179,* 250–8.

The Problem of Physical Treatment in Psychiatry

3

> I know that most men – not only those considered clever, but even those who are very clever and capable of understanding most difficult scientific, mathematical, or philosophic, problems – can seldom discern even the simplest and most obvious truth if it be such as obliges them to admit the falsity of conclusions they have formed, perhaps with much difficulty – conclusions of which they are proud, which they have taught to others, and on which they have built their lives.
>
> Leo Tolstoy, *What Is Art and Essays on Art*

Armed with antidepressants and antipsychotics the popular view of psychiatry is that of a progressive medical speciality with effective pharmacological interventions for the most common and serious forms of mental illness. The prefix 'anti' resonates strongly with drugs in other fields of medicine – anti-inflammatory, anti-tuberculous, anticoagulant, anticonvulsant, antihypertensive and so on. It creates an image of psychiatry as a science-based medical speciality whose drugs have emerged from years of painstaking laboratory research into the biological basis of conditions like schizophrenia and depression. The truth, as Joanna Moncrieff points out, couldn't be more different. Her most recent book, *The Bitterest Pills* (Moncrieff, 2013), examines how neuroleptic drugs became the frontline treatment for people diagnosed with schizophrenia and other forms of psychosis.

The first neuroleptic, chlorpromazine, started out life as an antihistamine drug for use in anaesthesia for surgery. Right from the outset it was noticed that it induced a deep state of indifference and tranquillity in those who took it. At the time it was believed that this state of 'hibernation' might be useful in reducing the risk of shock during surgery. Henri Laborit, the French surgeon who was investigating its use, was so taken with its tranquillising properties that he suggested to his psychiatrist colleagues that they might find it useful to calm agitated and over-aroused patients. When they did so in 1952, they were so impressed by the results that the use of the drug in psychiatry rapidly took off. In those early years chlorpromazine was not called an antipsychotic. According to Joanna Moncrieff (2013), this word first appeared in the medical literature ten years later, when a paper by Mapp and Nodine (1962), made the distinction between an antipsychotic drug that 'antagonised' psychotic symptoms, and tranquillisers that reduced anxiety. By that time commercial factors had taken over as the pharmaceutical industry realised that a vast new market was opening up.

This brief sketch is important for a number of reasons. It challenges the idealised view of psychiatry as a scientific medical speciality. Neuroleptic drugs and antidepressants rose to prominence despite the absence of a genuine scientific understanding about the biological basis of psychosis. Neuroleptics do have the property of damping down the experiences of psychosis, but this has nothing to do with elaborately constructed theories of chemical imbalances. The background context to this chapter is the lack of evidence for the effectiveness of psychiatric drugs used in the treatment of people diagnosed with depression or schizophrenia. The same holds for ECT, but there is neither the time nor space for proper consideration here. Those interested can follow this up in a recent paper by John Read and Richard Bentall (2010). In depression we consider two widely used interventions: the class of drugs known as selective serotonin reuptake inhibitors (SSRIs) and cognitive behavioural therapy (CBT). The neuroleptic drugs[1] are the treatment of choice for people suffering from schizophrenia, and we will examine the evidence used to justify this. But before that, a word is necessary about the scientific methods that are used to establish the efficacy of any intervention in medicine today, and which are at the heart of evidence-based medicine.

Evidence-Based Medicine and the Placebo Effect

Over the last thirty years the rigorous methods of scientific inquiry spread from the laboratory to the consulting room. Evidence-based medicine (EBM) is the '… conscientious, explicit and judicious use of the current best evidence in making decisions about the care of individual patients' (Sackett et al, 1996: 71). This was a '… new paradigm …' for medicine, that moves practice away from '… intuition, unsystematic clinical experience, and pathophysiologic rationale … to the examination of evidence from clinical research …' (Evidence-Based Medicine Working Group (EBMWG), 1992: 2420). It is a scientific method in its own right,

---

1. These drugs are more commonly referred to as 'antipsychotics'. For reasons that will become clear later on, this is misleading. They have no specific 'anti'-psychosis properties. The word 'neuroleptic' literally means to seize the neuron, which is a more truthful reflection of the powerful effects these drugs have on the central nervous system. For similar reasons, I prefer not to use the word 'antidepressant'. Drugs belonging to the tricyclic and SSRI families have a wide range of effects on the central nervous system, but we will see that there is no evidence they are specifically 'anti' depression.

rooted in a scientific view of human experience, and a major component of the technological paradigm through which mental health professionals understand and engage with suffering (Thomas *et al*, 2012), and which we considered in the previous chapter. However, it has a small difficulty. Something else is inextricably bound up with the act of treating someone, whether it is with tablets, injections, ECT, or even surgical procedures. This something simply does not fit with the technological paradigm. It sticks out like a sore thumb, and any attempt to establish the therapeutic value of a new drug has to take it into account.

The medical anthropologist Moerman (2002) points out that in Western medicine, doctors have been aware for centuries that patients get better after taking pills that contain no active ingredients. The phrase used to describe this – the placebo effect – has changed its meaning over the centuries. The word *placebo* is the first person singular of the Latin verb *placere*, to please. It means, literally, 'I shall please' (*SOED*, 2007).[2] But in the nineteenth century the word was used by physicians to apply to any medication used to please rather than benefit the patient. Moerman shows how the formal properties of placebos, their colour, the form in which they are given (tablet, capsule or injection) influence their potency. The majority of these formal properties are heavily dependent on culture. For example, two Italian studies used different-coloured placebos to induce sleep (Moerman, 2002: 49). The results indicated that Italian women fall asleep much more quickly and sleep longer when given blue placebos, but the opposite happens in Italian men. Moerman points out that for Italian women blue signifies the colour of the Virgin Mary's dress. The Mother of God is a powerfully reassuring figure for women living in a Catholic culture. For men, however, blue is the *Azzurro Savoia* of the national football team, and is thus associated with power, strength and excitement. It is generally acknowledged that the placebo effect is so powerful (it extends beyond drugs to surgical and physical procedures) that it is necessary to demonstrate the effectiveness of new drugs against the non-specific beneficial properties of placebo.

The medical profession has evolved an elaborate method to control for the confounding influence of the placebo effect. In its simplest form, the double blind, randomised, placebo-controlled trial (DBRCT, usually abbreviated to RCT) involves randomly allocating patients to one of two treatment groups, active treatment (the drug under investigation) and placebo (inert, or dummy tablets). The tablets in both groups appear identical, but patients and doctors are unaware of which group the patient is in, hence double blind. This awareness could interfere with any effect of the active drug. If both parties are aware which group the patient is in this could bias the patient's subjective reports of progress and the objective clinical ratings made by the doctor. In any case, the very act of giving a patient a placebo will result in the patient's condition improving because

---

2. According to Moerman, in medieval English it took on the meaning of a flatterer or sycophant; Chaucer names such a character in the *Canterbury Tales* 'Placebo'.

of non-specific factors such as hope and the quality of the relationship between patient and doctor. For this reason it is important to be clear whether or not the active drug confers any additional benefits over and above placebo.

In RCTs, patients are randomly allocated, so that all patients in the trial stand an equal chance of receiving either active treatment or placebo. It is also necessary to maintain blindness to treatment condition in both patients and doctors. Part of the difficulty here is that psychiatric interventions such as drugs and ECT have powerful side effects.[3] This means that it is highly likely that participants will guess whether active treatment or placebo is being taken. We will see that this makes it particularly difficult to interpret the results of RCTs in psychiatric interventions.

The most recent development in EBM has been the introduction of the meta-analysis. Over the years, thousands of RCTs have been conducted to assess the efficacy of a wide range of psychiatric drugs and psychological therapies. A meta-analysis involves carefully pooling data from many studies and re-analysing the results using a variety of statistical procedures. The more observations (patients) there are in a statistical analysis, the more robust the conclusions that can be drawn from the results. Such analyses are not without their drawbacks, particularly the difficulty of ensuring that the studies included are sufficiently similar in terms of patient selection, severity of illness, and outcome measures used.

The evidence gleaned from RCTs and meta-analyses is not the final word on the value of a drug in clinical settings. There are three concepts that are helpful here. *Efficacy* concerns that which can be measured, usually over a short period of time within the restricted context of an RCT. In psychiatry it is indicated by changes in scores on rating scales that purport to measure mood, voices and so on. A treatment may be shown to be efficacious in a trial (the changes in scores of the rating scales in patients given active treatment are significantly greater than those given placebo), but this does not mean that the drug is effective. *Effectiveness* refers to whether or not a drug works in real clinical situations, and over a longer period of time (most RCTs last only a few weeks). Finally, both efficacy and effectiveness may have little relationship with patient *satisfaction*. For example, the ratings of symptoms that are used to measure efficacy in RCTs of interventions for people who are diagnosed with depression or schizophrenia may have little if any relevance to the lived experiences of the people who are subjects in these studies. They will have quite different expectations and views about what improvement and recovery mean. This in part is to be understood in terms of the different values held by different groups. With all this in mind, what does the technological paradigm in psychiatry have to say about interventions for 'depression' and 'schizophrenia'?

---

3. People also experience side effects on placebos. A review of over 100 DBRCTs (Rosenzweig *et al*, 1993) found that 19 per cent of subjects taking placebos spontaneously reported side effects. These included headache (7%), drowsiness (5%), and tiredness (4%).

Drug and Other Therapies for Depression

We will now consider the evidence in relation to drugs and cognitive behavioural therapy (CBT).

Drugs

Antidepressants are believed to work because they have specific effects on neuro-transmitters in the brain. The most influential biological theory of depression to emerge over the last fifty years has been the monoamine theory. In this view, the experiences that lead to a diagnosis of depressive disorder are believed to arise from a reduction in the levels of certain neurotransmitters, especially serotonin (or 5-hydroxytryptamine) and noradrenaline. For this reason depression is sometimes referred to popularly as a 'chemical imbalance', one that is rectified by drugs. This is a gross over-simplification. There is no clear evidence that such chemical imbalances exist. The introduction of drugs to treat depression was not an innovation that followed on from years of painstaking laboratory research into the biological basis of depressive disorders. The story of these drugs is one of serendipity. The drug iproniazid was originally introduced to treat tuberculosis, but it was noticed that many patients became 'inappropriately happy' when taking it and thus it was used to treat depression as the first monoamine oxidase inhibitor. The story of these chance developments is fascinating in its own right, and has been detailed by Healy (1997) and Moncrieff (2008, see especially Chapter 8, 'The Construction of the "Antidepressant"').

Drugs like Prozac are believed to work because they increase the levels of the neurotransmitter 5-hydroxytryptamine. However, of late the evidence suggests that any clinical benefit that arises from their use is as much related to the placebo effect. Drug trials for depression show an unusually large placebo effect compared with active treatment in a series of meta-analyses carried out in Australia and New Zealand (Andrews, 2001). The placebo groups achieved 60 per cent of the improvement seen in active treatment groups. Andrews (2001) concluded that a number of factors might account for this, including spontaneous remission, and encouragement, or hope, brought about by being on treatment. Kirsch and Sapirstein's (1998) review of nineteen placebo-controlled trials found that the placebo group averaged 75 per cent of the improvement seen in active treatment groups. They suggested that the improvement in active treatment groups could partly be accounted for by unblinding, that is to say, by people guessing correctly that they were on active treatment because of their side effects. We will look at this shortly.

Kirsch and Sapirstein (1998), in a meta-analysis of data from studies in which over 2,300 patients were randomly assigned to antidepressants or placebos, found that as a proportion of the drug response the placebo response was constant across different types of medication (75%), and the correlation between placebo effect and drug effect was .90. This indicates that virtually all the variation in the size of the drug effect was due to placebo. They concluded that although antidepressants were generally superior to placebo, most of the benefit from these drugs could be explained by the placebo effect. It is now accepted that the size of the placebo response in drug trials of new antidepressants is sufficiently large to justify the continued use of placebos (Khan *et al*, 2000). This is not the case in other branches of medicine. We (Thomas *et al*, 2012) made a simple comparison with other medical treatments through the 'Gems of the month' section in the Cochrane library. The first review of placebo-controlled RCTs in April 2009 was a meta-analysis of antibiotics for infection control following colorectal surgery (Nelson *et al*, 2009). Compared to placebo, the risk of infection was reduced by 70 per cent in the active treatment group. In absolute terms, an infection rate of about 30 per cent in operations for those taking placebo dropped to 10 per cent for those taking antibiotics, a highly significant and clinically meaningful finding. Non-specific factors (placebo response) may play a small role in preventing post-operative infections, but this is nowhere near as prominent as it is in the treatment of depression.

There are several reasons why the results of in excess of 1,000 RCTs investigating the efficacy of antidepressants are open to misinterpretation. Here, I only have space to deal with what might broadly be called 'innocent' mis-interpretations that arise from the methodological complexities of RCTs. There are many less 'innocent' misinterpretations that are claimed by some to be cynical manipulations and distortions of the evidence wrought by the pharmaceutical industry and academic psychiatrists in their pay. The purpose here is a tendency to distort and 'spin' the evidence in favour of their products, either by making them appear more effective than they actually are, or to obscure the risks and dangers associated with their use. Joanna Moncrieff's *Maudsley Discussion Paper No. 13* sets out these problems in detail (Moncrieff, 2003). She also points out (Moncrieff, 2007) that rating scales used to 'measure' depression commonly used in drug trials contain items like poor sleep, anxiety and agitation that are not specific to depression, and that respond in any case to the non-specific sedative properties of drugs used to treat depression. Improvements on the scores of these items in RCTs thus reflect non-specific improvements, not a primary improvement in mood as is claimed by the technological paradigm. In any case, there is no agreement as to what constitutes a clinically significant (as opposed to a statistically significant) change in the scores that are used to measure depression (Moncrieff & Kirsch, 2005). This relates to the distinction we considered earlier between efficacy and effectiveness.

There is also the problem of unblinding in RCTs. Moncrieff and Kirsch (2005) point out that drugs used to treat depression have many side effects, and because of this patients (and their doctors) are likely to guess they are on active treatment. This may increase their expectation and hope of improvement, and Moncrieff *et al*'s (1998) meta-analysis supports this. The effect size of antidepressant drugs in non-active placebo trials fell from 0.50 to 0.21 in trials that used atropine as an active placebo. Atropine induces subjective side effects similar to those caused by antidepressants. In other words, patients improve if they experience side effects, because they believe that they are receiving active treatment, even if this is not so.

It is possible that the failure to show a clear difference between antidepressants and placebo is because of the recruitment of less severely depressed people into clinical trials who respond less favourably to antidepressants. This relates to the long-held belief that what was once called endogenous depression (severe) responded better to antidepressants than neurotic depression (mild). Moncrieff and Kirsch (2005) reviewed several meta-analyses in their study and found little evidence in support of the view that people with more severe forms of depression respond better to antidepressants. Kirsch *et al*'s (2008) examination of FDA data found that drug–placebo differences in outcome for depression did indeed increase as a function of initial severity, but these differences were small, and only reached criteria for clinical significance in patients at the upper end of the very severely depressed category. However, this relationship was attributable to the decreased responsiveness of severely depressed patients to placebo, rather than the fact that they responded preferentially to active treatment. Using the National Institute for Health and Care Excellence (NICE) criterion for judging clinical effectiveness, Kirsch *et al* (2008) concluded that the additional benefit of antidepressants over placebo was not clinically significant.

Psychotherapy for depression

The most widely evaluated form of psychotherapy for depression is cognitive behavioural therapy (CBT). This fits well with the technological paradigm because its proponents argue that it rectifies specific psychological 'faults' in cognition or thinking processes that are considered important in causing depression (Beck, 1993). Despite this, several studies have shown that it is possible to dispense with most of the specific elements of CBT without adversely affecting outcome (Jacobson *et al*, 1996; Longmore & Worrell, 2007). One detailed review of studies of the effectiveness of different components of CBT concluded that there is '… little evidence that specific cognitive interventions significantly increase the effectiveness of the therapy' (Longmore & Worrell, 2007: 173). It is true that some studies found in favour of CBT as a specific intervention, but the number in favour is no more than one would expect from chance alone. So whilst supporters of CBT may point to fifteen studies that show that it is superior to other forms of psychotherapy, there are over 2,000 studies that find no difference (Wampold, 2001).

The same holds for other forms of psychotherapy. One of the largest trials ever undertaken to compare the efficacy of different therapies was the National Institute of Mental Health's Treatment of Depression Collaborative Research Project (TDCRP). It compared the efficacy of CBT, inter-personal therapy (IPT), antidepressants, and placebo. Follow-up assessments were made at 6, 12 and 18 months after treatment. Of all patients who entered the trial and were followed up to the end, the proportion who recovered and remained well during follow-up did not differ significantly among the four treatments (Elkin *et al*, 1989; Shea *et al*, 1992). The best predictor of outcome across all four groups was the quality of the relationship between patient and therapist as seen by the patient early in treatment (Shea *et al*, 1992). Recent meta-analyses have also highlighted the importance of the therapeutic relationship in positive outcome. It is up to seven times more influential in promoting change than the treatment model (Duncan *et al*, 2004; Wampold, 2001). This, together with '... the observed superior value, across numerous studies, of clients' assessment of the relationship in predicting the outcome' (Bachelor & Horvath, 1999: 140), is a strong indication that non-specific aspects of psychotherapy, especially a strong therapeutic alliance, are more important than the specific techniques used. Wampold concludes from his review of the literature that 'Decades of psychotherapy research have failed to find a scintilla of evidence that any specific ingredient is necessary for therapeutic change' (Wampold, 2001: 204). This provides a strong empirical case for putting the patient's values and preferences, rather than the therapist's technical model, in the 'driver's seat' of therapy.

Schizophrenia

For many years the view that schizophrenia is a biological disorder requiring long-term treatment with neuroleptic drugs has dominated psychiatric care and mental health policy. Belief in the effectiveness of these drugs gave rise to claims by some psychiatrists that community care would not have been possible were it not for their introduction. The fifth edition of Sargant and Slater's (1972) book on physical treatments in psychiatry implies that introduction of chlorpromazine revolutionised the treatment of people suffering from schizophrenia, making it possible to care for them in the community, and greatly reducing the duration of hospital admission:

> The use of chlorpromazine has had far-reaching effects on the attitudes of psychiatrists towards their patients and on the setting in which treatment is given. It has been possible to relax security arrangements; and physical restraints have been almost abolished. Patients who previously would have needed admission to a mental hospital can now be taken into the open wards of general hospitals, with the sense of freedom given by ready access to the coming and going in the corridors and in the street outside. (Sargant & Slater, 1972: 20-1)

The evidence we are about to consider renders these claims in a different light. Neuroleptic drugs do not 'cure' schizophrenia, but they do subdue and tranquillise acutely psychotic people, making it easier to manage them in the community. Thus there is a sense in which it is possible to claim that neuroleptics contributed to community care, but only through their properties in providing pharmacological restraint and control, not through 'curing' schizophrenia as the profession claimed. Despite this, the narrative of progress to community care through 'effective' treatment has continued to dominate psychiatric attitudes about the role of the profession in the community, exemplified by the growth of early intervention services.

In the technological paradigm referred to in Chapter 2, the experiences that lead to a diagnosis of schizophrenia (hearing voices, unusual beliefs, disturbances in thinking processes) are believed to be caused by specific disturbances in brain function. The dopamine theory maintains that the condition is caused by overactivity of neurons that rely on the neurotransmitter dopamine. Neuroleptic drugs are believed to work because they rectify the specific disturbance in brain function that causes the experiences that lead to the diagnosis. In addition, by ridding the person of psychotic experiences it is widely believed that they help to maintain social function. Once on drugs it is necessary to stay on them for a long time in order to make sure that the condition does not 'relapse'. If people stop taking drugs there is a high risk that this will happen, because once off the medication the underlying disturbances in brain function are no longer controlled. Despite the central position of the dopamine hypothesis and its more recent variants as the rationale for the use of neuroleptic drugs, Joanna Moncrieff's recent review of the literature failed to find evidence that the experiences of psychosis or schizophrenia are related to dopamine overactivity (Moncrieff, 2009).

In the last chapter we saw that there is no evidence that people given a diagnosis of schizophrenia are different biologically in any way from people who do not have the diagnosis. With this in mind, I want to examine three claims that are made for the use of neuroleptics in acute psychosis: that they are effective in the short-term management of the condition; that their long-term use improves outcome; that they are safe.[4]

Are neuroleptics effective in short-term management?

The view that neuroleptics are effective in the treatment of schizophrenia is deeply ingrained in the minds of psychiatrists, mental health professionals, health managers and politicians. It is reinforced by evidence in clinical practice guidelines, like the NICE guidelines used in England and Wales. This has important consequences for the human rights and civil liberties of people who are said to be suffering from schizophrenia. It provides the justification for forcing them to take neuroleptic drugs against their wishes, whether in hospital,

---

4. It is helpful here to keep in mind the evidence concerning the natural history of the condition called schizophrenia from the previous chapter.

or in the community following the introduction of community treatment orders in 2008. But on what evidence is this view based? Taken at face value, most RCTs appear to suggest that neuroleptics are superior to placebo in the short-term management of schizophrenia. However, as Moncrieff (2008) points out, most of these studies last only a few weeks, whereas most episodes of psychosis last at least a few months, so it is very difficult to draw any conclusions about the value of these drugs in the short to medium term. In other words this problem is that of the distinction between efficacy and effectiveness made earlier (p. 52).

Moncrieff points out that evidence from RCTs that follow up patients for at least a year provide a more realistic view about the clinical effectiveness of these drugs. The problem here is that out of the many hundreds of RCTs investigating the efficacy of neuroleptics in the short to medium term, only three followed up people for a year or longer. There is a dearth of evidence that is helpful in deciding how long people should remain on these drugs after a single acute episode of psychosis. Schooler et al (1967) found that one year on, the placebo group had significantly fewer hospital admissions than the active drug group. Rappaport et al's (1978) RCT followed up eighty young men in their first or second episodes of schizophrenia over three years. They found that at one-year follow-up only 27 per cent of the placebo group had been readmitted, compared with 62 per cent of people on active treatment. These figures stand in marked contrast to those from Kraepelin (see Chapter 2, p. 45). Those who were given placebo and remained off active treatment over the follow-up period showed greater clinical improvement and better adjustment in the community compared with active treatment groups. May et al (1981), carried out a large-scale study of neuroleptics with placebo, psychotherapy and milieu therapy (admission to a well-staffed acute inpatient unit). Although the neuroleptic group did better early on in terms of symptom reduction, these differences disappeared over the three to five years of follow-up. Between 15 per cent and 44 per cent of patients who were not allocated to neuroleptic treatment on inclusion into the study remained off these drugs for at least three years.

Bola and colleagues (2012) searched the Cochrane Schizophrenia Group Register to identify RCTs that investigated the effectiveness of neuroleptic drugs in first- and early episode schizophrenia. They identified and assessed 681 studies, of which only six met their inclusion criteria. There were three main reasons why studies were excluded: they were not studies of treatment in an acute episode (i.e., they were carried out after patients' conditions had stabilised); they did not have a non-medication arm (i.e., they simply compared one neuroleptic drug with another, without a placebo comparison group); they did not use random allocation (John Bola, personal communication, 14th February 2012). The main finding from the six studies that met their inclusion criteria was that people who were given neuroleptics were less likely to leave the study early than those given placebo. They concluded that these data were too limited to assess the efficacy of neuroleptics in first-episode schizophrenia. This stands in contraposition to the confident assertion that neuroleptics have proven efficacy, and that they should be the first line treatment for schizophrenia. This discrepancy can only be rectified by large-scale independent clinical trials of these drugs.

There is now compelling evidence that some people who experience acute psychosis do well without receiving neuroleptic drugs. Bola *et al* (2009) compared studies with at least quasi-experimental design in which psychosocial interventions with postponement of neuroleptic medication were compared with immediate neuroleptic treatment in the acute episode, and where follow-up of subjects for at least one year was recorded. They identified five studies (Bola & Mosher, 2003; Ciompi *et al*, 1992; Cullberg *et al*, 2002; Lehtinen *et al*, 2000; Rappaport *et al*, 1978) involving 261 subjects.[5] All five studies reported moderately better outcomes for the psychosocial groups. In addition most people in the psychosocial group were not receiving medication two or three years after initial assessment. These results support the view that some people with a diagnosis of schizophrenia do well without neuroleptics in early episodes.

One of the most elegant pieces of evidence that there are people diagnosed with schizophrenia for whom medication is unnecessary comes from a study by Vaughn and Leff (1976), who examined the interaction between drug treatment and expressed emotion (EE). This is a measure of the level of criticism and anxious over-concern within a family, usually directed at a member who has been diagnosed with schizophrenia. Work in the 1970s indicated that it had an important influence on the course of the condition called schizophrenia, with people living in families characterised by high levels of EE tending to have more frequent 'relapses' and readmissions to hospital. They allocated people in their first episodes of schizophrenia into high and low EE households, and estimated

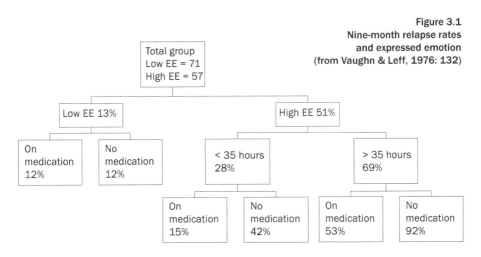

Figure 3.1
Nine-month relapse rates
and expressed emotion
(from Vaughn & Leff, 1976: 132)

---

5. We will encounter most of these studies in Chapter 12, where we consider minimal medication alternatives to treatment as usual for people who experience psychosis.

the number of hours of direct contact they had with their close relatives each week. The level of expressed emotion in the household on admission had a strong influence on the nine-month 'relapse' rates. Of people living in high EE households, 51 per cent relapsed in the nine months following discharge, compared with 13 per cent in low EE households. There was a particularly striking interaction between EE, medication and relapse (Figure 3.1).

Relapse rates after discharge were much lower for people living in low EE households (13%) than high EE households (51%). In addition, medication has little influence on nine-month relapse rates for those living in low EE households (12% for those on medication, 15% for those not on medication). It only appeared to make a difference for people living in high EE households. These data fit quite well with the early accounts of the mode of action of neuroleptics which we considered briefly at the start of this chapter.

These drugs induce a state of tranquil indifference, making it easier for a psychotic person and the family to co-exist, especially in situations where the atmosphere may become quite tense. Whether this is justifiable is of course a completely different matter. Overall these figures indicate that for a significant proportion of people diagnosed with schizophrenia, medication has little effect on outcome in the first nine months. Joanna Moncrieff concludes that although neuroleptics may reduce the symptoms of schizophrenia in the short term, '... there is little to suggest that this has any ultimate benefit' (2008: 77), and she also refers to other studies that reveal that neuroleptics are no more effective than benzodiazepines in the short-term management of schizophrenia. Wolkowitz and Pickar (1991) reviewed fourteen RCTs comparing neuroleptics and benzodiazepines. In seven out of the ten studies that reported robust clinical outcome measures, benzodiazepines were as effective as neuroleptics in reducing psychotic symptoms. This evidence indirectly contradicts a central assumption of the technological paradigm – that 'schizophrenia' is an illness caused by a specific disturbance in brain function which can be rectified by neuroleptics.

Are neuroleptics more effective than placebo in the long term?

Claims for the efficacy of neuroleptics in preventing relapse in the long term are based in discontinuation studies. These involve the selection of a group of patients whose condition is stable, and then randomly allocating them to one of two groups. One remains on active treatment, whilst the other is placed on placebo tablets or injection. The problem here, as Moncrieff (2008) points out, is that the switch to placebo is usually made rapidly over the course of a few days, and this places these subjects at risk of adverse effects of discontinuation. This makes it impossible to know if any subsequent deterioration in mental state is a true 'relapse', which, had the person remained on active drugs, would not have occurred. However, there are ways of looking at the data from discontinuation studies that offer a clue. There is no reason beforehand to assume that a genuine 'relapse' on stopping medication should be distributed anything other than evenly over time after the discontinuation. In other words someone experiencing a 'true' relapse, and not just adverse effects of discontinuation (whatever they might be) is just as likely to have a relapse in the second, third or fourth three-month period after stopping as they are in the first.

Gilbert *et al* (1995) reviewed 66 discontinuation studies involving over 4,000 patients. They found that recurrence of symptoms on discontinuation was more likely in people who had been on higher doses of neuroleptics prior to stopping, and also when discontinuation was more rapid (i.e., took place over less than two weeks). Ten months after stopping 53 per cent of patients had experienced a recurrence of psychosis, compared with only 16 per cent of people who remained on active medication. Taken at face value this would appear to suggest that neuroleptics are effective in preventing 'relapse'. But was this genuine 'relapse'? Using the same data as Gilbert, Baldessarini and Viguera (1995) found that half of those whose symptoms recurred did so within three months of stopping active treatment. As time since discontinuation passed, the risk of symptom recurrence fell away. A further meta-analysis of twenty-eight discontinuation studies by Viguera *et al* (1997) found that 54 per cent of subjects experienced recurrence in the twelve months following discontinuation, but only 2 per cent did so in the second year. This suggests that whatever it is that happens when people stop taking medication, it is not simply a 'relapse of schizophrenia'. The fact that changes in mental state tend to cluster in the three months after stopping is strong evidence that something else is going on.

Harrow and Jobe (2013) also point out that evidence from long-term studies of neuroleptic treatment, especially double-blind discontinuation studies, indicates that the risk of relapse is significantly greater in the six to ten months following discontinuation. This adds weight to the possibility that the re-emergence of psychotic experiences on discontinuation is more than just a 'recurrence' of a schizophrenic illness. The higher rate of relapse shortly after discontinuation may arise as a consequence of the long-term effects of neuroleptic drugs on receptor sensitivity. Their own long-term studies (Harrow & Jobe, 2007; Harrow *et al*, 2012) suggest that most people who remain on neuroleptics continue to experience psychosis, and have poor social function. Robert Whitaker, who had reviewed the evidence from these studies, draws the following conclusions:

> Thus, in this review, they sum up the big puzzle regarding the evidence base for antipsychotics. Do they show efficacy over the short term? Yes. Do patients withdrawn from the drugs relapse at higher rates than those maintained on the medications? Yes. But is there evidence that over the long term, the drugs may worsen outcomes? Yes. (Whitaker, 2013)

One way of interpreting this evidence is that so-called 'relapse' on discontinuation of neuroleptics is a form of drug-withdrawal state. The existence of such states has been recognised as a problem with benzodiazepines for many years. Another possibility is that it is a form of receptor supersensitivity syndrome. The administration of drugs that suppress dopamine transmission bring about compensatory changes in the body, with an increase in the number and sensitivity of dopamine receptors in the brain. If the drugs are discontinued rapidly, this results in a sudden excess of dopaminergic activity (see Moncrieff, 2006; Thomas, 1997, especially Chapter 6).

Moncrieff (2008) points out that studies of long-term neuroleptic treatment in schizophrenia emphasise the importance of symptom recurrence as an indicator of 'relapse' at the expense of other outcomes, such as quality of life, social and occupational function, or subjective experiences. This reinforces what she calls the disease-centred model of drug action. Her review of the literature fails to find evidence in support of the 'extravagant' claims made for the use of long-term neuroleptics in improving outcome. Indeed, the most robust finding to emerge from international comparisons of the outcome of schizophrenia in different cultures is that people diagnosed with schizophrenia in non-Western countries have a much better outcome. In these countries neuroleptic drugs are used much less frequently, and this has led some commentators, most notably Whitaker (2002), to suggest that neuroleptic drugs may contribute to worse outcome in the West. This is supported by studies that show that people who avoid long-term, or any, treatment with neuroleptics do better (Bola & Mosher, 2003; Harrow & Jobe, 2007; Lehtinen et al, 2000). For example, Harrow and Jobe (2007) found that at fifteen-year follow-up, 40 per cent of people with a diagnosis of schizophrenia who were not on medication had recovered, compared with between 5 and 17 per cent of those on medication.

It remains unclear how many people gain additional benefit by taking neuroleptics. It is also impossible to say how many people gain benefit from their long-term use because of the difficulties in interpreting the results of discontinuation studies. In Chicago, Michael Harrow and colleagues are carrying out one of the longest prospective studies of the role of neuroleptic drugs in the long-term management of people diagnosed with schizophrenia. They have followed up a group of patients diagnosed with schizophrenia and bipolar disorder for twenty years. The original sample consisted of 145 people who were comprehensively assessed on induction to the study in the early 1990s, and then followed up on five subsequent occasions, when their symptoms status (positive and negative symptom measures), social function (work history and family function), medication history and hospital admission rates were reassessed. Most were young (mean age 22.9 years) and had had few, if any, previous hospital admissions. Fifteen years later they were able to complete assessments on over three-quarters of the original sample (Harrow & Jobe, 2007). From their longitudinal assessments they derived an indicator of recovery for each person, based on the absence of psychotic symptoms or adequate psychical function over the previous year.

The important feature of this study is that it was naturalistic. It observed the natural progress of patients over time. There was no uniform treatment plan for all patients over the years, and in this sense it is more representative of what happens to large numbers of people diagnosed with schizophrenia and followed up in outpatient clinics in the US and elsewhere. At the fifteen-year follow-up 61 per cent of people diagnosed with schizophrenia were taking neuroleptics. Of those who weren't taking neuroleptics, 29 per cent had been taking them at the two-year follow-up point. Overall, individual patients had complex patterns of neuroleptic drug use over time.

They found large and significant differences in global (social) function between those on and those not on medication at four of the five follow-up points:

> Patients with schizophrenia who had removed themselves or been removed from antipsychotic medications showed *significantly better global functioning and outcome than those still being treated with antipsychotics*. (Harrow & Jobe, 2007: 409, emphasis added)

Similar findings emerged for patients with non-schizophrenic psychoses. Although at fifteen years only a small proportion of people with schizophrenia met their recovery criteria, most of these were not taking medication. People not taking medication were also more likely than the medicated group to have met the criteria for recovery at earlier assessment points. Further analysis of their data supported the view that those who were not on medication were different from the other group, and may have self-selected to stop taking their medication by virtue of having better earlier prognostic and developmental potential.

They comment that their results appear to be in conflict with the day-to-day experiences of many psychiatrists who tend to see patients only when they are in treatment either consistently or sporadically. It stands to reason that people who come off medication and do well tend to remain outside mental health services, so that psychiatrists' expectations of the outcome of people diagnosed with schizophrenia are skewed towards those who struggle. Overall, their results identify the existence of a subgroup of people with the diagnosis of schizophrenia who do well off neuroleptic medication, do not relapse, and experience sustained periods of recovery. Not all people with the diagnosis need to take neuroleptics continually. The same group have recently confirmed this in the same cohort followed up at twenty years (Harrow *et al*, 2012).

In contrast, Wunderink *et al* (2013) investigated the role of long-term neuroleptic treatment using a different methodology. They carried out a seven-year follow-up study of patients diagnosed with schizophrenia, who were later randomly assigned to maintenance therapy (MT), or dose reduction/discontinuation (DR). They compared the rate of recovery between the two groups. They recruited over 80 per cent (103/128) of the original trial at seven years, and after ensuring that all those who entered this trial had experienced at least six months without psychosis, they randomly allocated individuals to MT or DR groups for eighteen months. The main outcome measure was the rate of recovery defined in terms of the absence of psychotic symptoms as assessed by a widely used rating scale, and social function as assessed by a social disability schedule. The recovery rate in the DR groups was over twice as high (40.4%) as that in the MT group (17.6%). This was largely accounted for by a higher rate of social recovery in the DR group. There were no differences in terms of symptom ratings between the two. In addition the DR group received significantly lower doses of neuroleptic medication over the two-year follow-up period. This is the first study to confirm that dose reduction strategies result in better outcome than maintenance therapy with neuroleptics.

Are Neuroleptics Safe?

There are two sources of evidence here: the reduced life expectancy and risk of sudden cardiac death in people with a diagnosis of schizophrenia, and the effects that neuroleptic drugs have on brain structure.

Reduced life expectancy and sudden cardiac death

There is evidence that people diagnosed with schizophrenia are more likely to suffer from serious medical conditions, and have reduced life expectancy compared with age-matched controls. A recent literature review (Casey et al, 2011) found that the diagnosis of schizophrenia was associated with significant medical mortality, especially from diabetes and cardiovascular disease. The interpretation of these studies is not an easy matter. Reduced life expectancy is almost certainly the outcome of a number of many different influences that impact adversely on health, including lack of exercise, poor diet, smoking, the effects of stress and life in poor urban areas, as well as receiving poor quality care in primary health care and other hospital settings. Wildgust et al (2010) found that the life expectancy of people with a diagnosis of schizophrenia is reduced on average by between 15 to 25 years, with hypertension, smoking, obesity, raised blood glucose levels, and physical inactivity particular problems. Chang et al (2011) investigated the impact of serious mental illness (SMI) on life expectancy at birth in 31,719 people on the Maudsley Hospital case register. Between January 2007 and December 2008 there were 1,370 deaths. They calculated that for men with a diagnosis of schizophrenia life expectancy was reduced by an average of 14.6 years (9.8 years for women). They identified poor diet, physical inactivity, smoking, illicit drug use, and long-term neuroleptic use as the main risk factors for reduced life expectancy in these groups.

However, there are two specific risks associated with the use of neuroleptic drugs that may play an important role in mediating the reduced life expectancy of people with a diagnosis of schizophrenia: obesity and sudden cardiac death. It has been known for many years that people on long-term neuroleptic medication tend to put on weight and carry a risk of maturity-onset diabetes. This problem became more acute twenty years ago following the introduction of the so-called 'novel' neuroleptics, particularly clozapine. Epidemiological studies suggested that the use of atypical neuroleptics increased the risk of developing diabetes mellitus by a third (Sernyak *et al*, 2002), a serious condition that has important implications for long-term health and life expectancy. Other evidence points to a role for neuroleptic drugs in reducing life expectancy through cardiovascular disease (Laursen *et al*, 2012). The cardiovascular hazards of neuroleptic drugs have been recognised since the 1960s when it was found that they induced ECG changes known to be associated with the risk of sudden death through cardiac arrhythmias. In the United States, the drug company Abbott Labs withdrew its application for approval of sertindole, a neuroleptic drug, because of the risk of sudden death brought about by ECG abnormalities caused by the drug. In one trial involving 2,000 people, 27 died unexpectedly, and 13 of the deaths were sudden (WHO, 1998).

Hennessy *et al* (2002) examined data from nearly 100,000 patients involved in trials of typical and atypical neuroleptic drugs. They compared the incidence of serious cardiovascular complications in these patients with that in two other groups of people on long-term medication for glaucoma and psoriasis. The rate of serious cardiac problems including cardiac arrest was between two to five times higher in people with a diagnosis of schizophrenia. Ray *et al* (2009) calculated the adjusted incidence of sudden cardiac death in people taking neuroleptic drugs in the Texas Medicaid health insurance programme. They compared over 44,000 people on typical, and 46,000 people on atypical, neuroleptic drugs, with 186,000 matched control subjects. Both neuroleptic groups had twice the risk of sudden cardiac death. This risk doubled when people on high doses of neuroleptics were compared with those on low doses. There was no evidence to support the claim that atypical neuroleptics are safer than typicals.

Brain volume and neuroleptics

The idea that there are fundamental physical differences in the brains of people diagnosed with schizophrenia can be traced back to Kraepelin. He believed that the poor prognosis of dementia praecox was related to an underlying degenerative process affecting the brain in much the same way that neurosyphilis caused psychosis and dementia. Over thirty years ago the results of early studies using X-ray computed tomography (CT) scans did indeed suggest that some patients with schizophrenia had brain shrinkage and increased ventricular volume, but methodological problems made it difficult to interpret the significance of the results. For example, most studies grouped together people in their first episode with those who had had the condition for many years, making it difficult to know whether any differences were due to the illness, or factors associated with the length of time they had been ill, such as medication and other physical treatments.

The precise relationship between the diagnosis of schizophrenia and loss of brain tissue is unclear. One view has been that 'schizophrenia' is a neuro-developmental condition in which the brain fails to develop normally. If this is so, then one would expect to find evidence of physical differences in the brains of people who have the diagnosis when they first present with the condition, usually in early adulthood. Another view is that once the condition appears, brain tissue is gradually lost and this becomes more severe as time passes. Recent studies have relied on nuclear magnetic resonance (NMR) scans. Steen *et al* (2006) reviewed the results of 66 such studies involving nearly 2,000 patients; most were of relatively small numbers of patients, and only a small proportion studied people in their first episodes. Those studies that did find significant reductions in brain volume were rarely replicated, and few findings were robustly significant. However, Steen *et al* did not entertain the possibility that neuroleptic medication or other treatment-related factors might be associated with reduced brain volume. Research from animal studies shows that the long-term administration of neuroleptics can reduce brain volume. In order to establish whether reduction in brain volume over time in people given the diagnosis of schizophrenia is an intrinsic feature of the condition, or an iatrogenic problem related to treatment with neuroleptic drugs, we must study brain volume in the first episode and then follow it up over time, gather accurate estimates of medication use, and then see whether changes in brain volume are related to medication. Another approach is to identify a group of people with schizophrenia who have never received neuroleptic drugs, and compare their brain volumes with carefully matched people with schizophrenia who have been treated with these drugs. Lieberman *et al* (2005) conducted a double blind RCT with people in their first episode of schizophrenia treated either with haloperidol or olanzapine. All patients had initial NMR scans and at least one subsequent scan over the two-year follow-up. Patients in the haloperidol group had significant decreases in brain volume (grey matter) compared with the olanzapine group. Although this establishes a link between reduced brain volume and neuroleptics, the results are inconclusive. Ho *et al* (2011) examined four potential predictors of change in brain volume – length and severity of illness, and history of drug misuse and neuroleptic treatment – in 211 people with a diagnosis of schizophrenia who had an average of three NMR scans over a mean period of 7.2 years. They found a significant correlation between reduced brain volume and length of follow-up. Controlling for the effects of the other three factors, they found that reductions in brain volume were correlated with the level of neuroleptic drug treatment. They concluded that: '… antipsychotics have a subtle but measurable influence on brain tissue over time, suggesting the importance of careful risk–benefit review of dosage and duration of treatment as well as their off-label use' (*ibid*: 128).

Moncrieff and Leo's (2010) systematic review attempted to answer directly the question of whether neuroleptics cause a reduction in brain volume, and also whether these drugs contribute to structural changes in the brain that are usually attributed to the disease process. They identified fourteen longitudinal studies where there was evidence that brain volume decreased or ventricular volume increased during the course of neuroleptic treatment. Studies of untreated patients either did not detect, or did not report, changes in brain volume. This included three studies of untreated patients with long-term illnesses:

> The results suggest that the brain changes found in some first episode studies may be attributable to drug treatment, especially because some studies suggest that structural changes may occur after short periods of treatment. (Moncrieff & Leo, 2010: 1415)

They conclude that there is clear evidence that neuroleptics play a part in reducing brain volume and increased ventricular volume.

Conclusions

As far as the treatment of depression is concerned, the evidence indicates that much of the effectiveness attributed to the specific properties of drugs used to treat depression arises from a non-specific factor, the placebo effect. The same applies to the use of CBT in depression. Much of the effectiveness of this intervention relates to non-specific factors, especially the quality of the therapeutic relationship as seen by the patient. There are serious problems in trying to interpret the results of studies that claim to show that neuroleptics are effective. On balance, the evidence suggests that these drugs may reduce symptom levels in the short term for some people. How this happens is far from clear, but we can be fairly certain that it is not because these drugs work specifically by rectifying an underlying chemical imbalance in dopamine transmission. Joanna Moncrieff's drug-centred model (Moncrieff, 2008, 2013) offers the most rational way of understanding how some people may gain short-term benefit from these drugs. This proposes that they change brain function in such a way as to induce an abnormal mental state (disengagement, disinterest, tranquillity) in which distress and agitation related to the experiences of psychosis are damped down. Most of these studies are of low quality, and the great majority are simply insufficiently long to draw any firm conclusions about the effectiveness of these drugs over months and years. In particular it is impossible to draw any clear conclusions as to whether the use of neuroleptics in the short term helps or hinders recovery in the longer term.

The evidence from the small number of studies that follow up patients over months or years indicates that many do well without neuroleptic drugs. Careful analysis of discontinuation studies designed to assess the effectiveness of neuroleptics in preventing 'relapse' in the long-term management of people diagnosed with schizophrenia suggests that these drugs may actually make the outcome worse. There is growing evidence that as well as not being particularly effective, neuroleptic drugs are harmful. Their use is known to contribute to poor physical health and increased mortality in people given a diagnosis of schizophrenia; to increase the risk of sudden death from irregularities of the heart beat; and to lead to brain damage indicated by loss of brain tissue.

All this begs the question: why have such ineffective and harmful procedures been visited on psychiatric patients? I propose three reasons. First, in the absence of properly validated scientific theories about psychosis it becomes relatively easy to justify an intervention for which there is no evidential basis. Second, psychiatrists are medical practitioners, and a number of factors lead them to feel that something must be done to 'cure' psychosis. These factors range from the altruistic – a genuine concern for the suffering of patients – to the selfish, i.e., the need to show that psychiatry is just as scientific as the rest of medicine. This may in part relate to the low prestige of psychiatry as a speciality in medicine, and more than that, the low social status of psychiatric patients, which in the past and present has meant that they have been forced to endure indignities, and have experienced curtailment of their civil and human rights. Worse, as Robert Whitaker has described (2002), throughout history they have been subjected to invasive and dangerous interventions under the guise of medical treatment that are in truth a threat to life. As a matter of urgency psychiatry must find other ways of helping people who experience psychosis. Neuroleptic drugs may have a limited role to play in this for short periods of time (a few weeks, maximum), something which will be considered in Chapters 12 and 14.

Recommended Reading

Bola, J. & Mosher, L. (2003) Treatment of acute psychosis without neuroleptics: Two-year outcomes from the Soteria project. *Journal of Nervous and Mental Disease, 191,* 219–29.

Moerman, D. (2002) *Meaning, Medicine and the 'Placebo Effect'.* Cambridge: Cambridge University Press.

Moncrieff, J. (2003) *Is Psychiatry for Sale? An examination of the influence of the pharmaceutical industry on academic and practical psychiatry.* Maudsley Discussion Paper No. 13. London: Institute of Psychiatry. Accessed on 24th May 2012 at http://www.critpsynet.freeuk.com/pharmaceuticalindustry.htm

Moncrieff, J. (2008) *The Myth of the Chemical Cure: A critique of psychiatric drug treatment.* Basingstoke: Palgrave Macmillan. (See especially Chapter 6, Are neuroleptics effective and specific? A review of the evidence, pp. 76–99.)

Moncrieff, J. (2013) *The Bitterest Pills: The troubling story of antipsychotic drugs.* Basingstoke: Palgrave Macmillan.

Read, J. & Bentall, R.P. (2010) The effectiveness of electroconvulsive therapy: A literature review. *Epidemiologia e Psichiatria Sociale, 19,* 333–47.

Thomas, P., Bracken, P. & Timimi, P. (2012) The limits of evidence-based medicine in psychiatry. *Philosophy, Psychiatry and Psychology, 19,* 295–308.

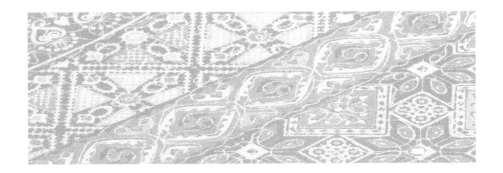

Section 2

Science and the
Contexts of Psychosis

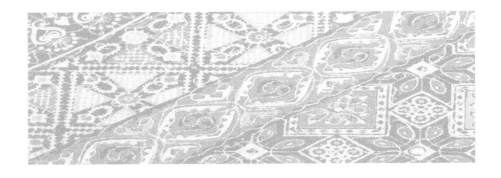

Scientific Models of Psychosis I: The Moral Implications of Childhood Adversity

4

The scientific models that we have examined in the last two chapters have failed to deliver an explanation of psychosis and distress that has much value as far as the diagnosis and treatment of these states is concerned. In this chapter and the one that follows I want to examine a different type of scientific knowledge that sheds light on a range of factors that are important not simply in explaining psychosis and why some people are at greater risk of developing it than others, but also in helping us to understand the experiences that constitute psychosis. This evidence largely comes from epidemiology: the study of patterns of illness and disease in populations or other large groups of people identifiable in some specific way. The value of this knowledge is that it draws attention to the wide range of contexts in which psychosis and other forms of distress originate. In addition, it helps us to establish links between the specific nature of these contexts, and the meaning or personal significance of the experiences of psychosis. This is important because in Chapter 6 we will see that one of the main weaknesses of neuroscience is that it is incapable of engaging with these contexts, and for this reason disregards them. The work to be presented in this chapter and the following one thus sets out the ground for later chapters where we consider the sort of help and support that pays serious attention to the contexts and meaning of psychosis and distress.

There is another reason why contexts are so important. Psychiatrists and mental health professionals belong to the same society as those they try to help. We share these contexts with them. No matter how much we would prefer to ignore this, it is important that we recognise this fact. Our work as members of respected professions brings us prestige, social standing and financial reward. We are fortunate to enjoy high social status as a result of our work. This is in marked contrast to most people who use mental health services. Our therapeutic endeavours take place against and within the context of inequality that we will consider in detail in this chapter. The same holds for the context of racism and the history of colonialism and slavery to be dealt with in the next chapter.

It is necessary to be clear about the role that contexts play, and why I consider them to be so important. I am not claiming that socio-economic inequalities (in this chapter) or racism (in the next) cause psychosis, although there are those who make such claims. My reluctance to do this is in part because to use the verb 'cause' implies a return to scientific modes of thought, which is something I am keen to avoid for reasons that will become clear later on. Nevertheless, there is scientific evidence that draws attention to the role of contexts in psychosis and distress. The difficulty is that causal models of the relationship between, say, childhood adversity and psychosis focus attention on mechanisms within the individual, usually elaborated in terms of stress. The difficulty with this is that it overlooks the extent to which the context of childhood adversity is ultimately a political problem that requires social and political action. A vital outcome of the next two chapters, then, is to raise a series of questions about mental health work in the light of the contexts that we are about to consider. Essentially, these questions concern the moral implications of psychiatric theory and practice. This view has significant implications for the role of psychiatrists, mental health professionals, and therapists.

The main question addressed in this chapter is relatively straightforward: what happens if we disregard the context of childhood adversity that features prominently in the lives of many people who use mental health services? Scientific research in epidemiology and psychology has drawn attention to the frequency with which childhood adversity figures in the lives of people who experience psychosis and distress. Epidemiological research has revealed the impact of socio-economic factors, particularly income inequality, on health and wellbeing. This influence is apparent in the earliest years of *all* our lives, and continues to operate throughout our childhoods, influencing our wellbeing and shaping our future risk of ill health (physical and mental). Psychological research has revealed the impact of childhood abuse on adult mental health, including the risk of schizophrenia and other psychoses. Both sets of evidence yield scientific models that identify stress as the fulcrum around which the relationship between childhood adversity and adult mental health pivots. The danger of this is that we respond solely through interventions intended to change the individual's sensitivity to stress, either through drugs or therapy of one sort or another. At best such approaches are partial. This is because having gone to the trouble of adducing evidence that social, economic and political factors are central to our understanding of a wide range of mental health problems, those factors are then left unattended. The logic of scientific models is that we end up developing 'better', 'more sophisticated' and 'more effective' interventions aimed at regulating the individual's response to stress through psychopharmacological or psychotherapeutic means. But the underlying political and social contexts remain unchallenged. For too long many psychiatrists and mental health professionals have turned a blind eye to this. We have baulked at rising to the challenge that social justice presents to our scientific theories and models. It is too easy to say we cannot change society, or that tackling social injustice is not a part of our job description.

If we accept that adversity linked to inequality is an important context in understanding psychosis and distress, especially the individual experiences of suffering that arise from this, then it follows that we must rethink our role in trying to help those who suffer. What does it mean to care for someone under these circumstances? What is care really about? How can mental health professionals rise to challenge injustice and inequality as they affect people who use mental health services? I won't be answering these questions here; rather I raise them for consideration later in this book.

We start this chapter with the evidence that income inequality is closely related to a wide range of outcomes in health, wellbeing and social cohesiveness. Although there is a sense in which we may think of income inequality as a hard scientific fact – it is relatively easy to measure and manipulate mathematically – this should not obscure the fact that it is also a proxy for a wide range of adverse social and environmental circumstances that are the key to understanding of the impact of childhood adversity and abuse on personal experiences of psychosis and distress. As Jacqui Dillon has written, this is precisely where the personal is the political (Dillon, 2011). Then we move on to consider the links between childhood adversity and psychosis. Much of this work has focused on sexual abuse in childhood, and although the evidence indicates that this is a potent and important factor in psychosis, it is at the same time part of a range of adverse experiences including physical and emotional abuse that occur inside and outside the family. What happens to our children in the classroom, in the playground, on the streets, by text message, Twitter or on Facebook is just as important as what happens to them in the family. Bullying by peers has been linked to the development of psychotic experiences in children. We then consider an important lesson from history to set the scene for the final section on the moral implications of scientific models of psychosis and distress.

Childhood Adversity, Income Inequality and Mental Health

Nearly twenty years ago, when I was writing *The Dialectics of Schizophrenia*, I wanted to draw attention to the importance of social adversity, especially poverty, in relation to psychosis. People have known about the link between schizophrenia and social class ever since Faris and Dunham's pioneering work during the Depression of the 1930s. They found that the frequency of first admissions to hospitals in Chicago for schizophrenia gradually decreased as you moved away from the poor inner-city areas to the more prosperous suburbs (Faris & Dunham, 1939, 1965). In London, Thornicroft *et al* (1992) studied over 200 patients admitted to hospital with chronic and serious mental illnesses over the course of four years. They found a fourfold variation in admission rates in the seven health authorities that admitted to the two hospitals in which the study was based. The most socially deprived district, at that time Islington, accumulated patients at a rate of eleven patients a year, per 100,000 population. This rate was four times greater than that of the least socially deprived district, West Essex. There was a significant correlation between the rate of accumulation of people with chronic illnesses and measures of deprivation, such as overcrowding, unemployment and membership of social class five.[1] This, and similar studies, suggested that poverty may be important in mediating the relationship between socio-economic and psychiatric status. Support for this view came from an American study (Bruce *et al*, 1991), which found that people who met the poverty criteria had a significantly increased risk of mental ill health. At follow-up interview six months after initial assessment, people living in poverty were almost twice as likely to have developed some form of mental health problem than those not living in poverty.

Like many people in the 1980s I had been deeply influenced by the *Black Report* (Black *et al*, 1982),[2] which drew attention to the strong relationship between social class and health. Back then the view was that the role of public health was to raise the overall standards of health of the population as a whole. Health inequalities were generally considered to be a marginal issue, a political matter which the medical profession, if it had any sense, was well-advised to avoid. The *Black Report* challenged that by drawing attention to the importance of poverty in relation to health inequalities. Since then, advances in epidemiology, especially the cross-fertilisation between epidemiology and economics, have cast the relationship between poverty and health in a slightly different light. It is now clear that in the economically advantaged (EA) countries it is no longer *absolute* poverty that appears to be important in relation to health and wellbeing, but *relative* poverty. In addition, it is not just health that is affected by this relationship, but a wide range of factors that relate broadly to social cohesiveness and individual wellbeing. The most detailed and thorough exploration of these relationships is to be found in the work of Richard Wilkinson and Kate Pickett, particularly in their book *The Spirit Level* (Wilkinson & Pickett, 2009).

Their book argues that differences in social status closely related to income

---

1. This is one of the systems of classifying the population by socio-economic groupings used by the Office for National Statistics (ONS). Social class five are people who have 'routine' or 'semi-routine' occupations, or what was once called manual labour. People in social class one have higher managerial, administrative and professional occupations. (See http://www.ons.gov.uk/ons/guide-method/classifications/current-standard-classifications/soc2010/soc2010-volume-3-ns-sec--rebased-on-soc2010--user-manual/index.html#7. Accessed on 12th February 2014.)

2. I must confess a personal interest in the *Black Report*. Its main author, the late Professor Sir Douglas Black, was a nephrologist and Professor of Medicine at Manchester University where I studied medicine in the late 1960s. The very first exposure to real patients in my third year was under his supervision when I was attached to his firm. He was a man of great compassion whose interest in the family and social circumstances of his patients' lives had a great influence on my development as a doctor. The story of the *Black Report*, originally commissioned by the Callaghan government in 1977, is an indictment of the tendency of politicians to attend only to scientific evidence that suits their values and beliefs. The report was ready for publication and distribution in May, 1980, when Margaret Thatcher came to power, but the incoming government suppressed it.

permeate society, spreading out into the family where they shape the child's physical, emotional and psychological development and well-being. The single most important feature of the argument developed in *The Spirit Level* is that it is *relational*. What is meant by this? Earlier work on poverty and health saw the relationship in terms of the direct effect of material and physical factors related to income, such as diet or quality of housing, on the individual's health. In this view, people whose income is low in absolute terms are unable to eat healthily, and live in crowded, poor quality housing. These factors adversely affect their health. The evidence presented by Wilkinson and Pickett indicates that absolute poverty alone cannot account for the relationship between health and social status. More important is how we see ourselves as individuals in relation to those around us. This is a more complex set of relationships, in which social and psychological factors, particularly social status and how we see our social position in relation to others, mediate the effects of income inequality on health and wellbeing. This is especially important for mental health.

In societies like the USA and UK, two of the most unequal in the world as far as income distribution is concerned, relative income inequality has the greatest impact on health. This is because it has a profound and corrosive influence on the quality of family, community and social relationships. Countries that have high levels of income inequality have societies that have lower levels of trust and mutuality. Mutuality refers to the extent to which individuals in a society feel comfortable with each other, trust each other, and recognise that working and cooperating together serves common interests that can combat loneliness, isolation and social adversity. In broad terms it corresponds to what Putnam (2000) calls 'social capital'. The evidence presented by Wilkinson and Pickett suggests that this sense of trust and mutuality has a powerful influence on family life, and thus childhood. Children living in low-income-inequality nations like Japan and the Scandinavian countries do better at school. Fewer children drop out of education, and there are lower rates of teenage pregnancy and births in these countries. Children brought up in these countries experience higher levels of wellbeing (Figure 4.1 overleaf) and lower levels of conflict (bullying and harassment). It is not surprising that adults in these countries have lower rates of mental illness, including psychosis.

Wilkinson and Pickett begin by showing that there are limits to the progress that societies can make in terms of improving health through economic growth.[3]

---

3. Their figures come from a variety of respected independent organisations including the World Bank, World Health Organization, United Nations and the Organisation for Economic Co-operation and Development. It is worth noting in passing that this aspect of their argument has implications for an economic system built upon the maximisation of profit and exploitation of the planet's resources. The health of the greatest proportion of the population of the earth will not be maximised through economic growth through transnational capitalism and the free market, but through an economic system aimed at developing and sustaining greater equality between and within nations.

Figure 4.1*

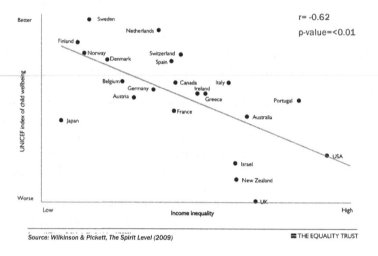

Child wellbeing is better in more equal rich countries

Source: Wilkinson & Pickett, The Spirit Level (2009)   ☰ THE EQUALITY TRUST

Figure 4.2*
We apologise for the poor quality of the graphic in this figure. It is included to show the shape of the distribution rather than the identity of each point.

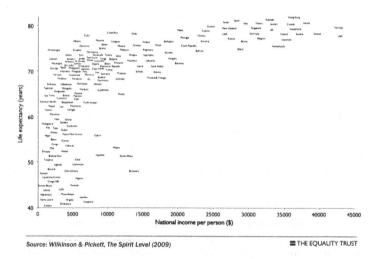

Income per head and life expectancy: rich and poor countries

Source: Wilkinson & Pickett, The Spirit Level (2009)   ☰ THE EQUALITY TRUST

* There are problems in reproducing these detailed graphs (Figs 4.1, 4.2, 4.3 & 4.4) in print. For best resolution view them online at http://www.equalitytrust.org.uk/sites/default/files/attachments/resources/SpiritLevel-jpg_0.pdf or a print copy of *The Spirit Level* (Penguin).

If we examine national income per head of the population against life expectancy (Figure 4.2) across a large number of nations we find that life expectancy increases with income, but beyond a certain point the relationship levels off. There is a ceiling effect, as increasing the wealth of affluent, or economically advantaged (EA), countries beyond this point has no effect on life expectancy.

A similar relationship exists for levels of reported happiness in countries, as they become wealthier. Levels of happiness increase with income to a certain point, beyond which further increases in income have no effect on happiness. This means that for economically disadvantaged (ED) countries economic growth can bring real benefits for health and wellbeing, but once a country reaches a certain minimum level of affluence further economic growth has little effect.

However, if we examine the relationship between income and health within EA countries rather than between them, a different picture emerges. Within EA countries, death rates are closely related to income. People with higher incomes have lower death rates than people with lower incomes. The wealthy tend to be healthier and happier than the poor, a relationship that holds across all the more affluent countries.

It is relatively straightforward to measure a country's income inequality using a number of economic indicators. The measure used by Wilkinson and Pickett calculates the ratio of the level of income of the top 20 per cent of the population and the bottom 20 per cent. On this measure Japan and the Scandinavian nations have relatively low levels of income inequality. In these countries the richest 20 per cent are less than four times richer than the poorest 20 per cent. In the most unequal countries (the USA, UK, Singapore and Portugal) the wealthiest

Figure 4.3

Health and social problems are worse in more unequal countries

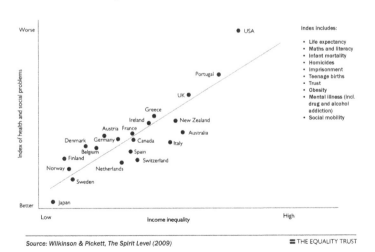

Source: Wilkinson & Pickett, The Spirit Level (2009)   THE EQUALITY TRUST

20 per cent have on average an annual income approximately nine times greater than the poorest 20 per cent. Another measure, the Gini coefficient, assesses inequality across an entire society. A society with a coefficient of 1.0 is one in which *maximum inequality* exists – all the income goes to one individual, and everyone else gets nothing. A coefficient of zero indicates *perfect equality*, where income is shared equally between all members of society so everyone receives the same amount. On this measure, most EA nations score between 0.3 and 0.5. Wilkinson and Pickett examine levels of income inequality in relation to a wide range of measures of health, wellbeing and social cohesiveness. Figure 4.3 shows that in EA countries there is a close relationship between income inequality and a composite index of health and social problems. These include the perceived levels of trust within a society, levels of mental illness, life expectancy and infant mortality, obesity, children's educational attainment, levels of teenage births, levels of social mobility, homicides and rates of imprisonment. That such a wide range of seemingly unrelated phenomena is related to income inequality suggests that the cause, whatever it might be, extends beyond the material circumstances of our lives. Of course factors such as diet, the quality of our home environments, and the healthiness of our life styles are important to a point. Some of these factors are influenced by absolute levels of income. But the message that emerges from Figure 4.3 (p. 77) is that relative, not absolute, income is the key variable. This suggests that whatever is at work here concerns some sort of interaction or relationship between the individual and the wider society in which she or he lives.

Figure 4.4

The prevalence of mental illness is higher in more unequal rich countries

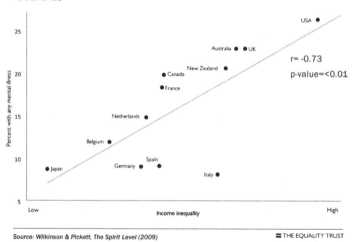

Source: Wilkinson & Pickett, The Spirit Level (2009)   THE EQUALITY TRUST

Wilkinson and Pickett point out that the relationship in Figure 4.3 is statistically robust. We would hardly ever expect to see such a strong relationship through chance alone.[4] This is not an artefact brought about by statistical legerdemain. It is strong evidence that the level of income inequality in a country is related to the prevalence of health and social problems.

Similar relationships are seen for rates of mental illness. The World Health Organization set up the World Mental Health Study Consortium to estimate the numbers of people in different countries who developed mental illnesses, as well as the severity of those illnesses. Data are available for twelve of the twenty-one EA countries examined in the other graphs. Figure 4.4 shows that there is a strong relationship between levels of income inequality and the proportion of people in those countries who developed a mental illness in the preceding twelve months. Again, this relationship is highly unlikely to have arisen through chance. For countries with relatively low levels of income inequality like Japan, Germany and Spain, less than 10 per cent of the population had experienced mental ill health in the previous twelve months. In high-inequality countries the rates were over twice as high, over 20 per cent in the UK and 25 per cent in the USA. These figures refer to the prevalence of anxiety and depression, as well as being an index of serious mental illness (psychoses). All were particularly strongly related to levels of income inequality.

To summarise, income inequality is linked to a wide range of health, mental health (including psychosis) and social problems in EA countries. It is also closely related to the experience of childhood adversity.[5] These findings complement an important body of research that has emerged over the last ten to fifteen years about the role of specific types of childhood adversity, especially child abuse, in relation to psychosis.

Childhood Adversity and Psychosis

When we consider the relationship between childhood adversity and psychosis, the first point to remember is that this is a field dominated by biological science. Despite this, it has been known for many years that childhood adversity is an important factor in a wide variety of adult mental health problems, including

---

4. In *The Spirit Level* they show that the same relationships between income inequality and health and social wellbeing are found in 50 of the 51 US states, using the Gini index. This further strengthens the claims they make for the importance of income inequality.

5. Wilkinson and Pickett are careful about the claims that can be made on the basis of correlations between variables, and it is important to be clear about this. Correlations simply reflect mathematical relationships between measures that represent different variables. They do not establish a causal relationship. It is possible, for example, that an unknown intervening variable that is related to the two variables being examined is responsible. However, the fact that so many different variables concerning health, wellbeing and social problems are related to income inequality suggests that the validity of these observations is robust.

schizophrenia and other psychoses. Earlier studies tended to rely on samples drawn from inpatient populations of people who had already received psychiatric diagnoses. The results of such studies can be difficult to interpret, for although they reveal important information about the prevalence of childhood adversity in people who are already admitted to hospital, it is difficult to draw any firm conclusions about the relevance of this finding more generally. This is because people who develop psychoses and have experienced childhood adversity may be more likely to be admitted to hospital for other reasons. For example, it is possible that they may have fewer social supports and it is this that results in them being admitted. For this reason recent epidemiological studies have focused on large samples of people drawn from the community. In these studies subjects are screened for psychiatric disorders and their experiences of childhood using standardised interview schedules.

These studies raise a different set of problems. They have to recruit very large numbers of people if they are to identify a sufficient number with mental health problems. This is especially so for psychosis, which is relatively less common than depression and anxiety. Even then it is not possible to say for certain that childhood adversity causes psychosis (see footnote 5, p. 79). This is a problem that faces any retrospective study – one that looks back in time to examine what past circumstances might have given rise to an illness in the present. The only way we can overcome this problem is a prospective study that selects a large group of people at random, assesses the extent to which they face adversity in childhood, and then follows them to see what happens to them as adults. The problem here, as Eleanor Longden *et al* (2011) point out, is that it would be impossible to undertake such a study for ethical reasons, since researchers, like everyone else, have a duty to report abuse when it occurs. Longden *et al* (2011) also refer to the problems that arise if we ask adults to report their childhood experiences. A number of factors, including infantile amnesia, retrospective bias associated with the presence of depression, and the controversial issue of false memory syndrome, can make it difficult to interpret any relationships that emerge.[6]

Despite the difficulties, the link between childhood adversity and a wide range of mental and physical health problems in adulthood has been established beyond doubt. This evidence has been comprehensively reviewed by John Read and colleagues (Read *et al*, 2001, 2005, 2009) and Longden and colleagues (Longden *et al*, 2011). Read *et al* (2009) found 59 studies in which on average 65

---

6. Nevertheless, a number of studies also reviewed by Eleanor Longden and colleagues (2011) indicate that the personal accounts of childhood adversity and trauma by adults with serious mental health problems are both valid (Parker, 1990; Fisher *et al*, 2011; Bifulco *et al*, 2005), and reliable (Meyer *et al*, 1996; Goodman *et al*, 1999). If anything, the evidence they review indicates that psychiatric patients under-report abuse (Dill *et al*, 1991; Wurr & Partridge, 1996; Read, 1997; Spataro *et al*, 2004; Fisher *et al*, 2011).

per cent of women and 55 per cent of men admitted to psychiatric hospitals had experienced sexual or physical abuse in childhood. Four large-scale community survey studies, two in the USA (Kendler *et al*, 2000; Green *et al*, 2010), one in Canada (MacMillan *et al*, 2001), and one in England (Jonas *et al*, 2011), involving over 25,000 people, have confirmed that there is a strong relationship between childhood adversity and a wide range of adult mental health problems, including major depressive disorder, anxiety disorder, panic disorder, OCD, bulimia, substance and alcohol misuse, and PTSD. None of these studies, however, looked specifically at the relationship between childhood adversity and schizophrenia.[7]

Read *et al* (2005) carried out another review that specifically investigated the relationship between child abuse, psychosis and schizophrenia. They consider abuse more specifically in terms of trauma, pointing out that the diagnosis of post-traumatic stress disorder (PTSD) has drawn attention to the importance of trauma in a wide range of psychiatric disorders, although the main focus of this work has been on non-psychotic conditions. Relatively little attention has been paid to the relationship between trauma and psychosis or schizophrenia. Despite this they found clear evidence of a link between child sexual abuse (CSA) and schizophrenia in the studies they reviewed, and a particularly strong relationship between childhood abuse and hearing voices that extended *across* diagnostic boundaries from schizophrenia to bipolar disorder. They also found a strong relationship between CSA and delusional beliefs. Some studies indicated that the content of delusional beliefs and auditory hallucinations in people with a history of CSA was related to the abuse. For example, references to 'evil' or 'the devil' in psychotic experiences was more common in people who had been sexually abused.

They also refer to three major studies published in 2004, which they describe as a 'watershed' year. All three investigated the relationship between CSA and schizophrenia or psychosis with '… much larger samples and more sophisticated methodologies' (Read *et al*, 2005: 337). One, by Spartaro *et al* (2004), found a non-statistically significant increased risk of schizophrenia in abused women and men. The two other studies, one by Bebbington *et al* (2004) with over 8,500 adults, and one by Janssen *et al* (2004) with over 4,000 adults, found strong correlations between CSA, as well as other varieties of childhood adversity, and psychosis. Bebbington *et al*'s retrospective study found that a history of sexual abuse was 3.9 times more common than in people who had no psychiatric diagnosis. The experience of domestic violence was twice as common, and running away from home 2.9 times more common, in people with psychiatric diagnoses. Janssen *et al*'s study was prospective in the limited sense that they followed up a group of people who at the time of initial assessment had no psychiatric diagnosis,

---

7. There may be a number of reasons for this. These include the domination of theories of schizophrenia and psychosis by the biomedical model, a desire to avoid 'blaming' families, and the re-diagnosis from schizophrenia to PTSD or dissociative state once a history of abuse is revealed (Read, 1997).

but who over the course of the study period (two years) went on to develop a psychosis. People who had experienced abuse before the age of sixteen were 11.5 times more likely to develop psychosis.

In their later review, Read *et al* (2009) identified a total of eleven epidemiological studies that investigated the relationship between psychosis and childhood adversity in the general population, ten of which found significant associations between childhood ill-treatment and psychosis. The evidence indicates that the relationship between psychosis, schizophrenia and childhood abuse and neglect is at least as strong as it is for more common psychiatric conditions. The large-scale population studies suggest that the link may be a causal one, that the more severe and persistent the abuse, and the more varied it is, the stronger the relationship with adult psychosis.

Before moving on, I want to examine briefly the picture of childhood adversity that emerges from these studies. To what extent does it correspond to the sort of childhood adversity described by Wilkinson and Pickett in their work? Many studies investigating the relationship between adult psychoses and childhood adversity have focused on a single form of adversity, such as sexual abuse. The assumption is that such an overwhelmingly terrible experience must have profound implications for adult wellbeing and health. Whilst this is of course true, childhood adversity is a complex phenomenon consisting of a variety of different experiences that may occur singly or together in different combinations and over extended periods of time. There have been relatively few studies of the impact of multiple forms of childhood adversity upon health. The question here is whether isolated incidents of adversity are sufficient to have an impact upon adult health, or whether repeated exposure to a wide range of adverse experiences, including physical, emotional and sexual abuse, has a cumulatively greater impact. This is important because one implication of *The Spirit Level* is that income inequality is associated with a wide range of adverse experiences in childhood, whereas many of the psychological studies have restricted themselves to a single, albeit severe, form of abuse, such as sexual abuse.

Felitti *et al* (1998) studied the long-term impact of abuse and household dysfunction in childhood on disease risk factors, quality of life, health care use, and mortality in 9,508 people in an American health care plan. All subjects were asked standardised questions to assess psychological and physical abuse during childhood as well as violence against respondents' mothers. They also adapted four questions from a standardised instrument to assess sexual abuse in childhood, and they gathered information about exposure to alcohol or drug abuse during childhood. The most common form of childhood adversity was exposure to substance abuse in the household (25.6%). Over half of their respondents (52%) experienced more than one category of adverse childhood exposure, and 6.2 per cent reported more than four exposures in one or more categories. There was a strong relationship between the extent of childhood exposure and the number of health risk factors for leading causes of death in adults, and a strong relationship between the breadth of exposure to abuse or household dysfunction and multiple risk factors for several of the leading causes of death in adults. Overall, their results show that it is common for people who have experienced adversity to experience more than one form of it. Experiences of adversity tend to cluster. In addition, the impact of these experiences on adult health status is cumulative. There is a strong relationship between the range of exposure to adversity and an increasing risk of serious health problems in adulthood.

Similar results emerge from one of the community studies referred to earlier. Green *et al* (2010) investigated the relationship between adult psychiatric disorder and twelve different categories of childhood adversity, falling into four broad categories: childhood loss (parental death, parental divorce, other separation from parents and caregivers), parental maladjustment (mental illness, substance misuse, criminality and violence), maltreatment (physical abuse, sexual abuse and neglect), other (life-threatening childhood illness, extreme childhood family socio-economic adversity). In their representative sample of 9,282 American adults they found that childhood adversity clustered within individuals. Children who experienced adversity commonly did so in more than one, and often in three or four, categories; it was uncommon for children to experience a single category of adversity. In particular, child neglect nearly always occurred alongside other forms of adversity. It is important to bear this in mind when considering the wider sociopolitical correlates of adversity, and especially the consequences of income inequality described by Wilkinson and Pickett. Green *et al* also identified what they called a 'maladaptive family functioning cluster' of parental mental illness, substance abuse, criminality, family violence, physical abuse, sexual abuse and neglect. This was strongly correlated with the first onset of psychiatric disorder. There were, however, no clear relationships between specific forms of adversity and particular psychiatric diagnoses. They concluded that childhood adversity has '... powerful and often subadditive associations with the onset of many types of largely primary mental disorders throughout the life course' (Green *et al*, 2010: 113).

These studies draw attention to the importance not just of sexual abuse, but also of a wide range of adverse childhood experiences for mental disorders commonly found in adults. Although there is a widely held view that the risk of sexual abuse comes from strangers outside the family, abuse commonly occurs within it. Recent figures published by the National Society for the Prevention of Cruelty to Children (NSPCC) show that reported rates of abuse and maltreatment perpetrated by adults or siblings living within the family (24.5%) are twice as high as those perpetrated by people from outside (12.8%) (Radford *et al*, 2011). But abuse and maltreatment occur outside the family as well; at school, in the playground, on the streets, on Facebook and Twitter. Two recent studies (Lataster *et al*, 2006; Campbell & Morrison, 2007) found associations between bullying and nonclinical psychotic experiences, including hallucinations, paranoid beliefs and dissociation in adolescents. Schreier *et al*'s (2009) study examined the relationship between bullying (repeated peer victimisation), childhood adversity and psychotic symptoms in early adolescence, controlling for factors such as prior psychopathology and IQ. They found that bullying was a moderate-to-strong predictor of psychotic symptoms by the age of 12.9 years. Those who had been exposed, at age 8 or 10, to either overt bullying or relational bullying (rejection by peers) were twice as likely to experience psychotic symptoms at age 12; while those who were victims of both types of bullying were 4.7 times more likely to experience psychotic symptoms. Victimisation reported by children, parents, or teachers was a significant predictor of psychotic experiences, and this effect was cumulative. In other words there was a dose – response relationship between severity or chronicity of peer victimisation exposure and the development of psychotic symptoms.

> This finding of a dose-response relationship is consistent with findings of the relationship between other forms of abuse of power such as sexual or physical abuse of children with psychosis and other mental disorders. (Schreier et al, 2009: 532)

A Lesson from History

Although the discipline of psychiatry has clung tenaciously to the belief that schizophrenia is a biological disorder, it is also important to recognise that until relatively recently there was a strong tradition that tried to understand psychosis in terms of psychological and social factors, as well as the biological. The biopsychosocial model is usually associated with the work of the American psychiatrists, George Engel (1977) and Adolph Meyer (1957); see Double (2007). However, in recent years this model has metamorphosed into what is called the stress–vulnerability model (Zubin & Spring, 1977; Norman & Malla, 1993). This variant has become highly influential in research into schizophrenia. It proposes that psychoses like schizophrenia can be understood in terms of an interaction between environmental factors, such as life events and social adversity, and an underlying biological vulnerability.

The difficulty with this, as John Read and colleagues (2001) point out, is that vulnerability, especially a biological view of what constitutes vulnerability (and one dominated by genetic theories), has overshadowed the role of social factors in schizophrenia. Vulnerability has increasingly come to mean genetic predisposition, to the extent that this has dominated research into schizophrenia and other psychoses. In addition to this, the social and psychological components of what was formerly the biopsychosocial model, such as life events, trauma and social adversity, have been lumped together under the rubric 'stress'. In common parlance the word 'stress' has many meanings,[8] but no longer in psychiatry where genetic and neuroscience research completely dominate the stress–vulnerability

---

8. Footnote 8 opposite.

model. This indicates that in psychiatry there has been a fundamental shift in the meaning of the word. Rather than dealing with a range of social factors in relation to psychosis, 'stress' is now more narrowly understood in biological terms, and particularly in terms of the hypothalamic–pituitary–adrenal (HPA) axis.[9]

Table 4.1
Percentage of biological and psychosocial research studies in schizophrenia published since 1961

Research Category	Total 33,648	1961–1970 2,014	1971–1980 5,854	1981–1990 10,663	1991–2000 15,117
Genetics	3.8	2.7	3.4	4.5	3.7
Biochemistry	2.5	4.7	3.3	2.4	1.9
Neuro-pyschology	1.5	0	0.3	1.1	2.4
Socio-economic status	0.3	0.6	0.6	0.3	0.2
Child-rearing practices	0.8	1.6	1.4	0.8	0.4
Child abuse	0.1	0	0	0.1	0.1

From Read *et al*, 2001: 321

Read *et al* (2001) produce empirical evidence to support this claim. They analysed the content of research into schizophrenia published over the preceding fifty years, from which it is clear that biological hypotheses and theories dominate (Table 4.1). Studies of the role of stress peaked at a lowly 1.2 per cent in the 1980s then fell away. By the end of the twentieth century, the proportion of studies

---

8. The *Shorter Oxford English Dictionary* gives nine different senses to the word, including '… hardship, adversity or affliction …' and '… force, pressure or violence against a person for the purpose of compulsion' (*SOED*, 2007). These of course concern the social and interpersonal factors that act on the individual from outside. Only relatively recently has the word come to be associated with '… a condition or adverse circumstances that disturb, or are likely to disturb, the normal physiological or psychological functioning of the individual' (*ibid*: 3057). At least as far as our wider culture is concerned, the meaning of stress encompasses our social, physiological and psychological worlds.

9. The HPA axis is concerned with the neuroendocrine regulation of stress. It consists of various nuclei in the hypothalamus, nerve tracts from there to the adjacent pituitary gland, a number of hormonal feedback mechanisms, and the adrenal glands (situated above the kidneys) and are responsible for the secretion of the body's main stress hormone, cortisol. As well as being important in preparing the body for 'fight or flight', the system also plays an important role in regulating diurnal rhythms and the immune system.

investigating the role of socio-economic factors in the condition had fallen to 0.2 per cent, from a peak of 0.6 per cent in the 1960s and 1970s. Studies of child-rearing practices peaked at 1.6 per cent in the 1960s, a time when interest in the influence of family life on the origins and course of schizophrenia was at its zenith. Overall this supports the view that even in studies that adopt scientific methodologies, interest in social, economic and family contexts relevant to understanding psychosis has been on the wane for decades.

But there is another feature of this biological preoccupation with vulnerability that has further constrained interest in social and environmental factors in schizophrenia. Most biological studies have been concerned with the role of events and stressors at two specific points in the lifespan of the individual: the months immediately before and after birth, and the months leading up to the first appearance of psychosis. For example, there have been many biological studies of the role of very early events in the lives of people who develop schizophrenia, such as maternal viral infections in pregnancy, perinatal events like birth injury, and postnatal events like viral infections (see, for example, Crow *et al*, 1994; Jones *et al*, 1994). But the focus in these studies is inexorably biological. Most have ignored what happens throughout the life of the growing, developing child, especially in terms of the quality of family life. One reason for this is that most researchers and the bodies who fund them assume that schizophrenia is a biological disorder, and so they have only looked at those periods in the individual's life where, according to biological theories, events are likely to have an impact, usually in the earliest stages of development. Another reason is the distinction between form and content of experience proposed by Karl Jaspers (1963). This has been enormously influential in psychiatry. Bracken and Thomas (2005, see especially pp. 120–2) have drawn attention to the consequences of this distinction, particularly the way it separates phenomenology as a scientific approach to the detailed description of the contents of consciousness, from hermeneutics and attempts to engage with the interpretation, and thus meaning of, the contents of consciousness (voices, severe distress, unusual beliefs and so on).

Researchers have been so blinded by their assumptions about the biological basis of schizophrenia that they have overlooked the possible significance of non-biological factors in the condition.[10] This raises the question: what about the life that continues between these two points? In particular, is there anything about the quality of the social and emotional environment during childhood years that might be important in relation to adult psychosis?

It is in biological studies of the relationship between traumatic brain injuries

---

10. This, as Read *et al* (2001) have pointed out, is an example of the preoccupation with 'normal science' described by Thomas Kuhn (1962). In normal science, the prevailing theory, or paradigm, sets out how scientific data should be used. Scientists engaged in research within the established paradigm are generally not involved in work that tests the paradigm, which is taken for granted. Instead they are solving puzzles related to the paradigm.

(TBIs) and schizophrenia that we find the most egregious instances where researchers' devotion to investigating the biological basis of schizophrenia has morally blinded them to the significance of the most extreme forms of childhood adversity. Malaspina *et al* (2001) wanted to establish whether exposure to TBI in people with a family history of schizophrenia increased their risk of developing the condition, and whether any increased risk was related primarily to the genetic risk, or whether TBI contributed to the risk independently. They found a significantly increased risk of TBI in people given a diagnosis of schizophrenia, and that in those individuals who had more than one relative with a diagnosis of schizophrenia the risk of both schizophrenia and TBI was greater. They write: 'Perhaps increased exposure to traumatic brain injury is a consequence of an inherited diathesis of attentional abnormality in schizophrenia families ... Schizophrenia genes may increase exposure to head trauma, with head trauma further increasing the risk for schizophrenia' (Malaspina *et al*, 2001: 444). In other words one's risk of both schizophrenia and head injuries is to be explained on the basis of genetic factors.

Now it is of course possible that TBI occurs by chance in road traffic accidents, or in young men through alcohol-related fights. It is even conceivable that clumsiness in childhood, which may have a genetic basis, may increase the chances of a child suffering a TBI. The Malaspina study had access to details of the ages at which subjects sustained their injuries, as well as the number, frequency and severity of injuries. From this information it should have been possible to have made a judgement as to whether the injury was accidental or non-accidental, but there is no reference to this anywhere in the paper, despite the evidence elsewhere that the most likely cause of these injuries was violence by a parent or other adult. One in eight American children aged between ten to sixteen years has experienced aggravated assault (Boney-McCoy & Finkelhor, 1995). This partial interpretation of their results limits the credibility of the paper, and contributes to a misrepresentation of a complex set of relationships.

In the middle of the nineteenth century, Auguste Ambroise Tardieu was professor of forensic medicine in the University of Paris. Labbé (2005) has recently drawn attention to the importance of his work on child abuse, which has been widely neglected. Tardieu's duties included performing autopsies in the Paris morgue under instruction from the courts. He investigated thousands of crimes, and over the years was shocked at the large numbers of young children whom he had to examine. His *Forensic Study on Cruelty and the Ill-treatment of Children* (Tardieu, 1860), is a classic description of the battered-child syndrome. In twenty-one of the thirty-two cases he reported, the perpetrators of these crimes were the parents. Three years earlier he published the first edition of his book *Étude Médico-Légale sur les Attentats aux Moeurs* (literally *Forensic Study on Offences against Morals*). It is almost certainly the first systematic account in the medical literature of the sexual abuse of young children, particularly young girls,[11] and went through seven editions until 1878. It presents a detailed analysis of 632 cases of sexual abuse in girls, and a further 302 in males. In the 1878 edition Tardieu clearly states that the evidence from his work indicated that fathers sexually abused their daughters:

> Ce qui est plus triste encore, c'est de voir que les liens du sang, loin d'opposer une barrière à coupables entraînements, ne servent trop souvent qu'à les favoriser. Des pères abusent de leurs filles, des frères de leurs soeurs.
> [What is even sadder is to see that ties of blood, far from constituting a barrier to these guilty drives, are too often used to support them. Fathers abuse their daughters, brothers their sisters.] (Tardieu, 1859: 43)

Labbé points out that Tardieu's work met with a great deal of hostility and was ignored by his colleagues. Parisian society at the time was reluctant to accept that such terrible deeds occurred in the families of the (mainly) poor, and thus the importance of sexual and physical abuse remained unacknowledged. Masson (1984) also refers to Tardieu's work in his book describing Freud's about-turn on the seduction theory of neurosis. In contrast to Labbé, he suggests that awareness of child abuse, especially sexual abuse, was a notable feature of Parisian medical life towards the end of the nineteenth century.[12] The important point here is to draw attention to a persistent failure of the scientific community (Freud regarded himself primarily as a scientist) to acknowledge the role of the most extreme forms of childhood adversity in relation to psychosis, whether it be by the founder of psychoanalysis or contemporary biological research into schizophrenia.

Moving Beyond Models

The work of Richard Wilkinson and Kate Pickett, and that of John Read, is important because they draw attention to the impact of income inequality and social adversity on childhood, and in turn the negative influence of childhood adversity on adult wellbeing and mental health. One way of interpreting these

---

11. The book is in three parts. The first has the title *Outrages publics à la pudeur* (An outrage to public modesty); the second, *Viols et attentats à la pudeur* (The shame of rape and attacks); the third, *De la pédérasty et de la sodomie*, requires no translation. It is worth noting that the language of this book, written by an eminent academic and doctor, is dominated by words like 'shame' and 'outrage'. It suggests that at that time the issue of child abuse was spoken about in language that carried powerful moral judgements.

12. It seems improbable that when Freud went to Paris to work with Charcot in 1885, just seven years after the publication of the seventh edition of Tardieu's book, that he would have been unaware of the controversy that shrouded Tardieu's work. Freud's early ideas about sexual seduction in hysteria were, as Masson argues, influenced by the view that the sexual abuse of children was well-established. But in 1897 he abandoned this theory, replacing it instead with the view that reports by female patients of childhood sexual activity were fantasies.

relationships is in terms of social justice – the extent to which society is fair and just. I have tried to set this out in Figure 4.5, which draws on some of the key relationships described by Wilkinson and Pickett. There are two elements running at ninety degrees to each other through the figure. As we move from left to right we move along a gradient in social justice, from societies that are fair and equal (in terms of income distribution) to societies that are characterised by high levels of income inequality. As we move up from the bottom of the figure, these differences are reflected in measures of social cohesiveness, childhood experiences and health. But as we move from bottom to top, we also move from the moral concept of social justice, through the nature of the society and communities we live in, then into the family and the quality of the child's early relationships, to end up finally at the top with the impact of all this on the individual's wellbeing and mental health. The point here is that in the light of the evidence presented above, we cannot conceive of adult mental health without taking into account the background contexts of family life and childhood, community and ultimately the extent to which the societies in which we live are fair and just.

Figure 4.5

Social Justice and Wellbeing

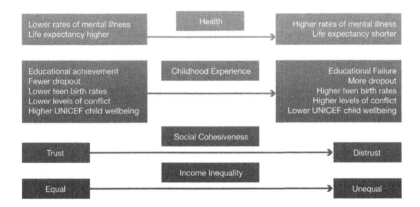

Childhood experience is the key to these relationships. Not what happens in and around birth, not what happens in the weeks leading up to the first appearance of a psychosis in a seventeen-year-old, but the quality of life throughout childhood. It is the extent to which a child is loved unconditionally, valued and nurtured in a safe and secure family environment.

But there is another way of thinking about these relationships, a scientific way that constructs a model of how the different elements fit together. Such models have appeared regularly in the scientific literature in recent years. Brunner (1997) proposed an ethological model based on primate research to develop a biological explanation of the relationship between health and socio-economic circumstances. Stress and the neuro-endocrine 'fight or flight' response are at its centre. Schreier *et al* (2009) also place stress and the HPA axis at the centre of their explanation of the relationship between bullying and psychotic experiences in childhood. Wilkinson and Pickett turn to evolutionary psychology at the end of *The Spirit Level* to explain the relationships between social adversity and health in terms of stress related to social status, shame and humiliation. Again the HPA axis figures prominently. Read *et al* (2001) have developed a traumagenic neuro-developmental (TN) model of the relationship between childhood adversity and psychosis, in which stress mediated by the HPA features prominently.

Figure 4.6

Childhood Adversity and Wellbeing

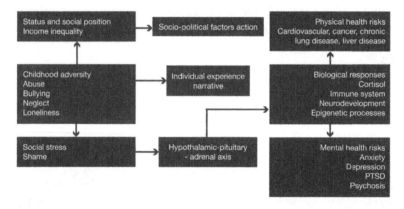

Figure 4.6 summarises the main features of these models. Stress and the HPA axis are held to be the vital elements in explaining the relationship between childhood adversity and poor mental and physical health. In biological terms, stress originating in childhood adversity triggers a number of responses. The release of cortisol and changes in the immune system increase health risks for a variety of diseases, including cardiovascular conditions and cancer. At the same time, stress acting through the HPA system may have an impact on neurodevelopmental and epigenetic processes[13] leading ultimately to psychosis in adults.

Models are helpful, there is no denying that. They enable us to make sense of complex realities in ways that help us to develop new hypotheses that can be tested through scientific methods. In time this may lead to new technological forms of help through the development of more effective and safer therapeutic interventions. In other words models like those set out above are important in helping us to overcome the failures and shortcomings of existing models and

---

13. Footnote 13 opposite

theories about psychosis, and the interventions that arise from them.

But models have their limitations. It can take a long time for new theories to filter through into better interventions. The situation for people who use mental health services is urgent and pressing right now. All that is on offer to them are dangerous and largely ineffective drugs and physical treatments. There is an urgent need for safer ways of helping people. But there is a more fundamental problem. Figure 4.5 draws attention to the importance of contexts in understanding psychosis and distress – contexts of social justice, of childhood adversity tied to income inequality. But the scientific model in Figure 4.6 explains these relationships in terms of biological phenomena. And what arises from this is that the focus of our interventions is way downstream on individual 'vulnerability', far removed from the origins of stress in our social conditions, and cast in terms that have little to do with social justice. Read and others (2009) are correct to draw attention to the need to move away from a 'bio-bio-bio' model of psychosis to one in which psychological and epigenetic factors are given due prominence. But the anxiety is that we end up developing new psychological and pharmacological therapies aimed at rectifying the 'faulty' individual's brain/mind, rather than confronting the injustices linked to the problem in the first place. This project is already well underway as can be seen in the rapidly expanding research into the neurobiology of childhood adversity (see, for example, Tyrka *et al*, 2013).

The value base of scientific psychiatry is the reduction of suffering and the restoration of health, coupled with the belief that rational decision-making based on scientific methods is the best way of achieving this (Thomas *et al*, 2012). Throughout his book *Mad in America*, Robert Whitaker (2002) catalogues the harmful psychiatric interventions that have been visited upon the mad. He intones a litany of abusive and damaging practices, including spinning chairs, cold baths, blood-letting, metrazole-induced convulsions, surgical procedures that include the removal of women's ovaries and uteri, insulin coma, ECT, lobotomy and, most recently, neuroleptic drugs. All these interventions were justified in their time because of two reasons. First, they were considered to be scientific; second, the moral imperative that doctors feel they are under to do good. The value of beneficence is a very powerful one in medicine, but its position is questionable.

---

13. Epigenetic processes represent interactions between genes and environmental factors, so that the latter may inhibit or encourage the expression of genetic information. It can be seen most clearly in the idea that certain environmental influences may switch particular genes on or off. Recognition of the importance of these processes has resulted in our understanding of the role of genetics in relation to human characteristics, moving away from the idea that we are what our genes have determined. It means that we have to understand human physical and natural characteristics as the outcome of a complex series of interactions between genes and environments. This has immense implications for even the most sophisticated of current genetic models of psychosis, predicated upon genes of variable penetrance, or multiple gene effects. It makes the search for biological factors in psychosis infinitely more difficult and complex, a point well made by Steven Rose (2001).

Whilst most agree that there is an absolute injunction upon doctors to do no harm, it is debatable whether the same holds for beneficence (Gillon, 1985). As Whitaker points out, beneficence can be tragically misguided.

This isn't an argument for abandoning the value of beneficence. The reduction of suffering and the restoration of health have been central to the practice of medicine since the time of Hippocrates. But the recent history of scientific psychiatry has not been a happy one. Some, especially those engaged in researching the neurobiology of trauma and its long-term consequences, may construe what I have said in the chapter as an attack on their work. That is not my intention. I am not opposed to the TN model. It represents an important move away from the oppressively harmful category of schizophrenia. But my fear is that we may replace one set of oppressive and harmful practices with yet more, as Robert Whitaker and others have so powerfully and tragically documented. If we are not to ruin more lives, there is a duty on all of us, particularly those who advocate for any new scientific model in the field of mental health, to be clear about the safeguards, checks and balances that should be in place. How will any interventions that might arise from the TN model be used? How will their safety and effectiveness be evaluated? Who will be involved in this, and how transparent will these evaluations be? How will the model and the practices based in it stand in relation to other ways of understanding and responding to psychosis?

The evidence presented in this chapter indicates that scientific models and technological interventions should only be a part of our response to trauma and adversity. Our work as mental health professionals can benefit enormously if it is augmented by a set of values that also acknowledges the importance of social justice in health and wellbeing. The widening gap between rich and poor means that it is essential that our work also recognises the importance of these values alongside the more traditional values of medical and psychiatric practice. If we are serious about the need to reconfigure the help and support that is available to people who experience psychosis and distress, then this analysis helps us to be clear about the direction we should be moving in. At the centre of Figure 4.6 is not the HPA axis, but two elements that are directly related to the contexts of social injustice that give rise to stress in the first place – individual experience and social action. These elements unite, to use Jacqui Dillon's words, the personal and the political (Dillon, 2011). Through narrative, individuals negotiate meaning and understanding of experiences rooted in adversity and oppression. Social action, embodied by the work of the survivor/service user movements, brings individuals together. Narrative and social action are at the heart of service user and survivor activism. The skill and art of psychiatry will in future be found in ways that enable us to work with and alongside these elements. Narrative psychiatry and community development open up ways in which we can achieve this.

Recommended Reading

Labbé, J. (2005) Ambroise Tardieu: The man and his work on child maltreatment a century before Kempe. *Child Abuse and Neglect, 29,* 311–24.

Longden, E., Madill, A. & Waterman, M. (2011) Dissociation, trauma, and the role of lived experience: Toward a new conceptualization of voice hearing. *Psychological Bulletin, 138,* 28–76. doi: 10.1037/a0025995.

Read, J., Bentall, R. & Fosse, R. (2009) Time to abandon the bio-bio-bio model of psychosis: Exploring the epigenetic and psychological mechanisms by which adverse life events lead to psychotic symptoms. *Epidemiologia e Psichiatria Sociale, 18*(4), 299–310.

Read J., Perry B.D., Moskowitz, A. & Connolly J. (2001) The contribution of early traumatic events to schizophrenia in some patients: A traumagenic neurodevelopmental model. *Psychiatry, 64,* 319–45.

Read, J., van Os, J., Morrison, A. & Ross, C. (2005) Childhood trauma, psychosis and schizophrenia: A literature review with theoretical and clinical implications. *Acta Psychiatrica Scandinavica, 112,* 330–50. doi: 10.1111/j.1600-0447.2005.00634.x.

Wilkinson, R. & Pickett, K. (2009) *The Spirit Level: Why equality is better for everyone.* London: Penguin Books.

Scientific Models of Psychosis II: Racism, Psychiatry and the Experience of Black People

5

An African-Caribbean teenager is attacked and murdered by a gang of five white youths at a bus stop in south-east London for no reason other than the colour of his skin. They shout 'What – what, nigger' before forcing him to the ground and stabbing him (*The Guardian*, 2011). The Metropolitan Police fail to investigate the crime properly because of institutional racism. Almost twenty years later, in 2011, the Crown Prosecution Service finally manages to prosecute and convict two men of his murder.

An article appears on the website of an extreme right-wing organisation under the title 'Shock as Government Report Claims Schizophrenia is "Epidemic" Amongst Africans in Britain' (BNP, 2009).

A thirty-eight-year-old African-Caribbean man dies in a secure psychiatric unit after he is forcibly medicated and restrained by four members of staff following a row with a white patient over the use of the ward telephone. The report into his death concludes that on the evening he died he '… was not treated by the nurses as if he were capable of being talked to like a rational human being, but was treated as if he was a "lesser being" … who should be ordered about and not be given a chance to put his own views about the situation …' (NSC NHS Strategic Health Authority, 2003: 25).

An eminent professor of psychiatry is quoted by an article in *The Guardian* (Britain's leading left-of-centre newspaper) as referring to the results of a major study of schizophrenia in black people[1] as evidence of an 'epidemic' (Lewin, 2009).

A metropolitan police officer is suspended for saying a black man resembled a monkey. He claims it had nothing to do with the man's race, but '… he was pointing him out in a discussion about evolution …' (*The Guardian*, 2012b). He is subsequently cleared of racially aggravated harassment by a court.

The chairman of a campaign to combat racism in football stands down from

1. 'Black' throughout refers to people who trace their origins and heritage to Africa, then via slavery to the Caribbean, and then through migration symbolised by the MV *Empire Windrush* to Britain. It also refers to people from Africa who migrated in order to avoid persecution and genocide in the continent over the last fifty years.

the sport's governing body after attacking the Football Association, the Premier League and two clubs, Chelsea and Liverpool, for a failure of 'morality' and 'leadership' over the way they handled instances of racial abuse by two prominent players (*The Guardian*, 2012c).

The British National Party (BNP) article about the 'epidemic' of schizophrenia in black people ends with a plug for a book ('recommended reading') by Rushton (1995) with the title *Race, Evolution and Behaviour: A Life History Perspective*. The article has this to say about it:

> Using evidence from psychology, anthropology, sociology and other scientific disciplines, this book shows that race is a reality and that there are recognisable profiles for the three major racial groups in terms of brain size, intelligence, personality and temperament, sexual behaviour, and rates of fertility, maturation, and longevity.
>
> The profiles reveal that, on average:
>
> - Orientals and their descendants around the world fall at one end of the continuum
> - Blacks and their descendants around the world fall at the other end of the continuum
> - Whites regularly fall in between.
>
> This worldwide pattern implies evolutionary and genetic, rather than purely social, political, economic, or cultural, causes.

This chapter is concerned with the relationship between black people and British psychiatry, a relationship best exemplified through the apparently raised incidence of 'schizophrenia' in young black men. But it is inconceivable to consider this relationship without setting it within the wider context of the relationship between black people and white people in British society. This context is not simply a contemporary issue; it is not simply a matter of how the two groups live alongside each other in multicultural Britain. There is much more to it than that. If we are to understand the fear and anxiety that psychiatry evokes in the heart of black communities, it is necessary for us to engage with the tragic history of slavery, and the role played by medical and scientific knowledge in this.

At the core of this chapter is a snapshot of British psychiatry's attempts to explain 'black schizophrenia' from the 1960s through to the end of the 1980s. Why? Because the profession's enthusiastic search for the biological basis of the phenomenon occurred at a time of great social and political ferment in black communities. The 1980s and 90s were marked by disorder on the streets of English cities, in Brixton, Tottenham, Toxteth, Moss Side and elsewhere. Young (mainly) black men protested against unemployment, the use of the 'sus'[2] law by the police,

---

2. From 'suspected person', a law dating back to the early nineteenth century that allowed the police to stop, search and arrest any person on the streets whom they suspected of having the intent to commit a crime.

their loss of hope (the same hope that brought their parents to this country), and in white eyes everywhere the gaze of superiority and hostility. At the end of this chapter we will see that there has been a shift in the way that British psychiatry has tried to make sense of psychosis in black people, but as the recession deepens and income inequality increases, the plight of young black men worsens. One in four of black sixteen- to twenty-four-year-olds is unemployed. Young black men are more likely to be out of a job than any other ethnic group (*The Guardian*, 2012d).

We cannot understand the significance of recent biological research into 'black schizophrenia' without reference to the role played by medical and scientific theories in classifying human beings into different races. This is because, in its most basic terms, these theories have for 300 years been used to paint a picture of humankind in which to be black is to be inferior, subhuman or degenerate in comparison with white. It may be true to say that we have moved beyond the crude racial science that was used to justify the Holocaust, but a shadow lingers in the minds of people of African-Caribbean heritage: the distant presence of slavery and standing behind this the role of science in justifying an earlier Holocaust.

This chapter begins by examining the origins of scientific theories about differences between racial groups, especially differences in their brains, intellectual capacity and cultural characteristics. These were used to justify the view that black people are inferior to white people. Attempts to prove scientifically the superiority of white Europeans can be traced back at least as far as the Enlightenment. But in Britain it is the history of racism, aided and abetted by biological theories of racial difference and racial science, that set the context for the complex and difficult relationship between black and white, especially in mental health services.

Historically, the experiences of black people in mental health services differed markedly from those of white people. These experiences are considered through the accounts of black people. We also consider the evidence that they are much more likely than other groups to experience coercion in mental health care. This has been a matter of concern to the black community and speculation in the scientific community for many years. We also consider the evidence from within the psychiatric literature about the apparently raised incidence of schizophrenia in black people, paying particular attention to the scientific explanations for this. The early research can be seen as a quest for the biological basis of schizophrenia couched in terms of black people's increased 'vulnerability' for the condition. We will see that this vulnerability has been located in their brains, their genes, their family structures, and their culture. Either way, predominantly white researchers have construed the issue of black psychosis in terms of weakness or deficits that set black people apart from white. However, in recent years the interpretation of this evidence has changed. The chapter ends by considering recent scientific evidence that establishes a direct link between psychosis in black people and personal experiences of racism.

Slavery, Racial Difference and Science

Western thought has, since Christianity, been preoccupied with the idea of the single origin of humanity, and also with the ideal of purity signified by whiteness. The European Enlightenment upheld the Christian view of a single origin of humanity, epitomised by the slogan of the French Revolution, 'Liberty, Equality, Fraternity', and the opening words of the American Declaration of Independence: 'We hold these truths to be self-evident, that all men are created equal, that they are endowed by their Creator with certain unalienable Rights, that among these are Life, Liberty and the pursuit of Happiness'.[3] The term 'Caucasian' was coined by the German physician and naturalist Blumenbach in his system of classification of the human races. It represented an aesthetic ideal; he considered Georgian people (the doyen of the Caucasian race) to be great in beauty. He wrote 'The skin of the Georgians is white but it can easily degenerate to a blackish hue' (cited by Kohn, 1995: 28). By the end of the eighteenth century, Blumenbach had progressed to measuring skulls in an attempt to classify racial types, and thus founded the field of anthropometry. Superficially this suggests a progression towards a seemingly less value-laden, more 'objective' approach to the problem of the classification of human beings.

The work of the Swedish botanist and zoologist Linnaeus marks the origins of the scientific basis for the classification of plants and animals. His highly influential system of taxonomy was binominal, since each species is given two names, the first of which gives the genus, and the second identifies the species within the genus. Thus human beings belong to the genus *homo*, and to the species *sapiens*. In his *Systema Naturae* Linnaeus classified the human race into five groups, American, Asian, African, European and Monstrous (a mythological race of Patagonian giants). He did not order hierarchically the varieties of people he described, but his description of Europeans as 'governed by laws' and Africans as 'governed by caprice' (Baker, 2008: 93) nevertheless carries value judgements that set the scene for what was to follow.

Throughout the eighteenth and nineteenth centuries, naturalists and scientists became increasingly preoccupied with the idea that there were distinct biological differences between the various races. Seen through the lens of early European science it was inevitable that Europeans were held out as the ideal, the point of reference against which other races were to be compared. This work proceeded through three phases: aesthetic, anthropometric and psychological. Here we will focus on the first two, largely because they came to occupy a particularly important role in the justification of slavery. This is not to downplay the role of psychological science in the study of racial differences. This was, and remains, a highly controversial matter, but because my main concern is the role

---

3. Accessed on 10th December 2012 at http://www.archives.gov/exhibits/charters/declaration_transcript.html

of slavery in the relationship between black and white, and especially the part played by psychiatric and medical knowledge in justifying this, I do not plan to dwell on psychological theories of racial difference. By the time they started to become prominent in the second half of the nineteenth century, slavery had all but ended.

In the first phase it was simply assumed that European races were superior to others on aesthetic grounds. The Caucasian skull was widely regarded as the ideal, the most beautiful and perfectly formed. For example, the early French anthropologist Pierre Cratiolet wrote about Negroes thus:

> the cranium closes on the brain like a prison. It is no longer a temple divine ...
> but a sort of helmet for resisting heavy blows. (cited in Deutsch, 1944: 470)

The second phase was based on the view that measurement of the human skull, its dimensions and shapes, would make it possible to compare different races, so that conclusions could be drawn about their mental faculties, reason and intelligence. It began as a development from the aesthetic approach, by attempts to measure the extent to which the proportions and relationships between the different elements of the shape of the skull conformed to the aesthetic of the European ideal. But it also bears the influence of phrenology, the pseudoscience popular from the end of the eighteenth century. This purported to show that the measure of a person's intellectual and mental faculties could be gauged by the size of the bumps and indentations that were present on the surface of the skull. Anthropometry subsequently led to measurements of cranial capacity or volume, and thus estimates of brain size. The outcome of this work was the view that non-Europeans, especially African people, were phylogenetically closer to the primates and apes, and thus more 'primitive'.[4] This was because they were believed to have smaller skulls. Allied to this was the idea that black races had 'degenerated' from the white ideal, possibly through environmental factors. Either way, the implicit assumption was that white races were inherently superior to black.

Science and psychiatry in the service of slavery

Slavery was abolished in Britain in the first decade of the nineteenth century before the profession of psychiatry became established, and so it is in the US where we can see most clearly the role played by scientific knowledge and proto-psychiatry in arguing the case for the continuing enslavement of black people. The American Civil War was preceded by decades of argument and conflict about the abolition of slavery. In the face of growing calls for its abolition by the states north of the Mason–Dixon line, advocates of slavery, those in the south whose wealth and power was built on the forced labour of African people, became

---

4. Phylogenetics is the study of the evolutionary development of a species through a gradual progression of forms.

engaged in a desperate search for evidence to support the case for slavery. Deutsch[5] (1944) has described how pro-slavery preachers in the USA scoured the Bible for evidence in support of slavery. Papers arguing that slavery was a 'natural law' were published in learned journals, and economists warned of the financial ruin that would follow abolition. But the most influential arguments in support of slavery were scientific ones, based on early anthropology, or ethnology as it was then called, and psychiatrists were amongst the most enthusiastic advocates of these ideas. Ethnology was concerned not with culture, but with physical and mental differences between human beings. Deutsch continues:

> Essentially, the ethnological argument for slavery was based on the almost universally accepted belief that the Negro was biologically inferior to the white race. From this was deduced the corollary arguments that the Negro must always play a subordinate rôle in his relationships with whites, and that slavery was his natural status in this relationship. (Deutsch, 1944: 469)

This view, of course, ran counter to Thomas Jefferson's assertion in the Declaration of Independence that 'All men are created equal'. Deutsch shows how 'scientific' evidence that black people were inferior to white became important propaganda for the pro-slavery lobby. If science could prove that the position of black people was naturally one of inferiority and subservience to white, then black people were not entitled to status as human beings. They were subhuman, and thus excluded from the *Declaration of Independence*. One of the most influential works used to justify white supremacy was a book called *Types of Mankind*, written by Nott (a physician) and Gliddon (an English-born Egyptologist), published in 1854. This was widely cited by pro-slavery writers in the USA and elsewhere, as the '… Negro race was placed in the same category as domesticated animals such as horses, cattle, asses and "other brutes"' (Deutsch, 1944: 470).

The most egregious instance of science in the service of slavery is the work of the proto-psychiatrist Samuel Cartwright, whose work, as Deutsch points out, was widely cited in the pro-slavery literature in the middle of the nineteenth century. Cartwright was a medical practitioner in Mississippi who fought on the side of the Confederacy in the Civil War. In his essays he argued that the purported anatomical 'peculiarities' of black people indicated that they were closer to animals than other races of men. This was because their behaviour was governed by their '… instincts and animality … and less under the influence of his reflective faculties' (Cartwright, 1843). They were thus subhuman. This, as Deutsch points out, was pseudoscience. There was no empirical basis for such claims.

---

5. Deutsch was a campaigning journalist, who is probably better known in the USA for his series of newspaper articles exposing the appalling conditions in American public psychiatric hospitals in the 1940s, and published collectively in his book *The Shame of the States* (Weiss, 2011).

Deutsch gives a fascinating account of how the publication of the sixth US census in 1841 seemingly provided unexpected evidence for the view that slavery was of *benefit* to black people. The rate of mental disorder was found to be eleven times higher in free Negroes than it was in those who continued to endure enslavement. In addition it claimed to show that the rates of mental disorder in black people living north of the Mason–Dixon line were much higher than the rates of those living in the South. Slavery, it was argued, imposed a civilising and rationalising order upon black people. It was a benevolent institution, and masterhood the 'white man's burden'. Black madness, it was argued, was a moral evil arising from vicious habits and uncontrolled animal passions. Deutsch goes on to describe how subsequent detailed analysis of the census data upon which these claims were made proved that the data were fabricated. Most of the Northern towns in which these figures were based at the time had no black residents.

Suman Fernando (1991, see p. 37) was one of the first people to draw attention to *drapetomania* and Cartwright's work. The paper in which Cartwright described the condition was reprinted over a hundred years later (Cartwright, 1851, republished in Caplan *et al*, 1981). It begins by describing a wide variety of purported anatomical and physiological differences that set Negroes apart from other races, and the various physical illnesses to which they were prone as a result. What emerges, however, is that these ailments were believed to be related not only to these physical differences, but also to their customs and habits, in other words, their culture. For example, 'negro consumption' (tuberculosis) was popularly believed to arise from the habit of dirt eating. Cartwright argues that this is a mental malady, in part brought about by mismanagement of the slaves on the part of the master, and in part brought about by the Negroes' superstitious belief in witchcraft and magic – in other words, their culture, a vestige of African beliefs that had resisted eradication by the civilising influence of the white man.

He took the word *drapetomania* (a neologism concocted from the Greek word *drapetes* for a runaway slave) to refer to a form of madness seen in black people who escaped from slavery. He put the cause down to poor management on the part of the slave-masters, but it could be cured by establishing the correct way 'to govern negroes'. He warrants this with passages taken from the Old Testament, which he interprets to mean that black races must bow down before the white. In other words, black people must be kept in a position of subservience to white. A black person who escaped the 'civilising' influence of the slave-master was likely to experience madness as a consequence.

The other form of slave madness described by Cartwright was *dysaesthesia aethiopsis*, a condition called 'rascality' by overseers:

> From the careless movements of the individuals affected with the complaint, they are apt to do much mischief, which appears as if intentional, but is mostly owing to the stupidness of mind and insensibility of the nerves induced by the disease. (Cartwright, 1851: 321)

The condition led to wasteful and destructive behaviours, an utter disregard for property, crops and farm animals, theft, and generally disorganised behaviour. The condition was also associated with trouble and disturbances with other slaves and the overseers, and those afflicted seemed '... insensible to pain when subject to punishment ... the disease is the natural offspring of negro liberty – the liberty to be idle, to wallow in filth, and to indulge in improper food and drink' (*ibid*: 321). The implications are clear. In its natural state, black culture and the way of life of black people predisposed them to this form of madness. It was only through the 'civilising' influence of the white man and his superior culture and way of life, imposed for the black man's benefit through slavery, that these ailments could be prevented.

Cartwright's paper is a thinly disguised pamphlet in support of the supremacy of white over black, presented as an argument for the maintenance of slavery. White Europeans are superior biologically, mentally and culturally. This is true scientifically, he argues, and what's more, the Bible says so too. This justification for slavery was grounded in a bizarre mixture of pseudoscience (phrenology coupled to a curious and distorted view of human anatomy and physiology) and a highly selective reading of Biblical texts. It supported the view that slavery was a necessity for the black man and a burden for the white. It imposed a civilising influence on a phylogenetically more 'primitive' species. It served the advancement and improvement of black people.

Black people's experiences of mental health services

At the end of the eighteenth century, trade related to slavery accounted for 80 per cent of Britain's foreign income (Hague, 2007). But in March 1807, after a campaign lasting nearly thirty years, the Slave Trade Act received royal assent. This abolished the slave trade in the British Empire, although it wasn't until 1834 that the Slavery Abolition Act emancipated approximately 700,000 slaves in the West Indies.

Over 100 years later, at the end of the Second World War, Britain was an exhausted nation with a worn-out infrastructure in need of renewal and a shortage of labour to run essential public services and the newly promised National Health Service. Thousands of men and women from the Caribbean had fought for 'the mother country' in the armed services, and after the war it was natural that many saw in Britain a future of opportunity, hope and prosperity. On the 22nd June 1948 the MV *Empire Windrush* docked in Tilbury, carrying nearly 500 people from Jamaica, and thus began what was to become one of the most important social and cultural changes to affect the British Isles in the twentieth century. In the 1960s and 1970s the first wave of migrants from the Caribbean were settling down and raising their families, but something was wrong. Something terrible was happening to their children. A generation of young black people, young men in particular, disappeared from their homes, deserted the streets and churches, only to reappear in custody, in prisons, and, worst of all, in the psychiatric units that served the large cities.

Worse followed. In 1984, Michael Martin died in Broadmoor after being physically restrained by staff and forcibly given large doses of neuroleptic drugs. Four years later Joseph Watts also died in Broadmoor under similar circumstances. The verdict was accidental death. In 1991 Orville Blackwood died of heart failure after being forcibly injected with a combination of promazine and fluphenazine decanoate (both neuroleptics). The dose of both drugs was over the maximum level recommended by the *British National Formulary*. All three men were African-Caribbean. An inquiry (Special Hospitals Service Authority, 1993) suggested that the use of powerful drugs reflected crude stereotypes that black men were potentially dangerous. White health professionals found it difficult to conceal the fact that they perceived young black men as 'dangerous' or 'violent', and for this reason they were liable to receive higher doses of neuroleptic medication. According to MIND (2003) there were twenty-seven deaths of patients from black and minority ethnic (BME) communities in psychiatric care from 1980 until 2003. This list is almost certainly incomplete because no formal figures are kept.

Over time these personal tragedies contributed to a wider context of mistrust and fear in Britain's black communities towards mental health services. There is plenty of evidence to support this. The title of the report *Breaking the Circles of Fear*, published by the Sainsbury Centre for Mental Health (SCMH, 2002), captures this well:

> Service users become reluctant to ask for help or to comply with treatment, increasing the likelihood of a personal crisis, leading in some cases to self-harm or harm to others. In turn, prejudices are reinforced and provoke even more coercive responses, resulting in a downward spiral, which we call 'circles of fear', in which staff see service users as potentially dangerous and service users perceive services as harmful. (SCMH, 2002: 8)

The report presented the results of a qualitative study involving over thirty groups of black service users and carers in Lambeth, Haringey and Birmingham. These groups were facilitated by trained service users and carers, and the research team also conducted face-to-face interviews with psychiatrists. The results show that black people understood their negative experiences of psychiatry as part of a wider range of experiences of marginalisation and inequity related to racism in society. The experience of black people in many sectors of British society is unremittingly negative. There is, for example, plenty of evidence that black people endure poor-quality housing, lower pay and higher levels of unemployment than white people. Black children have higher rates of exclusion from school and referral to specialist services for behavioural problems (Modood *et al*, 1998).[6]

6. Footnote 6 overleaf.

It is clear from the report that for some people, coming into contact with psychiatry resonates powerfully with their negative experiences in other areas of society:

> Coming to mental health services was like the last straw ... you come to services disempowered already, they strip you of your dignity ... you become the dregs of society. (SCMH, 2002: 24, Service User)

This conveys powerfully the negative impact that contact with mental health services has upon the identity and sense of self of black service users. Others were so terrified that they were afraid their admission to psychiatric hospital would lead to their death: 'I remember when I first went into hospital ... I feared that I was going to die' (*ibid*: 24, Service User). Such fears are hardly surprising given the significant numbers of young black men who have died in psychiatric care. Carers expressed similar fears:

> I'm much more aware of the potential of the police, I'm afraid of informing the police in the wrong kind of circumstances. I don't want to know he's dead, I don't want to know he's committed some serious crime and he's ended up in Broadmoor or Rampton; I don't want that, that's what I'm trying to avoid. I can smell it on the horizon, but I'm trying my best to avoid it, that's why I do what I do. (*ibid*: 25, Carer)

Fear is the dominant tenor of the way service users and carers spoke about inpatient care. Ward environments were seen as 'impersonal, regimented and closed' (*ibid*: 40), with an obscure system of rules. Staff were seen as 'autocratic' and 'confrontational' in their attitudes, especially to young black people. Staff appeared too eager to resort to control, restraint and seclusion, and these actions took place without warning or discussion.

Black carers also described a sense of shame amplified by the effects of racism, especially a feeling that their families were in some way deviant and pathological. This may be because they were more likely to be broken up and their children taken into care on the basis of assessments by psychiatrists and social workers. Carers and family members in *Circles of Fear* reported that mental health professionals regarded them with suspicion and hostility. They were spoken down to and patronised, or worse, made to feel that they were a part of the problem. Overall, service users and families felt they were not respected as human beings within services. Indeed, they commonly felt they were not treated

---

6. It is perhaps worth noting in passing, and especially following the last chapter, that many white people have similar fears and negative experiences in relation to psychiatry and mental health services. My argument, however, is that the experiences of black people are qualitatively different from those of other groups because of the historical context of the relationship between black and white people in Britain, a history clouded by slavery and colonialism.

as equals, as human beings. The report expresses it as follows:

> As far as the experiences of families and carers are concerned, their response has now become a mantra: they 'are not treated with dignity and respect, not valued, not listened to or heard'. Much more serious is the allegation that they were not treated as though they were fellow human beings. In other words *they were treated as though they were subhuman.* (*ibid*: 63, emphasis added)

Such expressions, 'lesser beings', 'subhuman', resonate strongly with the way that black people have been described in the past by those who supported slavery. Despite the passage of nearly 200 years since its abolition in this country, it is difficult to escape the conclusion that black people still feel that white people see them as inferior, as not worthy of being treated with human dignity and respect.

Similar findings emerge from another study, *Real Voices* (Walls & Sashidharan, 2003) commissioned by the Department of Health in England. It reports a series of focus groups held in five cities in England, as part of a consultation to find out what improvements people from BME communities (Black, South Asian, Irish and Chinese) wanted in mental health services. Black people were particularly likely (78%) to report that staff racism within mental health services was a problem. The qualitative component of the study asked people about their experiences of racism. Although the report doesn't break down responses by the respondent's ethnic group, it is clear that racism covered a wide range of circumstances, including being stereotyped, and references to racially motivated verbal and physical abuse. In addition, people from BME communities were critical of care based in the biomedical model of distress, because they regarded it as irrelevant to their experiences of distress. It failed to engage with the social and cultural contexts of mental ill health that mattered to them. These experiences can be seen from a different perspective through research looking at differences in the way that mental health services diagnose and treat people from black communities.

Mental Health Services and Black People

Black people's attitudes towards psychiatry and mental health services are dominated by fear, suspicion and anger, and we can understand why this is, through the extensive research literature on how black people access and use mental health services. There are two main strands of evidence here. The first concerns the way that black people access mental health services, and what happens to them once inside. The second is the infamous role played by the diagnosis of schizophrenia, especially in young black men.

Access and treatment

The extensive literature here has been well summarised by Bhui and Bhugra (2002), who used Goldberg and Huxley's (1980) Pathways to Care model as a way of organising what is a complex array of studies. They modified the Goldberg and Huxley model slightly to address the issue of accessibility and service use by people from BME communities. In essence pathways to care sets out the different points through which people may access mental health services.[7] Most people receive help at level one, and never reach the attention of doctors. A lower proportion reach primary care (levels two and three), and fewer still are referred on to specialist mental health services (level four). Only a very small proportion of people who experience psychosis or distress ever find their way into level five, the specialist forensic mental health services that take referrals from the courts (criminal justice system), the police, and mental health services (usually inpatient units). The important point to note here is that at level five all patients will be on sections of the Mental Health Act. This, together with the fact that most are referred via the criminal justice system or police, indicates that their experience of mental health services is the most coercive – they have no choice about being in forensic services. In addition, it can be extremely difficult to get out of forensic services once you find yourself in them.

Bhui and Bhugra's work is helpful because it relates most of the recent research on the use of mental health services by people from BME communities to the different sites where they receive help, how they access these sites, and the extent to which their treatment is consensual or forced.

The research summarised in Table 5.1 covers people from a broad range of BME communities, but the focus in the text is specifically on black people. The most striking thing about this table is the extensive evidence that in contrast to people from other BME groups and white people, black people are over-represented at levels four and five. For example, African-Caribbean men are over-represented in forensic units, on remand and in prison. Admission rates to forensic units for black women are three times those of white women. Twenty per cent of people detained in secure units in England and Wales are African-Caribbean (relevant references in Table 5.1). Even at level four, black people's experiences of mental health services are more coercive than white people's.

---

7. The first level is the community, where the great majority of people who experience distress are located. Most of these people turn first to families and friends to discuss their problems. Some may also discuss their distress with spiritual and religious figures, such as priests, ministers and imams. It is as a result of such discussion that decisions are made to consult a GP, or some other source of help and advice, such as a traditional healer. The second level is primary care, where GPs are consulted, and many people treated (level three). Only a small proportion are referred on by GPs to specialist mental health services (level four), where they may be given treatment as outpatients or inpatients, and if the latter, informally or formally under the Mental Health Act. An even smaller minority is treated in specialist forensic settings (level five). People here are referred either from level four, or via the police or the criminal justice system.

**Table 5.1 Empirical research on BME inequalities
(adapted from Bhui & Bhugra, 2002)**

Level	Finding	Source
Level 1 Community	Black people more likely not to be registered with a GP compared to non-black people	Koffman *et al* (1997)
	40% of African-Caribbean people made contact with some helping agency in the week before admission, compared with 2% of general population	Harrison *et al* (1991)
Level 2 Presentation to Primary Care	Male Asians have higher GP consultation rate, but overall consultation for anxiety and depression lower in all BME groups	Gillam *et al* (1989)
	Black people had higher consultation rates in primary care, and more likely than white British to seek help from traditional healers	Kiev (1965)
	Black women less likely to be clear about what they want from GP, and were less satisfied with the consultation than white patients	Lloyd & St Louis (1996)
Level 3 Primary Care Action	GPs identify mental health problems in 26% of black and 34% of white patients.	Lloyd & St Louis (1996)
	Rate of detection of significant mental health problems in black people about half that of white people	Li *et al* (1994)
	African-Caribbean people with diagnosis of schizophrenia less likely than white people to be referred to mental health services by GP	Burnett *et al* (1999)
	No difference in detection of mental health problems by Asian GP in Asian and white people	Bhui *et al* (2001)
Level 4 Psychiatric Services	Higher rates for admission to psychiatric hospital for African-Caribbean than white patients	Bagley (1971); Bebbington *et al* (1991); Moodley & Perkins (1991); Wessely *et al* (1991); King *et al* (1994); Callan & Littlewood (1998); Davies *et al* (1996)
	Rates of admission for African-Caribbean men are 3 to 13 times higher than white men	Bebbington *et al* (1991); Moodley & Perkins (1991); King *et al* (1994); van Os *et al* (1996); Davies *et al* (1996)
	70% of African and African-Caribbean people and 50% of white comparison group had previously been detained under the MHA	
Level 5 Forensic Services	African-Caribbean men are over-represented in forensic units, on remand and in prison	Coid *et al* (2000)
	Admission rates to forensic units for black women are 3 times those of white women	Maden *et al* (1992)
	20% of people detained in secure units in England and Wales are African-Caribbean	Jones & Berry (1986)
	6% of African-Caribbean and 2% of white prisoners have mental health problems	Coid *et al* (2000)
	Black and Asian mentally disordered offenders have higher rates of schizophrenia	Bhui *et al* (1998)
	Black people (13%) are less likely to be granted bail than white people (37%) on basis of psychiatric reports	NACRO (1989)

The rates of admission for African-Caribbean men are three to thirteen times higher than white men, and 70 per cent of African and African-Caribbean people compared to 50 per cent of white patients have previously experienced detention under the Mental Health Act. At level three, GPs are twice as likely not to detect mental health problems in black people than white, and GPs are less likely to refer black people with a diagnosis of schizophrenia on to mental health services than white people. Overall these figures confirm the negative experiences of black people set out earlier. They indicate that black people are less likely to experience consensual treatment, and are more likely to be forced to receive treatment in secure environments.[8]

Psychiatry and 'black schizophrenia'

Psychiatrists have been aware of the link between migration and schizophrenia since a paper by Ødegaard (1932) which showed that Norwegian migrants to the USA had higher rates of schizophrenia than Norwegian people who remained in Norway. Interest in the issue in Britain first appeared in the early to mid-1960s just as the *Windrush generation* were settling into their new lives and starting to raise their children. These early studies were carried out in London, Birmingham, Nottingham and Manchester, all cities with growing black communities. They found that black people had rates of schizophrenia between 2.5 to 14.6 times higher than the white community (see Sashidharan, 1993 for an excellent overview of these early studies). In the main they concerned first-generation migrants from the Caribbean, but later on it emerged that the children of these first-generation migrants had even higher rates of psychiatric admission with the diagnosis of schizophrenia (see, for example, Wessely *et al*, 1991; Castle *et al*, 1991; Harrison *et al*, 1988; C. Thomas *et al*, 1993). Since then this evidence has continued to accumulate. One of the most recent studies was carried out by the Medical Research Council Aesop group (Fearon *et al*, 2006). This involved the identification of all people between the ages of 16 to 64 years admitted to psychiatric hospitals in south-east London, Nottingham and Bristol, a total of 568. They found higher rates for schizophrenic and manic psychoses in African-Caribbean people and black African men and women. The rates of schizophrenia were 9.1 times higher in African-Caribbean people, and 5.8 times higher in black African people.

Setting aside any reservations about the validity of the diagnosis of schizophrenia (in Chapter 2 serious reservations about the diagnosis were consi-dered), suspending our disbelief in the concept just for the moment, academic and clinical psychiatrists have puzzled over how best to account for these findings for some time. In broad terms they have come up with four theories to explain the raised incidence of 'schizophrenia' in black people, most of which can be seen as variations on the stress–vulnerability model we considered in the last chapter. The one exception is the idea that misdiagnosis may account for the

---

8. The evidence also indicates that black people are much more likely to be offered physical interventions like drugs and ECT than psychological therapies. One way of seeing this is in the light of the submerged beliefs white people hold about black people, that black people's feelings and emotions are cruder and less refined than those of white people, and that they are less intelligent, and thus overall much less likely to benefit from psychological therapies.

apparent increase in schizophrenia.[9] Sharpley *et al*'s (2001) review deals both with misdiagnosis, as well as with three other theories – biological, psychological and social. Psychological and social theories represent the 'stress' limb of the stress–vulnerability model, and I will have more to say about this at the end of the chapter. But for the time being I want to examine the pedigree of biological theories in some detail – the 'vulnerability' limb.

Foremost amongst biological theories of schizophrenia has been the search for a genetic basis for the condition. The finding of a much higher incidence of schizophrenia in African-Caribbean people living in Britain gave rise to the idea that in this group of people genetic factors might be important. In fact there is little if any evidence that this is the case, and those who have searched for the genetic basis of 'black schizophrenia' have concluded that environmental factors are more important. We will consider what these environmental factors are shortly. Sugarman and Craufurd (1994) compared the incidence of schizophrenia in the first-degree relatives of African-Caribbean people admitted to hospital with a diagnosis of schizophrenia, with the incidence in the first-degree relatives of white patients admitted with the same diagnosis. There were no differences in the risk for parents, but the brothers and sisters of the black patients had a much higher risk (15.9%) compared with white patients (1.8%). The risks were even higher in the brothers and sisters of second-generation African-Caribbean patients (27.3%). They concluded that although genetic factors may contribute to the risk of schizophrenia in black people, environmental factors play a significant role especially in young black men. Similar results emerged from a study by Hutchinson *et al* (1997), who found no difference in the risk of schizophrenia in the parents and siblings of first-generation African-Caribbean people and white people. However, the risk in the brothers and sisters of second-generation African-Caribbean people was seven times higher than that of the siblings of white patients. They concluded that second-generation African-Caribbean people in Britain are particularly vulnerable to an unknown environmental risk factor for the condition, or that some unknown environmental factor acts selectively on this group.

Early attempts to make sense of the higher rates of schizophrenia in migrants generally favoured psychosocial explanations involving stress. Migrants either were unsettled in their land of origin as part of the process of becoming mentally disordered, and this caused them to move, or alternatively, the stresses and strains

9. The misdiagnosis theory is partly supported by the finding that the rates of schizophrenia in people of Caribbean heritage in England are much higher than those of their peers back home. For example, Hickling and Rodgers-Johnson (1995) found that incidence rates for schizophrenia in Jamaica were lower than those reported in African-Caribbean immigrants in the UK and Holland, and within the reported range for other population groups worldwide. Similarly, Bhugra *et al* (1996) found the rates of schizophrenia in Trinidad were much lower than those of African-Caribbean people in London.

of adjusting to a new life in a strange culture were thought to be responsible. But by the 1980s, as the vogue for biological explanations of psychosis gained momentum, psychosocial explanations fell out of favour. Eagles commented on the '... dearth of evidence that psychosocial stress or disadvantage is of primary aetiological significance in schizophrenia' (1991: 784). He raised three possible biological explanations for the higher incidence of schizophrenia in West Indian migrants to Britain: maternal viral infections in pregnancy, obstetric factors and genetic factors. Epidemiological studies suggest that people diagnosed with schizophrenia are more likely to have been born in the winter months, and this has led some to suggest that seasonal variations in infectious diseases might somehow lead to an increased risk for schizophrenia. The evidence is far from convincing. A study in Finland found an excess of people admitted to hospital with a diagnosis of schizophrenia whose mothers would have been exposed to the 1957 influenza epidemic when pregnant, but a study from Edinburgh failed to find a similar relationship in Scotland.

Maternal viral infections and obstetric complications, although seemingly different, are believed to have adverse consequences for the developing brain, which may possibly predispose the individual to schizophrenia in late adolescence or early adulthood. Both are thought to contribute to what are called 'sporadic' cases of schizophrenia, in contrast to cases that are supposed to have a clear family history, and in which genetic factors are assumed to be important. The difficulty with these studies is that most of them are retrospective, or carried out on inpatient populations. This means that their results are extremely difficult to interpret for the reasons we considered in the last chapter. It is impossible to know whether it is a biological insult that increases the risk of schizophrenia, or associated non-biological factors. For example, epidemics like influenza spread more rapidly in poor urban populations where overcrowding is common. In addition such illnesses are likely to have more severe effects in poor people whose nutritional status is not as good as those who are better off. Likewise, immigrant women have higher rates of obstetric complications because they present later on in pregnancy and thus have less antenatal care. At the same time, such women are more likely to experience social adversity and poor health associated with poverty. It is therefore extremely difficult to disentangle these specific biological factors from the wider context of poverty and socio-economic adversity, factors that we know from the last chapter have enormous implications for the growing child's future mental health. It is hardly surprising, therefore, that Geddes and Lawrie's (1995) meta-analysis was inconclusive. Eagles (1991) also raised the possibility that genetic mutations may play a role in the increased risk of schizophrenia in black people in Britain. Whilst this might account for the higher incidence of schizophrenia in second-generation African-Caribbean people, again, there is no evidence to support this theory.

Reading Eagles' paper, written nearly a quarter of a century ago, at a time when black people were taking to the streets in a blaze of anger in Brixton, Toxteth and Moss Side, one is left with the image of psychiatry fiddling while inner-city England was aflame. It had to see the problem in terms of black people's brains, bodies, and ultimately their genes. Its remoteness from the lives of those affected made it extremely difficult, if not impossible, to engage with their experiences in order to understand them.

Jonathan Metzl (2009) draws attention to the tacit political role played by the diagnosis of schizophrenia in black men in the USA. He points out that coinciding with the rise of the Civil Rights Movement, there was a change in the demographics of schizophrenia (at least in the hospital in Michigan where his study was based). Until the 1950s the diagnosis in the hospital was largely one used in white, middle-class women. From the 1950s on, however, the diagnosis was increasingly applied to black men, as black people engaged in protest and civil disobedience against segregation and racist policies, and were seen by the white middle classes as potentially dangerous and violent.

The so-called cannabis psychosis is another attempt to explain black psychosis by problematising or pathologising black brains and black culture. The term has been widely used to refer to psychoses occurring in young people known to take the drug, particularly if they have African-Caribbean heritage. British psychiatry has been aware of the link between the drug and psychosis for over a hundred years (Warnock, 1903). Thornicroft's (1990) systematic review, however, found no clear evidence to support the existence of a distinct 'cannabis' psychosis, although very heavy use of the drug may bring about a 'schizophreniform' (i.e., schizophrenia-like) episode. He suggests that poor study design and selection bias may account for the apparent excess of psychoses related to cannabis in African-Caribbean people.

There is a view that the increased incidence of psychosis in some BME groups arises because they are more likely to experience income inequality and its associated socio-economic adversity. We saw in the last chapter how social injustice and childhood adversity are at the heart of psychosis for many people. But why is the incidence of schizophrenia in young black people so much higher than white groups who experience similar levels of income inequality? Why is it that their pathways to care and their experiences within mental health services are so negative and adverse in comparison with other groups who experience similar levels of social adversity? Is it to do with genetic and biological differences between racial groups as some have suggested? Is it to do with their early family environments and high rates of family breakup? Or is it something more complex: something that originates in the relationship between black people and white people, coloured by the history of slavery, a history that still resonates in the daily experiences of black people in England, and whose roots can still be discerned in scientific psychiatry's attempts to explain the psychosis of black people?

Racism and Psychosis

So far our discussion of the stress–vulnerability model in relation to 'black schizophrenia' has only dealt with biological vulnerability. We haven't yet considered stress. To end this chapter I want to return to this, with evidence that the most important form of stress for black people as far as the risk of psychosis is concerned is racism. Racism is a complex phenomenon that operates in a great variety of ways, overtly and covertly, through all levels of society from its institutions right down to the relationships between individuals. It is a specific form of discrimination based on perceived differences in terms of skin colour, language, dress, culture and religious affiliation. There are two forms of racism that are important in relation to the experiences of black people in mental health services: institutional and interpersonal. In his paper given at the Dialectics of Liberation conference in 1967, Stokely Carmichael made the distinction between individual racism and institutional racism, which he described as

> less overt, far more subtle, less identifiable [than individual racism] in terms of specific individuals committing the acts, but no less destructive in human life. [It] is more the overall operation of established and respected forces in society, and thus does not receive the condemnation that [individual racism] receives. (Carmichael, 1968: 151)

The *Macpherson Report* (TSO, 1999) defines institutional racism as:

> the collective failure of an organisation to provide an appropriate and professional service to people because of their colour, culture, or ethnic origin. It can be seen or detected in processes, attitudes and behaviour which amount to discrimination through unwitting prejudice, ignorance, thoughtlessness and racist stereotyping which disadvantage minority ethnic people. (TSO, 1999: 6.34)

There is a strong argument that institutional racism in the NHS is an important factor in the health inequalities experienced by people from black communities. Kwame McKenzie wrote as follows in the wake of the *Macpherson Report*:

> Health disparities are brought about and perpetuated not only by culture, class and socio-political forces external to medicine, but also by the ideology of the medical profession. This ideology leads to ineffective or no action in the face of disparities and to a lack of concerted effort to teach or discuss racism in medicine in undergraduate and postgraduate curriculums. Moreover, the emphasis on the biomedical model undermines the anthropological research which is need to properly document the perceptions, needs, and aspirations of minority ethnic groups. (McKenzie, 1999: 616–15)

At this point, however, we are primarily concerned with the experience of interpersonal racism, or what in essence are discriminatory interactions between individuals. Although this has been relatively little studied in relation to health, such experiences are an important everyday feature of life in England for many black people, for whom being made to feel different was routine (Chahal & Julienne, 1999). Given that this is so, some might argue that black people just have to get on with it, and that it shouldn't particularly affect their physical health or mental health. But the evidence indicates that this is not the case.

Nazroo (1998) points out that three aspects of the contexts of ethnicity have been widely disregarded in relation to health: the effects of disadvantage and adversity over the course of the individual's life, the ecological impact of living in deprived inner-city areas, and the effects of living in a racist society. Karlsen and Nazroo (2002) point out that little attention has been paid to the role of racially motivated verbal or physical attacks on the health and wellbeing of minority ethnic groups. They examined the relationship between racism, social position and health in ethnic minority groups in England in a representative sample of over 5,000 BME people and a comparison sample of nearly 3,000 white people. Personal experiences of racism and the perception of racism in wider society were both significantly associated with poor health. People who reported racial verbal abuse were 50 per cent more likely to describe their health as fair or poor compared with people who reported no such abuse. Those who reported racial physical attacks were 100 per cent more likely to describe their health as poor. There was a 150 per cent increase in estimated rates of depression and psychosis in people who reported verbal racial abuse.

The problem with this study is that the sample size was too small to separate out the impact of racism on mental health specifically in black people, compared with other BME groups, and the white control group didn't include Irish people, a group who also commonly experience racism. However, a subsequent study by Karlsen *et al* (2005) specifically examined the impact of racism on the mental health of different ethnic groups in England. They used data from a follow-up survey of a sample of people drawn from minority ethnic communities who had participated in the 1999 Health for England study, together with a white English sample. The minority community sample included 793 Irish, 691 Caribbean, 650 Bangladeshi, 648 Indian, and 724 Pakistani people. In addition to the two questions asked about experiences of racism in the Karlsen and Nazroo (2002) study, they also asked subjects if they had ever been refused a job or treated unfairly at work on grounds of race, colour, ethnicity or religion. Mental health was assessed on the basis of subjects' risks for developing significant anxiety or depression (i.e., becoming a clinical 'case') in the previous week, using a clinical interview schedule that gave *ICD-10* diagnoses. In addition, they made estimates of the annual prevalence of psychosis in the sample using a psychosis screening questionnaire.

African-Caribbean people were most likely to report racial harassment, followed by Pakistanis and Indians. The risk of psychosis was significantly associated with the experience of verbal racial abuse, physical assaults and work-place discrimination. Experiences of racial abuse (verbal or physical) doubled the risk of psychosis compared with those who had no such experiences. Work-place discrimination was also associated with an increased risk of psychosis, although this was not statistically significant. All these relationships were independent of age, gender, occupational and employment status. As the authors point out, it is difficult to draw any conclusions about the causes of psychosis because the design of this study was cross-sectional. It is impossible to know if racism causes psychosis, or whether having psychosis makes it more likely that the individual experiences, perceives or reports racism. Only a longitudinal study can clarify this.

This is exactly what Janssen *et al* (2003) did in Holland. They recruited a representative sample of 5,618 Dutch citizens (out of 7,076 invited to participate), assessed their mental states at the point of entry into the study, and then followed them up over three years before assessing them at the end (a total of 4,848 completed the study). These assessments were made using a standardised psychiatric interview schedule widely used in epidemiological research, which yielded *DSM-3R* diagnoses. When they entered the study all subjects were asked six questions about their experiences of discrimination, including racism and ethnicity. The rate of delusional beliefs in people who reported one instance of discrimination (0.9%) was nearly twice as high as the rate in those who reported none. In addition, 2.7 per cent of those who experienced discrimination in more than one domain showed evidence of delusional beliefs (but not hallucinations). These differences were statistically significant even when other (demographic factors) were accounted for. These results indicated that '... perceived discrimination predicts, in a dose-response fashion, incident delusional ideation' (Janssen *et al*, 2003: 73). This brings to mind the cumulative impact of experiences of abuse in childhood on the risk of adult psychosis in the previous chapter. The experience of racial discrimination is thus an important social factor associated with delusional beliefs. This is not to say that every black person who presents with delusional beliefs and psychosis does so because of racism, but it indicates that the experiences of racism do play an important role in the genesis of psychosis for some black people.

Conclusions

In Chapter 4 we set out the limitations of scientific models of psychosis in terms of a failure to engage with contexts that could best be seen as problems of social justice. Scientific models may deal with income inequality, social adversity and personal experiences of abuse to some extent, but ultimately they lead to technological responses that attempt to remedy problems or faults within the individual, through drugs or therapy. In the relationship between black people and psychiatry we see even more starkly the contexts in which black people are driven mad in British society. These are the same contexts in which psychiatrists and mental health services try to respond. This is a society in which a young black teenager is murdered simply because he is who he is; a society in which personal experiences of racism are accepted by black people as part of everyday life; where mental health services are institutionally racist, and young black men are more likely to be detained, drugged and diagnosed than their white peers. And black people are also less likely to be offered psychological, or 'talking', therapies. They are denied the opportunity to talk about their experiences once in mental health services. Maybe this is because we find it difficult to face up to what they might have to say were they given a chance to speak.

One of the most powerful moments in my life came a few years after I started work in my first consultant post in Manchester. I had started the process of building links with members of the city's black community. A few months into this they asked if I would join a group of them to watch a television documentary. A little curious I agreed, and turned up at a community centre a week later, where I was shown into a room. I was the only white person, and the dozen or so other people who had already gathered were prominent members of the local black community, most of whom I already knew. The documentary was a film called *Black*, a feature-length history of the suffering of black people in the Atlantic slave trade and on the plantations in the West Indies. It looked in some detail at the role played by the British people in this. When it finished we sat in silence for several minutes; I was too moved to say anything. Eventually, one of the others, a Jamaican woman who managed a hostel for young homeless black men turned to me and said that they had wanted me to see it because it spoke for them about their pain and suffering, and about the role that my people had played in that. They wanted me to know how they felt, and, more important, they wanted to be sure that I could accept their feelings; that I could face up to them, and that I wouldn't run away from them, deny them or act as though they were of no importance.

Kwame McKenzie has recently written as follows about how we should respond to the plight of black people in relation to mental health services:

> It is difficult not to accept the proposition that we should decrease racism and improve the environment of children, the socio-economic position of African and Caribbean people in the UK, social support, social capital and cohesion. (McKenzie, 2010: 736)

He argues that an implication of any analysis of the influence of personal experiences of racism and adversity on the mental health of black people in our society is that it draws attention to the importance of prevention through public health measures. But he goes on to point out that this raises a number of difficult questions, especially concerning the role of prevention. This was an important component of the government's policy Delivering Race Equality (DRE) (Department of Health, 2005b) and the work of the 500 community development workers the programme employed. DRE ran for five years and came to an end in 2010. Now there is anxiety that in the face of the recession, government work on equality and diversity has an even lower priority (*The Guardian*, 2012e). Health service budgets are being cut, and priorities moved away from innovative and creative prevention strategies back to the safe haven of treatment-based services focused on the individual. In the face of stasis and retreat, we back off from engaging with the social injustices experienced by black people. This is why narrative psychiatry and community development are more necessary than ever before.

Recommended Reading

Fernando, S. (1991) *Mental Health, Race and Culture*. London: Macmillan/MIND Publications.

Karlsen, S., Nazroo, J., McKenzie, K., Bhui, K. & Weich, S. (2005) Racism, psychosis and common mental disorder among ethnic minority groups in England. *Psychological Medicine, 35*, 1795–803. doi:10.1017/S0033291705005830.

Metzl, J. (2009) *The Protest Psychosis: How schizophrenia became a black disease*. Boston: Beacon Press.

Sashidharan, S. (1993) Afro-Caribbeans and schizophrenia: The ethnic vulnerability hypothesis re-examined. *International Review of Psychiatry, 5*, 129–44.

SCMH (2002) *Breaking the Circles of Fear: A review of the relationship between mental health services and African and Caribbean communities*. London: Sainsbury Centre for Mental Health.

Sharpley, M., Hutchinson, G., Murray, R. & McKenzie, K. (2001) Understanding the excess of psychosis among the African-Caribbean population in England: Review of current hypotheses. *British Journal of Psychiatry, 178*, s60–s68. doi: 10.1192/bjp.178.40.s60.

Walls, P. & Sashidharan, S. (2003) *Real Voices – Survey findings from a series of community consultation events involving black and minority ethnic groups in England*. London: Department of Health.

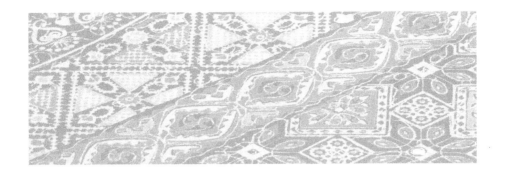

Section 3

On Neuroscience
and Narrative

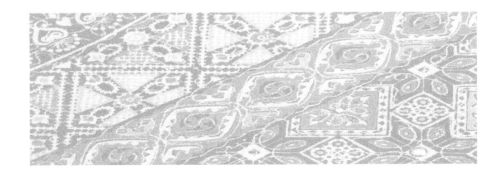

Why (Neuro)science Is Incapable of Explaining the Experiences of Psychosis

6

> Physical science, to which brain impulses ultimately belong, does not have any place for consciously experienced appearances. A neural account of consciousness is *a contradiction in terms*.
>
> Tallis, 2011: 94, original emphasis

There is a strong belief in some quarters that the failure of science to 'crack' the problem of psychosis will become a thing of the past, a temporary setback on the path to enlightenment. Science will at some unspecified future point establish psychiatry as a 'medicine of the brain'. Shortcomings of psychiatric diagnosis like the problem of validity will vanish as molecular genetics and neuroscience refashion the way we think about psychosis, shaping it into as-yet-unthought of forms. At least these are the claims we examined in Chapter 1, made by Craddock *et al* (2008) and Bullmore *et al* (2009). We are promised that these insights will yield novel and effective drug and physical treatments for people who experience psychosis and distress. Indeed, some are already abandoning categorical diagnosis in psychiatry and are turning instead to investigate the neurobiological sequelae of childhood abuse (Hart & Rubia, 2012). In Chapters 4 and 5 we found scientific evidence of the importance of contexts in understanding the experiences of people who suffer from psychosis. These include personal histories of trauma and adversity, especially in childhood, as well as other forms of oppression and abuse, such as racism and wider socio-economic contexts of inequality. The nature of these contexts raises moral and ethical questions about our work. They flag up important issues about values in psychiatry. What do we really believe to be important about what we do to help people who experience psychosis? Most psychiatrists will agree that contexts are important, and that we have a responsibility to bear witness to suffering and trauma. But they will also argue that ultimately these are things over which we have no control, so it is only right that we should resort to neuroscience to do all we can to ease the distress of individual patients. Isn't it right, they will argue, that if science offers even only a limited and imperfect view of suffering, we should use it to help the individual who has faced overwhelming adversity?

The purpose of this chapter is to scrutinise the claim that neuroscience will deliver new insights into psychosis that will help to ease suffering. Given the claims that have been made for neuroscience as guarantor of the future of psychiatry this is important. It is worth remembering that the scientific search for the biological basis of psychosis is at least 150 years old, and can be traced back to Griesinger (Marx, 1970). How do we know that we won't be in the same situation in another hundred years or so? Are we justified in pinning our hopes for the future of psychiatry on neuroscience? Can we justify the huge costs entailed in the research necessary to achieve this, noting that it is only wealthy Western nations that could afford such a project? What is the status of the technologies of neuroscience that feature in this task? Are there limits to this technology, and if so, what are they? The experiences of psychosis, voices, unusual beliefs, and intense distress are not properties of brains; they are the lived experiences of suffering individuals. More than that, the evidence from Chapters 4 and 5 indicates that these experiences are deeply enmeshed in personal stories, lives afflicted by trauma and adversity. In view of the high expectations placed upon neuroscience, we are entitled to ask: what assumptions does it make in its attempts to explain consciousness and experience, and what are the implications of these assumptions for a neuroscientific psychiatry? If there are indeed limits to neuroscience, then what are the consequences of this for the future direction of psychiatry? In essence, this is a critique of reductionism and determinism in neuroscientific investigations of subjective experience, the view that consciousness can be explained entirely with reference to physical states of the brain. In Chapter 14 we will see that there are signs that neuroscience is starting to move beyond such a limited and sterile position, by recognising the significance of the world in consciousness.

This chapter begins by describing the latest generation of brain-imaging technology, so we can understand what it can and cannot do. This preliminary examination reveals three problems: statistical, methodological and conceptual. However, these problems originate in more fundamental philosophical problems that face neuroscience in its attempts to investigate the neural basis of consciousness. As far as psychosis is concerned, there has been particular interest in studying brain activity when people who have psychiatric diagnoses (usually schizophrenia) hear voices. For this reason much of the focus in this chapter concerns functional imaging studies of verbal auditory hallucinations. The arguments developed, however, are relevant to neuroscientific studies of other experiences associated with psychosis. It is worth stating at the outset that the strategy adopted in this chapter is a conservative one. This is because this critique is primarily directed at the inadequacies of neuroscience in tackling consciousness.

'Seeing' Consciousness?

Developments in technology have revolutionised the practice of medicine over the last fifty years. In particular, the diagnosis and assessment of neurological disorders has benefited greatly from new techniques that make it possible to see the brain in much greater detail than was possible through conventional skull X-rays. Magnetic resonance imaging, a new method of visualising the internal structures of the body, was introduced in the early 1980s, and less than a decade later a variant of this technique made it possible to study the body's metabolic activity in vivo, by measuring the blood flow through tissues in real time. This technology, functional magnetic resonance imaging (fMRI), has since been widely used to study brain activity, opening up a new field of study in cognitive neuroscience research. Such has been the explosion in this field that Logothetis (2008) identified over 19,000 papers with 'fMRI' as a keyword published since 1991. Nearly one half of these are attempts to localise brain activity in relation to a wide range of cognitive tasks. And beyond serious scientific study there has been a frenzy of media interest in the field. Astonishing claims have been made about the ability of neuroscience to explain our most human experiences, as fMRI studies have infiltrated just about every human space there is, from investigations purporting to demonstrate the neural basis of romantic love (Bartels & Zeki, 2000), to the neurobiology of aesthetics in the appreciation of music (Salimpoor et al, 2013), and to the neurophilosophy of free will and criminal responsibility in criminology (Farahany, 2012). It is little surprise that some neuroscientists like Raymond Tallis (who is also a clinician) identify such cultural developments as 'neuromania'.

   One reason for the broad cultural appeal of this work is to be found in the popular belief that it enables us literally to 'see' consciousness, or at least the brain activity that appears to give rise to it. fMRI presents us with vivid and startling images of the brain, with multi-coloured lights flashing on and off indicating activity in different areas as the brain processes information necessary for consciousness. This for some is a 'pinball' view of the brain, and for many non-specialists, the neuroscientists who create and manipulate these images must indeed seem like pinball wizards. The assumption is that because we can now observe brain activity directly in real time this must tell us something fundamentally important about the neural basis of consciousness. It is very easy to be seduced into believing this. The origins of these images are shrouded in mystery for most, so they must represent the true nature of consciousness. But is this really the case? There are many steps, traps and pitfalls on the path from image of pinball brain and metabolic activity in brain tissue to conscious experience. In order to appreciate these obstacles it may be helpful to be clear about the basic principles upon which fMRI is based.

   When an area of the brain becomes active it has an increased need for oxygen and nutrients such as glucose, which it is incapable of storing, and as a consequence the blood supply to the area increases. Thus functional activity in an area of the brain can be detected by measuring its perfusion, the amount of blood passing through it. A number of techniques have been used to detect and measure changes in regional cerebral blood flow (or rCBF). Until recently positron emission tomography (PET) was widely used. This involves administering subjects a biologically active molecule such as glucose tagged with a radio-isotope. This carries a risk from ionising radiation (gamma rays) and for this reason fMRI has largely replaced PET in neuroscientific studies. fMRI exposes the subject's brain to a very powerful and constant magnetic field, which aligns all the nuclei in the atoms in the brain in the same direction. A second magnetic pulse is then briefly applied, which nudges the nuclei into a higher energy level. When the pulse ends the nuclei slowly return to their previous level and in doing so release a small amount of radio energy. This can be detected and measured to provide an indication of the positions of the nuclei. Oxygen-rich blood has different magnetic properties from deoxygenated blood, and this is used to indicate which areas of the brain have been active metabolically, and thus associated with the contents of consciousness under investigation. These data are then manipulated mathematically to generate a map of the brain showing the level of activity in different areas.

Seeing Voices in the Brain

Over the last twenty years there has been a rapid growth in studies that have used fMRI to investigate the neural basis of voice hearing, mostly in people who have received a diagnosis of schizophrenia. In general these studies compare the level of activity in the brain 'at rest', that is to say, when the person is sitting quietly in the scanner not hearing voices, with the activity when the person indicates to the experimenter that they are hearing voices. Subjects have a button which they are asked to press as soon as they hear voices, so the technician can operate the equipment. The activity in the resting state is then 'subtracted' from the activity measured when the person is hearing voices. The data are handled by complex mathematical and statistical procedures, which convert differences in brain activity between the two situations into a colour-coded map, the mysterious images that feature prominently in scientific papers, news reports and other media output. The assumption is that any difference in brain activity between the two states causes the voices heard by the person.

A recent review of brain-imaging studies of people with a diagnosis of schizophrenia who were hearing voices found '... insufficient neuroimaging evidence to fully understand the neurobiological substrate of [auditory hallucinations]' (Allen et al, 2012). The authors briefly acknowledge that the interpretation of these studies is complicated by a number of factors. Most include only very small numbers of subjects, making it difficult to draw firm conclusions about the relevance of the results more generally. Most fail to take into account the effects of medication. This is waltzing around the margins of the problem. There are major problems with these studies, which fall into three categories: statistical, methodological or empirical, and conceptual.

Statistical problems

A number of neuroscientists have drawn attention to the statistical limitations of functional brain imaging studies. Each observation (fMRI scan of a subject) generates a vast amount of data to be processed and analysed. This isn't a problem in itself, but it means that in order to be confident that the statistical analyses used are robust, each study requires a correspondingly large number of observations (i.e., cases). The difficulty here is that this is rarely the case. Most studies report findings on small numbers of subjects, and this raises the risk of a bias towards positive findings. Button *et al* (2013) describe in detail how a number of factors relating to study design, including the number of subjects, observations made, and the strength of the relationships under investigation, can exaggerate the power of a study and thus have a detrimental effect on the validity of the results. Although it is widely recognised in biomedical research that low statistical power reduces the likelihood of detecting a true effect, it is less well recognised that low power also reduces the likelihood that a statistically significant result represents a true effect. The statistical power of a study depends on two things: the size of the sample in the study, and the size or strength of the effect under investigation. If either or both of these are low, then this reduces the likelihood that a statistically significant finding represents a true difference. They examine these relationships across a wide range of neuroscientific studies, including fMRI studies in a literature search of papers published in 2011. They identified 48 papers that met their rigorous inclusion criteria, covering data from 730 primary studies. They extracted data from the meta-analyses that enabled them to calculate the power of each of the individual studies. They found that the actual number (349 of 730) of studies that claimed statistically significant findings was significantly higher than the number expected (250). Most of the meta-analyses had very low average power. Specifically they found that neuro-imaging studies based on very small numbers of subjects had very low power levels (8% across 461 studies), in 41 separate meta-analyses. If the low average power they found is typical, then this has profound implications, particularly that '... the likelihood that any nominally significant finding actually reflects a true effect is small ...' (Button *et al*, 2013: 371).

A more general problem that faces meta-analyses of scientific studies, particularly in medicine, is that of selective reporting. Researchers naturally want to publish their positive results. There is a tendency for negative results, such as a failure to find or confirm a statistically significant result, to be seen as less interesting. Consequently they may not bother to write up studies with negative findings, or to submit them for publication in scientific journals. Even if they do, journal editors may deem papers that report negative findings to be less interesting, and so reject them. Either way the outcome is that the published literature on which meta-analyses rely contain an unrepresentative excess of reports of positive findings.

David *et al* (2013) found evidence consistent with selective reporting bias in 94 meta-analyses of fMRI studies of brain activity. They identified a number of possible reasons for this. Many studies involved only a small number of subjects, which may exaggerate the numbers of areas of activity reported as being significant. In addition to this, small studies with negative or inconclusive results are probably not published, with the result that the published literature contains an excess of positive findings. Ioannidis (2011) analysed data from recent meta-analyses of brain volume abnormalities in patients with a variety of psychiatric conditions. He found that 31 per cent of these data (142 of 461 data sets) gave positive results when the expected number was only 78.5. He concluded that more studies than would be expected report statistically significant results, suggesting strong positive bias in the literature through the selective reporting and publication of studies that have positive results.

These statistical problems may not question the assumptions that neuroscientific studies of consciousness make, but they do cast serious doubt on their validity. It means that although a study may report a significant relationship between brain activity and an aspect of consciousness, we cannot assume that the relationship is true and robust. It might just be a chance finding. However, the empirical and conceptual difficulties raised by these studies lead to difficult questions about the assumptions that neuroscience makes about consciousness.

Empirical difficulties

At issue here as far as fMRI studies of people who hear voices are concerned, is the precise relationship between brain activity and voices. How do we know that the patterns of cortical activity that are seen when people hear voices actually reflect the underlying brain processes that cause the experience? This is important because the claim is that neuroscience will deliver causal accounts of experiences like voice hearing based on brain activity. The first and most obvious problem here is how we can be certain that the brain activity seen on an fMRI scan when someone hears voices is directly related to the experience, and not to some other brain activity related to the experimental condition. For example, subjects have to wait, listening vigilantly and ready to respond by pressing the button as soon as they hear a voice. This hardly represents a state in which the brain can be assumed to be at rest. Van Lutterveld *et al* (2013) tried to investigate these confounding factors through two meta-analyses of data, one of ten neuro-imaging studies of voice hearing (nine of these were studies of people with diagnoses of psychoses) and eleven studies involving auditory-stimulus detection tasks in healthy subjects with no psychiatric diagnoses. In the first set of studies, voice hearers indicated when exactly they were hearing voices by pressing a button. In the second set, subjects were required to press a button when they heard a non-speech target sound they had been asked to respond to. The authors used a variety of complex statistical procedures to compare patterns of brain activity in the two sets of studies. They claimed to have found evidence of brain activity in over a dozen brain areas that were believed to be specific for the experience of hearing voices, and not the auditory detection task.

The empirical problem with this can be posed as a question: how are we to understand the relationship between the observed brain activity and the voices that these studies assume are caused by the observed brain events? There are two closely related problems here: the relationship in time and in space between brain activity and conscious experience. Logothetis (2008) acknowledges that there are constraints in the spatial and temporal resolution of fMRI technology that limit the conclusions that can be drawn from these studies. The latest technology may well have greatly improved resolution, with voxel[1] sizes some two or three orders of magnitude smaller than earlier machines, but this doesn't make the task of interpreting the results of these studies any easier. A typical fMRI voxel contains over 5 million neurons, 2.2–5.5^{10} synapses, 22 kilometres of dendrites and 220 kilometres of axons (Logothetis, 2008). The technology creates images of the brain that consist of thousands of voxels.

The neuroscientist and philosopher Alva Noë (2009) points out that we have no way of knowing whether beyond current levels of discrimination there are groups of neurons that are active or inactive in a given task or situation. The spatial resolution of the technology is simply too blunt for us to be able to assume that there is a one-to-one equivalence between experience and brain activity in a specific area. In any case, let us assume that future technological advances make it possible for us to measure brain activity in every single neuron and axon across in the entire brain simultaneously. Would this enable us to explain the relationship between brain activity and the contents of consciousness? The answer must be no; we simply cannot understand a newspaper by trying to read it with an electron microscope. The second problem that we encounter here is that of the relationship in time between neuronal activity and perception. Neuronal activity occurs at the level of a few milliseconds, but it can take a much longer period of time, of the order of hundreds of milliseconds, to detect and process signals for the perception of images or hearing, and of a second or two for the emergence of conscious awareness.

The interpretation of these images is further clouded by the technique of normalisation. This is a procedure used to generate the multi-coloured images that accompany fMRI studies. Each human brain is unique in regard to size and

---

1. A voxel is the specification of a point in space widely used in imaging studies. Although not necessarily three-dimensional in itself, they are used to construct three-dimensional maps of organs like the brain.

shape. This makes it extremely difficult to relate the patterns of brain activity seen in one subject with those of a different subject engaged in the same task. Normalisation involves 'deforming' the data from a series of individual brain scans so that the observed activity corresponds to the same location across all the subjects' brains, irrespective of size and shape. This makes it possible to project the average activity across all subjects onto an idealised brain template. This means that the Fauvist-style images we see in scientific papers and elsewhere are not even those of a single real human being, but an idealised average. They don't even have the same relationship to the activity in a real person's brain that an identikit picture of a crime suspect has to a real person's face. fMRI studies leave unanswered the question precisely where in the brain is the physical site of the equivalence between brain activity and consciousness.

Finally, what exactly do the colours indicate? We are told they directly represent brain activity, but do they? Noë points out that they are actually based on physical measures of light (in the case of PET) or radio waves (fMRI), which in turn are assumed to represent metabolic activity in the area concerned. In reality, the final images of brain activity depicted by fMRI and PET studies are at least three levels of removal from brain activity. First, they are measures of cerebral blood flow; second, blood flow is assumed to correlate to metabolic activity; third, metabolic activity is assumed to correlate to mental activity. Stufflebeam and Bechtel (1997) make broadly similar points about PET. Each stage in the generation of these images involves transformation of the phenomena that can give rise to artefacts. In all, this makes it extremely difficult to interpret the significance of the empirical findings of these studies in terms of the conscious experiences they are said to cause.

Conceptual problems

There are two issues here. The first is an assumption at the heart of neuroscience, and without which its attempts to interpret the significance of functional brain imaging studies are meaningless. This is the assumption that mind has a modular structure. The second is an assumption about the 'resting state' of the brain, which is central to the design of fMRI subtraction studies widely used to study the experience of hearing voices. Modularity is the assumption that consciousness arises in a mind that consists of a set of discrete functional modules that process the information or data, which give rise to consciousness. This theory (and it is a theory) is associated with the work of the philosopher Jerry Fodor (1983), and it has played a vital role in cognitive theories and artificial intelligence that attempt to explain consciousness through mathematical processes and operations on sense data using the computer as an analogy, but it is also central to attempts to interpret the data from fMRI studies of brain activity associated with voice hearing. Logothetis (2008: 869) takes '... the modular organization of many brain systems as a well-established fact ...', but if, as Van Orden and Paap (1997) argue, it is wrong to assume that mind is organised along modular lines, then it becomes impossible to know how to interpret the results of these studies.

Noë (2009) argues that at best the images generated by fMRI scans represent a conjecture about what we think might be taking place in the brain. The basic problem here is how do we decide which aspect of brain activity is relevant to the mental phenomenon we are trying to understand. As far as studies of the experience of voice hearing are concerned we have seen that this involves what is called subtraction methodology. The activity in the brain when the subject indicates that she or he is hearing voices is subtracted from the activity when the person is lying quietly in the scanner and not hearing voices, the assumption being that under these conditions the brain is at rest. The difference in brain activity between the two conditions is assumed to be responsible for the experience of voice hearing. The different patterns of activity are then assumed to represent activity in specific 'modules' responsible for processing information that gives rise to the voices. Noë points out that given the current resolution of the equipment (see above) it is impossible to uphold the assumption that brain activity in a specific area corresponds to modular activity. It is almost certainly the case that neural organisation in the brain, and its associated activity are vastly more complex than could be accounted for by the assumed existence of brain modules. The assumption of modularity is a major claim about the nature of cognition that is impossible to verify empirically, and which has a powerful influence in shaping the interpretation of fMRI studies by neuroscientists. But it is an assumption too far.

The subtraction methodology begs another question. How do we know when the brain is at rest? More than that, how do we know what the activity of a resting brain is really like? In any case, how can we be sure that the level and patterns of activity of my brain at rest are more or less identical with yours? If we cannot be certain about the equivalence of brain resting states from one subject to another, then this makes the interpretation of the results of subtraction methodology studies all but impossible. A recent paper by Felicity Callard and colleagues (2012) raises serious questions about the assumptions made by many neuroscientists about the brain's 'resting' state, or the so-called default-mode network (DMN). They point out that historical assumptions about the nature of external task-based experiments in the 1990s defined the 'resting' state of the brain, or the DMN, in terms of neural regions that were not included in these studies. This makes it very difficult to interpret the nature of activity in the brain observed when it is supposed to be 'at rest'.

Neuroscience's Fundamental Flaw

Most of these problems are aspects of a matter that has preoccupied philosophers for millennia, the relationship between mind and body, or consciousness and brain. Elsewhere Pat Bracken and I have written about aspects of this, and the related issue of how it is possible for our minds to know about the world in which we find ourselves (Bracken & Thomas, 2000, 2002, 2005), and I will return to this shortly. As far as contemporary thought is concerned, both these questions can be traced back to the work of René Descartes, and his separation of body (a thing extended in space) from mind (a thinking thing). Since Descartes, dualisms of one form or another have had an enormous influence on philosophy, neuroscience, psychoanalysis, some forms of phenomenology, and psychology. However, in making the claim that neuroscience can explain consciousness in terms of natural processes and laws, it is important to recognise that this entails replacing the language of psychology with those of the natural sciences.[2] At the same time, cognitive scientists make the claim for a mental domain that is amenable to scientific study and investigation not through the natural sciences, but through mathematics and theories of information processing that liken the mind to a computer that consists of a hardware unit (the brain) running software (modular mind).

For the moment we are primarily concerned with the implications of separating body from mind, although we will have reason to return to mind–world dualism shortly. The work of Ray Tallis (2011) offers a sustained and vigorous analysis of the claim that neuroscience is capable of explaining consciousness. Tallis, who as a clinician was responsible for running a rehabilitation service for people recovering from cerebrovascular accidents, is also a neuroscientist and philosopher. He fully recognises the value of neuroscience in understanding neurological disorders, but at the same time is deeply sceptical about the claims made for its role in explaining consciousness. He does not attend to the problems of neuroscience in psychosis, but his account of the problems it encounters more generally in relation to consciousness illuminates its limits in psychiatry. We have already seen that some neuroscientists like Noë are suspicious about the claim that fMRI scans enable us to visualise brain activity responsible for conscious experience. Neuroscientific explanations of consciousness appeal to simplicity at one level, but they do so only because they are fundamentally flawed. In *Aping Mankind*, Tallis (2011) argues that this is because neuroscience fails to engage with one of (Western) philosophy's most difficult and enduring problems: the relationship between body and mind, or brain and consciousness. The problem can be posed as a question: what is the nature of the relationship between the physical events that occur in our brains (about which science has already revealed a great deal) and the contents of consciousness, our thoughts, emotions, beliefs, perceptions, memories and so on. Although neuroscience appears to address the problem of the body–mind relationship it cannot avoid a set of problems that concerns the relationship between brain and consciousness. These relate to

---

2. One might even be drawn to say that this has until recently been the primary goal of neuroscience, although some neuroscientists would dispute this.

the problem of the observer (or subject) in consciousness, the problem of the world (or contexts) in consciousness, the problem of sensation, the problem of intentionality of consciousness, and the problem of time and consciousness.

Before we set out on this I want to reiterate the point I made at the beginning of this chapter about the limited, or conservative, nature of this critique, which sees voices simply as contents of consciousness. If neuroscience can be shown to be inadequate in accounting for voices if seen in this way, then this has important consequences for a future psychiatry as a medicine of the brain. The key issue here is that neuroscience generates at best only a very limited view of the experiences of psychosis. It may be able to cast light on some of the necessary conditions for consciousness to emerge, but it fails to account for how biology, language, culture and other contexts come together to create experience.

The problem of the subject in consciousness

If we see particular areas of the brain light up when someone reports that they are hearing voices, we are wrong to assume that the activity seen on the brain scan is either the cause of the experience or identical to it. There may be a correlation between the two events, but this is not the same as saying that the two are the same thing (identical) or that one causes the other:

> Seeing correlations between event A (neural activity) and event B (say, reported experience) is not the same as seeing event B when you are seeing event A. Neuromaniacs,[3] however, argue, or rather assume, that the close relationship between events A and B means that they are essentially the same thing. (Tallis, 2011: 85)

Tallis argues that it follows from the identity argument (that consciousness and brain activity are identical, one and the same thing) that if I look at a yellow flower the experience I have of yellow should be the same as the activity in my brain. This is clearly nonsense. There is nothing 'yellow' about the nerve impulses and brain activity in the relevant parts of my visual cortex when I look at a daffodil. Or, to take another example, if someone has an fMRI scan when they hear the voice of God saying that the moon will crash into the Pacific Ocean tomorrow morning, then if the brain activity is identical to the experience, then the activity should have a divine quality about it. More than that, it should also have lunar and oceanic qualities, as well as an emotional quality of catastrophe and impending disaster. This is preposterous. The qualities of the conscious experience of hearing the voice of God saying that these things will happen, and those of the neural activities in the brain that appear to be associated with the

---

3. 'Neuromaniacs' is Tallis's expression for those who believe that ultimately all aspects of human experience will be explained in terms of the physical processes that take place in the brain.

experience, are entirely different.

One way around this in the philosophy of neuroscience is through the 'double aspect' theory. This states that although there is only one set of events in the brain, these events have two aspects: a neural or brain side, and an experiential or consciousness side. Tallis considers the philosopher John Searle's (1983) dual aspect theory. Searle argues that water is made up of molecules of H_2O (two atoms of hydrogen and one of oxygen), but the molecules are not wet, shiny and slippery like our experience of water is. This holds for the relationship between brain activity and consciousness. Consciousness consists of experiences (like the colour yellow, or hearing the voice of God) and although these may be nothing like the nerve impulses and brain activity that occur in association with the experience, the double aspect theory maintains that they are different aspects of the same thing.

Tallis unpicks this by asking what is meant by the word 'aspect'. For example, is it the same as an object like a house that possesses different aspects: front, side and rear? If so, it is impossible to think of any sort of 'thing' that has a mental or experiential front aspect, and a neural or material rear aspect. Double aspect theory breaks down because the different aspects of a house are nothing like the difference between a physical event – the patterns of cortical activation in the brain of someone hearing a voice – and the qualities that conscious experience has for the person. It only makes sense to talk of two aspects, or for that matter any aspect, of a house from the point of view of an observer or a subject who is free to vary her or his point of view on the object by walking around it, and thus see it from different angles:

> To invoke doubled aspects is to cheat: it smuggles consciousness in to explain how it is that neural activity, which does not look like experience, actually *is* such experience. (Tallis, 2011: 86, original emphasis)

Ultimately the double aspect theory of consciousness still maintains that brain events cause the experiences of consciousness. But we can't say that brain activity is the *same* as consciousness, and at the same time say that it *causes* consciousness. Cause and effect stand in a different relationship to identity and sameness. It simply doesn't make sense to say that the front aspect of a house causes the rear aspect. The key issue is that the relationship between the two requires something that neuroscience ignores or turns away from, an observer, a subject who is free to explore the house by walking around it. Neuroscientific accounts of consciousness disregard the significance of the conscious observer, the subject and perceiver of experience. The voice of God has the qualities it possesses only because a conscious subject is aware of it when she or he hears voices.

The problem of the world in consciousness

If consciousness is nothing more than brain activity, then we are entitled to ask the question: what role does the world play in consciousness? On the face of it there is strong evidence that the external world may be relatively unimportant as far as consciousness is concerned. The Canadian neurosurgeon Wilder Penfield treated severe epilepsy in the mid-twentieth century by surgically removing scar tissue in the cortex responsible for the focus of seizures, but to do this he had to make sure that he removed only the small area of damaged cortex responsible for the fits. He operated under local anaesthetic (brain tissue itself is insensitive to pain) and electrically stimulated the exposed cortex with his patients fully conscious. This was to make sure that he was not removing brain tissue essential to an important function such as motor activity, speech or sensation. When he did this in parts of the temporal lobes, patients reported vivid and complex experiences often relating to events from the past. It was as though they were watching a familiar scene from outside. But these experiences were generated entirely from within, through brain activity and without reference to what was happening in the world at the time. Another strand of evidence here is the changes in perception induced by drugs. Certain chemicals can bring about complex changes in perception. A literary example of this is to be found in Aldous Huxley's (1954) account of the effects of mescaline. The richness and complexity of these experiences arises directly from the action of the drug on the neurochemical processes responsible for consciousness, and without reference to the external world.

Such observations gave rise to a famous thought experiment in philosophy – the brain in a vat – proposed by Hilary Putnam (1982). This explores the proposition that if all our conscious experiences are caused by the neural activity of our brains, then it is entirely possible that we are deceived as to our true nature. For all I know I may be nothing more than a brain suspended in a vat of nutrient fluid, connected to a powerful computer that stimulates it in such a way that it gives rise to all the experiences that I have at the moment. In principle everything that I experience could directly arise from the way the computer stimulates my brain without reference to the external world. It would be impossible for me to know whether or not the world existed, or even if it did, it would be of no relevance to the contents of my consciousness. If such a situation were possible it would justify a wide range of sceptical positions about the world in which we live, our conscious experience of it, and in addition, the significance we attach to it in understanding ourselves as human beings.

The obvious flaw with this experiment, as Putnam points out, is that it is impossible to conceive of the idea that 'I am a brain in a vat' without a world that contained brains, vats, computers, laboratories and the scientists necessary to run the experiment. The very idea of such an experiment presupposes the existence of a world that contains all these things. Tallis points out that the experiment is valuable because it reveals the absurdity of claiming on the one hand that neural activity is correlated with conscious experience, and then claiming that brain activity causes conscious experience and indeed is the same thing as it; 'This way lies the madness of concluding that a stand-alone brain could sustain a sense of a world' (Tallis, 2011: 92). The fundamental problem with neuroscience[4] is its enthusiasm for accounting for consciousness in terms of representations that arise from physical processes in the brain, without reference to events in the world outside. It makes no difference if those representations originate in external stimuli in the here and now, or as we will see shortly, whether they are representations of memories, images and words from past experiences, as indeed was the case in Penfield's experiments. Their origins in worlds past or present are unimportant. What matters in this view are the mechanisms, processes and calculations carried out by the brain in processing the information that constitutes these experiences. This is the point at which neuroscience renders conscious experience meaningless because it is uncoupled from the world in which we exist.[5]

We have seen that there are close links between the experiences of psychosis and adversity, particularly childhood adversity. The content of voices is related to events and encounters with others that have taken place in the lives of people who hear voices. Neuroscientific accounts of voices generate explanations of these experiences that are detached and remote from these early events. The content of these experiences, their subjective qualities, their emotional tone, their symbolic functions, become irrelevant once we focus on the neural basis of the experience. Brains don't hear voices; human beings do.

The problem of sensation in consciousness

This is expressed by the question: how is it possible for the infinite variety of sensory experiences that I can have to be caused by neuronal activity? In contrast to the ever-changing richness of sensory experience, the repetitive firing of nerve cells and movement of action potentials down axons is fixed, monotonous and unvarying. The difficulty facing neuroscience is that the physical building blocks that constitute brain activity, the action potential, is the same in all areas of the brain. It always follows the same natural processes, rapid and reversible changes of the axon membrane's permeability to sodium and potassium ions. These

---

4. Strictly speaking, this problem is not primarily a feature of neuroscience, but of cognitivism. But, as we saw earlier in this chapter, neuroscience and cognitivism go hand in glove, through the assumption made by neuroscience that mind has a modular structure – an important part of cognitive theories that liken the mind to a computer.

5. Others too draw attention to the importance of seeing consciousness as standing in a relationship to a world. In recent years psychologists, philosophers and neuroscientists have written about the need for new ways of thinking about mind that engage with embodied consciousness situated in the world. Examples of this include Varela *et al* (1991) and Noë (2012).

electrophysiological processes are fixed and unvarying, so how is it possible for this singular process to give rise to the infinite changes in sensation that we continually experience? Neuroscience attempts to deal with this in two ways. One concerns the different locations in the cerebral cortex in which activity takes place. The other maintains that in addition to localisation, patterns of brain activity and their changes over time are important.

As far as localisation is concerned, it is clear that when I see colours, hear sounds, or have a memory, activity takes place in different parts of the brain. However, this doesn't account for the specific difference between these experiences. Why is it that if I perceive the colour yellow I have activity in one part of the brain, and activity only a matter of centimetres away might be associated with a completely different perception, such as hearing the flute being played. Localisation intrinsically just does not seem to account for the peculiarly specific nature of sensation, that is to say, its subjective nature. As Tallis puts it:

> Different wirings – to the eyes, to the ears or the nose – do not explain different experiences, particularly since, whatever energies land on sense endings, they are all translated into the same kind of energy: the electrochemical energy of nerve impulses. (Tallis, 2011: 98)

Others have argued that the peculiarly subjective nature of experience, the redness of red, for example, is explained by different patterns of activity that pass through the brain when we have such perceptions.[6] There is an infinite number of possible patterns of activity within the brain given the complexity of its wiring, but the argument Tallis used against localisation also applies here. It begs the question, why should particular patterns of brain activity correspond to particular experiences? Indeed, consciousness poses an even deeper problem. How is it possible for patterns of activity to come together in such a way that they recognise and interact with each other as is the case with conscious experience? For example, how is it possible for brain activity associated with the perception of the colour yellow, and that associated with a perceptual task such as shape recognition, in this case that of a flower, to come together in such a way that makes it possible for me to recognise a daffodil, whose appearance signifies the end of a long, cold winter, and the hope of mild spring days? The answer to this question is that recognition in the sense of meaning and significance is not a

---

6. In philosophy the term given to specific examples of such subjective experiences of consciousness is *qualia*, from the Latin, for 'what sort'. The physicist Erwin Schrödinger was deeply sceptical that the natural sciences could account for the subjective nature of experience: 'The sensation of colour cannot be accounted for by the physicist's objective picture of light-waves. Could the physiologist account for it, if he had fuller knowledge than he has of the processes in the retina and the nervous processes set up by them in the optical nerve bundles and in the brain? I do not think so ...' (Schrödinger, 1992: 154).

property of a brain but of a subject, a person who is immersed in a world, and who strives continually to interpret events in the world, to make sense of them, and to find meaning in them.

The problem of the intentionality of consciousness

Philosophers have long been preoccupied with the problem of consciousness. This is a vast area that I cannot hope to do justice to here, but there is one particular feature of consciousness that poses exceptionally difficult questions for those who maintain that physical processes in the brain cause it. The nineteenth century philosopher Franz Brentano proposed that mental states (and thus consciousness) are different from physical states because mental states are 'about' or 'towards' things (Brentano, 1874/1995). Our thoughts, perceptions and memories are about things. They are directed at objects, events or states of affairs in the world. This property is called intentionality, and it possesses a striking capacity to relate to events or objects that do not exist in the present. For example, I can see a tree through my window. It is mid-winter and it has no leaves. I can leave my study, go outside and walk around it, touch its bark, and shuffle my feet through the leaves on the ground that have fallen from its branches in recent weeks. The tree is 'out there', not in my head. Not only that, consciousness can be directed at things that are *not* in the physical world, such as unicorns, Mordor, or voices heard by a person in the absence of a physical stimulus.

Intentionality – the 'aboutness' and 'out-thereness' that our experience of the world possesses – poses real problems for neuroscience. Tallis argues that causal theories of perception based in the natural world and physical processes in the brain are incapable of accounting fully for these features of perception. Neuroscientific theories propose that our conscious experiences of the world are caused entirely by a chain of causal physical processes that extend from the world outside via our sense organs, and end in the brain. Let us again consider for a moment the tree outside my study. Light, in the form of photons that originated in the nuclear processes deep inside the sun, travels the 93 million miles across space, through the atmosphere, and interact with the atoms that make up the surface of the tree. Some of the photons are reflected back and enter my eye, where they interact with the receptors in my retina. This interaction gives rise to nerve impulses that pass through the optic nerve to the visual cortex at the back of the brain, where they give rise to complex patterns of brain activity locally, as well as more distant areas thought to be important in visual perception. These patterns of brain activity are caused by the transmission of nerve impulses down nerve fibres. In turn, these action potentials are caused by changes in the permeability of the membrane of the nerve fibre to sodium and potassium ions. Neuroscientific explanations of consciousness maintain that perception is entirely caused by these physical processes governed by natural laws. It is important to remember that the neuroscientific direction of causality, the chain of physical events that occur to bring about conscious experience, passes from outside to inside.

Intentionality poses this version of events a profound problem. The tree that I perceive as a result of these physical processes, I see *outside* me, in the world of which both it and I are a part. Although the processes that 'cause' my perception begin outside me, and continue within me, my conscious experience of the tree is not something I observe 'in here' inside my head. I experience it and see it out there in the world before me. There is, as Tallis points out, no way of explaining in causal terms this projection of my perception of the tree back into the external world. Our conscious experience of there being a world 'out there' defies explanation in causal scientific terms.

The problem of time and consciousness

Neural theories of consciousness are in conflict with some basic features of matter as we understand it. Time is central to our conscious experience. We are aware of the present emerging out of a past, and heading into a future. On the other hand, matter and physical systems in the natural world are outside time; they have no awareness of it.[7] Despite this, the idea that memory in some way is a physical process, like the marks left behind on a wax tablet, is an ancient tradition in philosophy and science exemplified by Plato's discussion, through Socrates, that such a view of memory is a false judgement. In neuroscience this view is represented by the idea that memory is an altered state in a physical object, the brain, brought about by the events that caused its altered state. But the events we recall through our memories are not identical with, or located in, the physical events and changes in the brain that appear to be associated with the memory, in much the same way that the physical events in the brain that are associated with the sensation of yellow do not have yellow properties. My memories are a part of me, of my consciousness. As Tallis points out, they possess a double 'dose' of intentionality. First, they point back in time to the experiences in consciousness that they are related to, and at the same time these contents of consciousness concern perceptions of events in the world.

> This double dose [of intentionality] reflects how memories are both in the present (they are presently experienced) and in the past (they are of something that was once experienced). *They are the presence of the past.* (Tallis, 2011: 125, emphasis added)

---

7. It is worth noting that in the final chapter of his book, Tallis tentatively proposes that the nature of consciousness is such a profound mystery for neuroscience that it may even force us to reconsider basic assumptions we have about the nature of matter. He refers to recent work by the philosopher Galen Strawson and others that entertains the possibility that matter might possess consciousness in a primitive form.

This is really important as far as the experience of hearing voices is concerned. Psychiatry describes such experiences as verbal auditory hallucinations (VAHs). The highly influential psychiatrist and phenomenologist Karl Jaspers defines hallucinations as '... actual *false* perceptions which are not in any way distortions of *real* perceptions but spring up on their own as something quite new and occur simultaneously with and alongside real perceptions' (Jaspers, 1963: 66, emphases added). The distinction Jaspers makes between false and real perceptions is based in the simpler view that hallucinations are perceptions without external stimuli. Thus VAHs are perceptions that occur in the absence of a physical event in the here and now responsible for triggering the perception. However, as we saw earlier, memories of past events share the property of intentionality with 'real' perceptions in the here and now. This is not to argue that hallucinations are nothing other than memories. There is a key sense in which the experience of hearing voices is quite different from remembering a conversation with a friend. Voices most frequently are experienced against the will of the individual who hears them. Memories concern events we are free to recall at will, 'about' past events that often bring pleasure. There are, however, certain types of memories that are well-recognised in psychiatry, such as those associated with the diagnosis of post-traumatic stress disorder. These include intrusive memories and subjective re-experiencing of past traumatic events. The intentionality of these experiences as memories is clear. They concern overwhelming and terrible events in the person's past. The issue here is that the double dose of intentionality of memory described by Tallis makes it possible to understand voices as contents of consciousness that may lack an external cause in the present, but as being tied to overwhelming events in the past. The fact that, unlike memories, people who experience psychosis find it impossible to exercise control or volition in relation to their voices[8] can be seen as symbolic of the sense of powerlessness that characterised their relationship to the events and people involved in the traumatic circumstances that occurred much earlier. However, in order to understand the *symbolic* function of voices means adopting a hermeneutic approach to understanding human experience. This emerges from an awareness of the challenge that temporality poses for natural-science accounts of human existence. A hermeneutic approach to human experience is comfortable with the issue of temporality, whereas neuroscience doesn't know where to start.

There is something very particular about our experience of time, the sense we have of a present moment extending back into a past, and opening out into a future of hopes, fears and uncertainties. The temporal depth of conscious experience is uniquely human and this raises all manner of problems for neuroscience. Ultimately we can pose this as a question: how is it possible for the

---

8. At least this is the case in the early stages of the experience. Romme and Escher's work (see Chapter 12) describes how, over time, voice hearers develop the ability to negotiate with their voices, asking them to go away, setting time aside to interact with them.

physical matter that constitutes our brains to generate and sustain the temporal depth that permeates consciousness? Tallis points out that these physical entities have no sense of a 'now' or a 'then', so how can they create the sense of time that we possess? Not only that, but because these elements are crowded together in the confines of the skull, how is it possible for them to maintain such a clear distinction between past, present and future? After all, I can flip between the three with ease and clarity without mixing them up. A memory of an event from the past is associated with a sense of it having taken place at a particular place in time. Although a memory is an event in my consciousness in the present, it explicitly involves something that is absent. The event that gave rise to the memory is absent by virtue of its presence in my past, not yours. My past – all our pasts are – as Tallis points out, extraordinarily complex, layered and elaborated aspects of personal (narrative) history, and collective history accessed through '... facts, through vague impressions, through images steeped in nostalgia. *This realm has no place in the physical world*' (2011: 124, original emphasis). Our subjective experience of time offers a fundamental objection to the view that neuroscience will explain consciousness.

Conclusions

To summarise, this philosophical critique has drawn attention to five key aspects of conscious experience that neuroscience is incapable of explaining. These are: first, the importance of the subject of experience, and of the conscious observer; second, the importance of the world in relation to consciousness; third, the richly varied and individual nature of sensation in consciousness; fourth, the 'aboutness' of consciousness, and especially the significance of the 'aboutness' of memory. This concerns not just memory, but also our imagination, and our ability to think and experience symbolically. Finally, there is the importance of time in consciousness, and the complexity of our relationship to time. Of all these things, time is the most vital when it comes to understanding ourselves. Our complex relationship to time transforms a critique about the limitations of neuroscience in consciousness into an understanding of the inability of neuroscience to grasp the significance of the experience of hearing voices. We may be able to 'see' voices in the brain, but these are silent, wordless voices that are disembodied and disconnected from the life histories in which they were embodied.

A future neuroscientific psychiatry, a 'medicine of the brain', would strip all richness, pain and complexity out of the experience of psychosis, because it has nothing to say about these aspects of experience. Voices may relate at one level to brain events, but we experience them irreducibly as parts of our lives. They are bound to the events and circumstances that we experience in the world, and through the complexity of memory and our ever-shifting experience of time, they become alive in the present. They are bound in our lives to experiences that are private and often unspeakable, the most intimate experiences of pain and suffering, to trauma and abuse (Corstens & Longden, 2013). They are tied to communal and cultural events that figure as great tragedies uniting us in grief and despair (Davies *et al*, 1999). In the next chapter we will see that one way in which a psychiatry of the future can engage with the meaningfulness of voices and the wider experiences of psychosis is through narrative.

Recommended Reading

Noë, A. (2009) *Out of Our Heads: Why you are not your brain, and other lessons from the biology of consciousness*. New York: Hill and Wang.

Tallis, R. (2011) *Aping Mankind: Neuromania, Darwinitis and the misrepresentation of humanity* (Chapter 3, pp. 73–146). Durham: Acumen.

Narrative Psychiatry: A Basis for Stories in Psychiatric Practice

7

This chapter sets out the basis of an attempt to answer a question frequently asked of critical psychiatrists: what difference does being a critical psychiatrist make to the way you work? There are as many different answers to this as there are critical psychiatrists, so what follows is a personal view. In order to understand the background to this it may help if I reflect for a moment on the process that led me to the position I now occupy. At no stage during my career did I sit down with the purpose of theorising about psychiatry, analysing its problems, and as a result deciding to work in a different way. There was never an intention to establish a new form of 'therapy' or a 'style' of clinical work. When Pat Bracken and I wrote the column 'Postpsychiatry' in *Open Mind* magazine from 1997 on, we were clear that we were not writing about a new form of expertise or therapy.

So, if I am not setting out a new form of 'therapy' what am I doing here? The process I have been involved in over the years can be seen as a form of archaeology, this time not in the Foucauldian sense. When I trained as a psychiatrist and sat the clinical part of the membership examination back in 1980 we were taught to present a formulation. Although diagnosis was a part of this, it was only a relatively small component. The formulation was a summary of the main features of the patient's story that drew together key elements from the person's life, especially childhood and other life events. It was an account of the events and circumstances that resulted in the patient coming to see the psychiatrist. This included an outline of the onset and development of the problems, and a summary of the key features of the person's life to that point, focusing especially on development, relationships and physical health (Greenberg *et al*, 1982). It attempted to answer two questions: why has this person presented at this particular time and in this particular way? So, there is a strong sense in which this chapter is not presenting anything radical or new. It is more an attempt to reinvigorate the spirit of something valuable that has been lost from psychiatric practice, at least in the psychiatry that I was trained to practise. I will follow the lead given by Brad Lewis (2011) in naming this way of working 'narrative psychiatry'. I am not claiming that I was 'trained' in any sense to use narrative in clinical work as a psychiatrist. But at that time there was a tacit assumption that it wasn't necessary to rely exclusively on diagnosis as is the case today, or for that matter on psychoanalytic, psychodynamic or psychological theories, to understand and makes sense of a patient's experiences. More important than anything else was the act of listening carefully to what the patient had to say, and attending to the patient's story. Looking back now, having had the opportunity to immerse myself in the literature on narrative in medicine, I can see that elements of narrative theory and practice featured in the way I was trained to work. But in those days it went under the more general heading of formulation.

There is, however, a little bit more to it than that. As we saw in the last chapter, developments in philosophy in the second half of the twentieth century have cast light on the limitations of science in our lives. In this chapter I intend to show that philosophy can also illuminate ways of understanding and engaging with psychosis that are grounded not in science, but in the humanities. Philosophy is especially useful in stripping away the assumptions that tint the way we see the world, assumptions that run so deep, and which we therefore take for granted, that we are no longer aware of them. The point here is that the way of working that I am about to set out is not one that sprang forth from this theory or that model. Indeed, it is this atheoretical stance that causes people the greatest difficulty in understanding the implications of critical psychiatry for clinical practice. Science cannot function without theories, models and hypotheses, so they must have a place in psychiatry if it is to be taken seriously as a scientific project. This is not to say that there is no place for science in psychiatry, not at all. We have seen in earlier chapters the value of Joanna Moncrieff's and John Read's work. Both are excellent examples of how clear scientific thought has re-examined evidence in new ways to draw attention to the limitations of existing theories.

However, Arthur Kleinman (2008) reminds us that medicine and psychiatry are more than science, and it follows that they must rely on more than theory. Theories and models are valuable in that they provide frameworks for members of different disciplines to communicate and investigate psychosis and distress, but they also constitute rules of engagement in interdisciplinary disputes over the right and authority to speak about psychosis and distress. The problem with psychiatry in recent years has been the proliferation of theories and models. Psychiatry has become overgrown with them. They compete with each other, choking out the light, obscuring what is really important – the stories of the suffering people we are trying to help. What I am about to describe in this chapter, narrative psychiatry, is something rarely encountered; a way of thinking about psychosis that is largely beyond theory, and certainly beyond models. This is because it originates not in science, but in the humanities.

It is important to remember that models and theories are not 'true' in the sense that they reflect a literal reality or state of affairs in the minds and brains of people who experience distress and psychosis. If we accept this we can see that scientific theories and models have value as one set of metaphors amongst many that may be helpful for patients and psychiatrists in trying to understand the experiences of psychosis. The reality is that individuals differ enormously in what they find helpful or unhelpful, and the greatest and most rewarding challenge in working as a psychiatrist is to try to work out with each person what exactly it is that she or he might find helpful. Narrative psychiatry offers a way of engaging with individual differences and preferences, and this it has in common with person-centred therapy and values-based practice. There is, as Brad Lewis (Lewis, 2011) points out, an additional benefit of narrative psychiatry. If we think about the practice of psychiatry as a form of narrative, it reconnects us with a long-standing view about medicine as an art, and this opens up the way for us to engage seriously with the valuable contribution that the humanities can make to our work and lives as doctors.

In the first section of this book we examined critically several aspects of psychiatric theory and practice, all of which raised the need for a different set of priorities and a different way of working in psychiatry. In broad terms we can summarise these new priorities as follows:

1. We must engage with meanings, contexts and diversity in clinical work.
2. We must engage with a wide variety of different ways of understanding psychosis and distress, and the varied responses that follow from these understandings. These different understandings do not exclude models that psychiatrists currently use within the technological paradigm (biomedical and cognitive), but they have to take their place alongside many others, including cultural, spiritual, political and philosophical.
3. We must engage with an endless variety of personal meanings of recovery.
4. We must engage with the moral and ethical complexities of psychiatric practice ('ethics before technology').

In what follows we will see how thinking about clinical psychiatry as narrative can help us to meet these objectives.

What Is Narrative?

The recent 'narrative turn' in the humanities originated in literary theory, and over the last forty years it has spread to the social sciences, law, theology and psychology, and more recently, medicine and psychotherapy. In these clinical fields (including narrative psychiatry) narrative stands at the intersection of a number of disciplines, including literary theory, phenomenology,[1] anthropology and sociology. In medicine, the use of narrative and narrative theory has been

1. Here I am referring to phenomenology as a hermeneutic process primarily concerned with interpretation and meaning. This is very different from the view of phenomenology as a descriptive tool that dominates psychiatry. For a more detailed excursion into this area, specifically with reference to the experience of hearing voices, see Thomas and Longden, 2013.

influential in general practice (Greenhalgh & Hurwitz, 1999), psychotherapy (Holmes, 2000) and family therapy (White & Epston, 1990). Some authorities see the use of narrative in clinical medicine as a way of dealing with the existential aspects of illness that have always been a central concern of the doctor (see Kleinman, 2008), but which evidence-based medicine doesn't address. Doctors are human beings, so when they take a history from a patient they are engaging in an act of interpretation (Greenhalgh & Hurwitz, 1999) that involves an attempt to understand the meaning of the patient's story. Interpretation and meaning are key aspects of the formal literary task of analysing narratives. But in medicine thinking about patients' stories in narrative terms opens up the possibility of engaging with the existential and moral aspects of illness and suffering.

It is no coincidence that some of the leading advocates of narrative in medicine in England are general practitioners like Trisha Greenhalgh, Brian Hurwitz and Iona Heath. Narrative understanding is particularly valuable in primary care where the complex human problems that are commonly encountered by general practitioners are not amenable to scientific solutions. In this respect psychiatry has a great deal in common with primary care. The difficulty is that the aspiration of psychiatry to be seen as a legitimate scientific branch of medicine has meant that it has attached little value to narrative understanding.

If we turn to narrative as a way of engaging with a patient's suffering we step back from the certainty afforded by EBM into a world of uncertainty and ambiguity. This is because the process of interpretation is a singularly individual one. Your interpretation of 'The Love Song of J. Alfred Prufrock' is likely to be quite different from mine. On the other hand this is its strength, because a fundamental concern of narrative in medicine and psychiatry is that it opens up the possibility of engaging with multiple meanings and interpretations. Iona Heath (2001) points out that the use of narrative in medicine is not a simple antidote to biomedical reductionism. Her use of a poem by Zbigniew Herbert not only draws attention to what she calls the 'uncertain clarity' of the use of narrative in general practice, but also highlights the value of the humanities in helping us to grapple with the ambiguities and complexity of medical practice. She writes:

> The great gift of what we do is that every day, if we allow ourselves not only to listen but to hear, we are brought face to face with what we do not know, with the limits of the understanding and the power of biomedical science. (Heath, 2001: 64)

Narrative medicine is now a well-established and valued enterprise that features prominently in academic life, clinical medicine and the output of journals like *Medical Humanities* in Britain, and *Literature and Medicine* in the USA. In subsequent chapters I will try to demonstrate that narrative offers a powerful way of engaging with patients in clinical psychiatry. But first we need to familiarise ourselves with some aspects of narrative theory.

The idea that we can think of a human life as a story may appear self-evident, but this deceptively simple idea has deep roots in philosophy. A number of philosophers wrote about narrative identity in the second half of the twentieth century, including Alasdair MacIntyre (1981), Paul Ricoeur (1984) and David Carr (1986). The figure who stands behind much of this work is Martin Heidegger (1962), a key insight of whose philosophy is that being, or human existence, is fundamentally temporal and historical. This opens up the possibility of thinking about human life in narrative terms. The argument is that if being is temporal, that is to say, if it is fundamentally grounded in our experience of time, then we may also think of being as narrative. Like a good story we can think of a human life as having a beginning, a middle and an end, enfolded by a plot. This doesn't mean to say that a human life can be summarised or captured as an ordered, flowing story. At the heart of the philosophical notion of narrative identity is the view that we live our lives tentatively, contingently, reflexively and 'pre-reflectively'. 'Reflexively' and pre-reflectively refer to quite different modes of being that complement each other. Our capacity for reflexivity concerns our ability to step back from ourselves to become aware of ourselves and to consider our actions and feelings in the context in which we find ourselves. In direct contrast to this mode of being, we are in the world pre-reflectively. Most of the time we don't step back and watch ourselves in the world; we simply are in the world, grappling with it, struggling to interpret it and make sense of how it seems to us. Although these modes of being are in a sense diametrically opposed, they complement each other.

Most of the time we live our lives pre-reflectively; we simply don't think of ourselves as stories. Nevertheless, we can think of our lives as work in progress, a great unfinished story. Our narratives only end when we die, and even then the story may not be complete. We leave loose threads behind which others try to gather up after we've left, as they continue to tell and re-tell stories as they remember us. What is important, as far as narrative identity is concerned, is our struggle to impose some sort of order on our inchoate and emergent experiences. Narrative, or telling a story about ourselves, is a powerful way of doing this. It assists us in our search for meaning and our attempts to understand our experiences. MacIntyre (1981) argues that human action is only understandable in so far as it is embedded in an historical context. It follows from this that history, human action and meaning must be related. How this happens has important consequences for understanding the role of narrative in psychiatry.

Holmes (2000), a psychiatrist and psychotherapist, uses the distinction between intentional and non-intentional causality (Bolton & Hill, 1996)[2] to

2. The distinction between intentional and non-intentional causality isn't as clear-cut as presented. Jeremy Holmes points out that even in medical conditions with clear-cut genetic causes (i.e., non-intentional causality) like Down's syndrome, stories remain important in understanding how the family copes, the love they have for the child, and the ambiguities of their own feelings about the situation they find themselves in. Intentional causality – the things that happen and arise as a consequence of the decisions we make as human beings – is fundamentally moral in nature.

understand the value of narrative in psychotherapy. Intentional causality is a feature of human agency, whereas non-intentional causality lies outside the realm of human life and has nothing to do with human agency. Non-intentional causality is a feature of science and the natural world. For example, we know that day follows night because of the rotation of the earth. We can understand what causes this to happen through the laws of physics. Before such a scientific understanding was available to us, we accepted that it happened as part of the will of God. Either way, the cause of day following night is out of our hands and has nothing to do with human intentions or actions. In contrast, last night I set my alarm clock because I had to get up early this morning for an important meeting. I didn't want to be late. The reason I carried out this action is understandable through my intention to be present at a meeting I wanted to attend. Human intentions lie behind human actions or agency. We will return to the narrative implications of the distinction between intentional and non-intentional causality later, through two narratives about voice hearing.

Being human means having agency, and thus having to face choices and make decisions to do things, or not to do things. The decisions we make have implications for others as well as ourselves – some good, some bad. Even when we have to face up to an event that arises from non-intentional causality and over which we have no control, such as a natural disaster that results in death and destruction, how we face up to this is still to an extent in our own hands, and thus subject to intentional agency. We may have no control over the event, but the path we tread subsequently in part is determined by decisions we make. In this way we can see that narrative and agency are central to understanding the meaning and significance of suffering.

Narrative and the Moral Basis of Suffering

If, as Iona Heath (2001) suggests, the use of narrative in medical (or psychiatric) practice takes us away from the relative certainty of EBM into the uncertainty and ambiguity of meaning and interpretation, it may be helpful if we can find a way of navigating around the narrative world. This is important if we are to understand the use of stories in clinical psychiatry. One of the most insightful approaches to narrative medicine has been set out by Arthur Frank (1995) in *The Wounded Storyteller*, based partly in his own experience of cancer. His work grapples with many issues including the problems of different forms of dualism, the issues of power and narrative legitimacy, and the ethical implications of illness narratives. This is a major work of compelling moral power that helps to clarify the problems that modernist (or technological) medicine pose for our understanding of suffering. His work on the use of stories in medical practice is for the most part directly relevant to their use in clinical psychiatry. There are important connections to be made between illness narratives and narratives of psychosis.

Frank sees illness as a call to narrative that takes place at two levels. First, we tell our family and our doctor about our illness. Second, we engage in storytelling to rebuild a life that has either been interrupted by illness, or fragmented by it. For this reason the stories we tell others about illness are attempts to salvage what he calls narrative wreckage. He distinguishes between taking a history and hearing the patient's story. When a doctor takes a history she or he may be listening to the patient, but in this context the patient has tacitly given the doctor permission to interrupt when necessary to ask more questions such as to clarify a symptom. The purpose of listening and narrative here is less to do with helping the patient to make sense of her experiences than it is to do with the doctor trying to make sense of it through the medical processes of history-taking and making a diagnosis. In contrast, hearing the patient's story means listening without interrupting, no matter how inchoate or disjointed the story might be. This is very important in clinical psychiatry, where patients' stories may be dismissed as meaningless because they show evidence of thought disorder.

Frank describes three types of illness narratives – restitution, chaos and quest. He sees the differences between them in moral terms, concerning the type of agency or moral choices each offers the ill person. In the restitution narrative the person's agency is restricted to accepting the diagnosis and treatment offered by the doctor and getting well again. In contrast the chaos and quest narratives involve understandings of illness that make a return to 'wellness', or the re-attainment of a way of life that existed before the illness, impossible as a moral choice. All three are valuable in relation to narrative psychiatry.

The restitution narrative

'Yesterday I was healthy, today I'm sick, but tomorrow I'll be healthy again' (Frank, 1995: 77) is a synopsis of the restitution narrative. This is a straightforward story about falling ill and regaining health. As a story, though, it has less to do with the patient and her moral agency than it has to do with technological psychiatry's ability to treat successfully. Indeed, this story fits hand-in-glove with a biomedical view of psychosis and distress, which sees the experience of hearing voices, for example, as arising out of a chemical imbalance that can be rectified by neuroleptic medication. The restitution narrative presupposes that technological psychiatry can deliver a successful remedy. In this narrative, illness is a mystery that becomes a puzzle to be solved by the doctor. The real hero is not the patient, but the doctor who solves the puzzle. Frank points out that modernist medicine cannot see a puzzle without wanting to solve it; but a puzzle solved is no longer a mystery. The only way that patients can deal with the mystery of illness is to face up to it, and wonder at it.

Setting aside the scientific 'causes' of disease, Frank uses the expression 'the founding act' to refer to the patient's understanding of the original reasons for the illness. The founding act is usually something that happened to the patient in the past, an accident perhaps (non-intentional), or a disappointment or loss (which could be intentional or non-intentional), or worse, a severe trauma (usually, but not always, intentional). This act, whatever it is, brings to the foreground the need for the patient to search for the moral basis of the illness and the suffering she or he experiences in order to understand it.

Our preoccupation with the importance of science in medicine and psychiatry rests in the expectation that the progress we make through science *will* ultimately make the world a better place at some future point, and that science is a sufficient response to suffering. This places us in a particular relationship with time, one in which the past is devalued as a place of darkness and ignorance, as we strive from the present towards an enlightened future. In this relationship how the person came to be in a state of suffering is unimportant. What matters is a future in which science will triumph by solving the puzzle of illness and suffering. The difficulty with this position, as Frank points out, is that if there is no remedy, if restitution is not possible, and the condition of illness must be endured for the rest of the patient's life; then the founding act – the past circumstances in which the illness arose – becomes extremely important. Under these circumstances trying to understand the meaning of the illness becomes a search for the moral origins of the condition: Was I to blame for my voices? If not, who was to blame? Why has this happened to me?

The chaos narrative

Chaos narratives are stories without plots, a seemingly random series of events lacking causal links. The teller of such stories is usually seen as not having a proper story to tell, an anti-narrative of disorder. Frank sees evidence of such narratives in the stories of Holocaust survivors, evidence that they are linked to trauma and the most extreme forms of adversity, suffering so intense that it is ineffable. For this reason silence often features in such stories:

> What cannot be evaded in stories told by Holocaust witnesses is the hole in the narrative that cannot be filled in, or to use Lacan's metaphor, cannot be sutured. (Frank, 1995: 98)

Chaos narratives are held by wounded storytellers, but the story can only be told once the person is able to step back from the immediacy of the suffering, because for as long as the suffering is being lived it is unspeakable. They are held in pre-reflective experience, overwhelmingly so, to the extent that it is impossible to step outside them in order to consider them reflexively. Attempts to put the story into words drive the narrative into a particular type of sentence structure described by Frank as 'and then and then and then' (*ibid*: 99). It is as though the person is so utterly overwhelmed by the enormity of what she or he has endured, that she is unable to use the more complex syntactical forms that enable us to express how our experiences are ordered in space, time, magnitude and relation: aspects of language use that are necessary in the construction of meaning through narrative. All we can do is to use the simplest form of sentence structure, that of clausal coordination (… and then … and then … and then …). Each clause is equipotent; we can discern no clear relationship between them.

These are the stories we most frequently encounter in clinical psychiatry. These are the fractured, inchoate narratives of people in crisis, overwhelmed by distress, suffering and psychosis. But it is difficult to engage with them for two reasons. They plunge us into meaninglessness and moral futility. What point can there be in the face of a litany of suffering? It is easier to turn away, retreat behind a wall of indifference, perhaps by classifying and ordering them through the language of psychopathology. Second, chaos narratives are the most embodied of stories. They are on the edge of great wounds brought about by unimaginable trauma, and they are also on the edge of speech. Chaos is unspeakable; it defies expression through language.

Despite this, Frank argues that it is important that we honour and respect chaos narratives, but the problem is that health professionals frequently respond in ways that make this difficult. They may turn away from the narrative, and in doing so they turn away from the person whose story it is. It is not possible to care for a person whose story has been denied in this way. Or they may try to drag them out of the story through some form of 'therapy'. This can be seen in the pressure experienced by some people to 'recover' from psychosis. We cannot and must not push people into recovery through 'recovery-based' practice or over-zealous interventions with drugs and ECT. Frank sees this as another example of modernism's failure to engage with suffering, which for many is a tragic reality that must be faced and accepted: 'There is no diagnosis, no modernist clinical category for "living a life of overwhelming trouble and suffering"' (*ibid*: 112). This is also true for psychiatry, and is why caring as an existential necessity is so important (Kleinman, 2008; Thomas & Longden, 2013). There is nothing to be done, other than to sit, to wait, to be with and available for the person in chaos, and to do our best to hear the story, and '… honour them for what they are being' (Frank, 1995: 112).[3] It is so much less painful for the psychiatrist to say that this person is schizophrenic, hallucinating or thought disordered. This is the point at which the diagnosis of schizophrenia renames a chaos narrative and in doing so silences the patient's narrative.

---

3. Frank points out that the worst thing that doctors can do to someone living a chaos narrative is to try to rush them out of it. Instead it is important that we accept the reality of chaos, no matter how uncomfortable it makes us feel. In part this means a wider acceptance in our culture for people whose lives are in chaos, through, for example, finding acceptable and valourised roles for them. This is where survivor groups, networks and activism are so vitally important. Ultimately there are strong affinities between chaos narratives and spirituality and religion. Many of the Psalms are chaos narratives.

The quest narrative

Quest narratives engage directly with illness in the belief that there is something to be learned from it. There is a sense in which illness is a journey or a search, although it may not be clear exactly what is being sought. Unlike restitution and chaos narratives, the quest narrative is the teller's to tell. Frank gives, as an example, involvement in patient advocacy, a particularly important example for people who experience psychosis and distress. As the ill person gradually regains a sense of purpose, the idea of illness as a journey begins to form. The meaning of the journey emerges recursively, because it is undertaken to find out what sort of journey the person is making. In part the answer to this is found in the company of others on similar quests. This is why peer relationships are so important for quest narratives. Despite the popularity of the journey metaphor in so-called new age culture, it has serious moral purpose. This can be seen in the value of perseverance, of determination to keep on trying to the end and not to give up in the face of doubt and uncertainty. Perseverance also implies a struggle against the odds, and the moral fortitude this brings. This is especially so given the adversity (especially stigma) that mental health survivors have to face.

Frank describes three types of quest narrative: the memoir, the automythology and the manifesto. Memoirs are gentle, non-linear reminiscences of past illness in the context of present life. The automythology concerns the re-emergence of a new self out of the ashes of the old. It is a rebirth, a phoenix. This is the metaphor of self-transformation following a great trauma, an act of personal change and rebirth. The manifesto quest is arguably the one that has the greatest significance for the view of recovery in psychosis, and is a powerful trope in survivor activism:

> Society is suppressing a truth about suffering, and that truth must be told. These writers do not want to go back to a former state of health, which is often viewed as a naive illusion. They want to use suffering to move others along with them. (Frank, 1995: 121)

This resonates powerfully in the work of survivor activists who see psychosis primarily in social and political terms.

Many survivor stories, or first-person narratives of psychosis, are quest narratives. They speak of discovering a new person through or after the experience of psychosis. Such stories stand as powerful moral beacons in the dark for other survivors. Frank points out that the moral purpose of engaging with such stories is '... *to witness a change of character through suffering* ...' (*ibid*: 128, original emphasis). In witnessing the story, the reader or listener reaffirms this change, which is one form of moral action, and at the same time incorporates it into his or her life as a possibility for change, which is another form of moral action.

Narrative Psychiatry

Stories are central to the practice of psychiatry. Psychiatrists have no diagnostic tests to turn to in understanding their patients' distress. They are entirely dependent on listening to the stories their patients have to tell them. The problem is, as Brad Lewis (2011) observes, that by and large psychiatrists are not well-versed in understanding stories beyond the immediacy of clinical practice. We can also be highly selective in what we listen to, attending to those aspects of the patient's story that fit our personal expectations and biases. Frank's work on illness narratives helps us to move beyond this, and to understand the moral value and purpose of those who experience psychosis and distress. Lewis (2011) describes that the primary objective of narrative psychiatry is to enable us to understand the person we are listening to:

> This narrative understanding brings patient and clinician together into a shared experience of the patient's world ... Narrative understanding is a deep appreciation of the person as a whole, what it feels like for this person, in this particular context, going through these particular problems. (Lewis, 2011: 65)

There are three basic elements of narrative that are valuable in understanding the use of narrative psychiatry in clinical practice: plot, metaphor and narrative identity. In telling a story the plot serves the function of drawing different elements together in a meaningful way. In psychiatry these elements may be phenomena or perspectives that may appear to be irreconcilable and to have little in common; nevertheless despite their incompatible and contradictory nature it may be important that they can be brought together within the person's story.

The second element is metaphor, the linguistic device in which the meaning of a word or phrase is attached to a different but similar object or action. A new meaning is thus created. Psychiatric theories abound with metaphor. Monoamine theories of depression propose that low mood is caused by relative underactivity of brain monoamines. There is no evidence that such underactivity is a reality in the brains of people who suffer from depression, and even if there were, that does not mean to say that it was causally linked to the subjective experience of depression. Nevertheless, for some people this is an attractive metaphor, especially if we say to a sad person that the medication we are prescribing will give them a 'lift'. Are we really talking about the level of monoamines in the brain or the patient's mood? It's not important, but the idea of a lift when you feel down is helpful. Indeed, as Lewis observes, the use of the chemical imbalance metaphor has become deeply embedded in contemporary Western culture. In medicine, diseases may represent scientific truths, but they too can be thought of as metaphors, and in this way convey meaning apart and distinct from any scientific truth. In the next chapter we will see that metaphor is the key to understanding how we talk about our inner states with others. If I feel depressed

I might say that I feel down, or blue, or low. If I am in a poetical frame of mind I might say my heart is full of sadness. I am not literally 'down', or 'blue', and no one believes for one moment that my heart is a container brimming with sadness, but everyone knows exactly how I feel.[4] Metaphors are also heavily contingent on cultural difference, which is why they are valuable when working with people from different cultural traditions.

The third element is narrative identity, which we have already considered. This is important in psychiatry because of the wide variety of identities that are available to us through the stories that we tell about ourselves. A consequence of the prominent role of science in society is that it has created new techno-identities that have implications for clinical practice. Nikolas Rose's (2003) account of the neurochemical self is one such example. Lewis points out that this form of identity is problematic because of the way it feeds into the commercial interests of the pharmaceutical industry. It may be trendy to think of one's sadness as reduced levels of monoamines, but the practice of narrative psychiatry means that we must negotiate such an understanding with a great deal of caution. We have to point to the lack of evidence that these drugs are effective, that they have many side effects, and that their use really serves the financial interests of the pharmaceutical industry.

Equally important here are the consequences of globalisation, especially the increase in cultural diversity of European nations as a result of mass migration to avoid war and persecution, or for economic reasons. As a result we encounter a staggering diversity of narrative identities in clinical practice in psychiatry – including scientific, religious and spiritual, existential, political, and cultural. Increasingly these identities are presenting in hybrid forms in individuals as a result of the processes of acculturation from one generation to the next. The point is that narrative makes it possible to chart an ethical course through these identities. It is important that as clinicians we are able to move rapidly and flexibly between these different narratives to suit the patient's needs.

Hearing Voices as Narrative

I will end this chapter with a thought experiment consisting of two short stories. They are largely fictional, but they also draw on elements of real people's stories to draw out particular points about narrative psychiatry that I want to emphasise. The stories concern two young women, Jackie and Jill, who have been referred to a psychiatrist for the very first time. Although they are largely fictitious they are typical of the stories of many people who present with psychosis.

---

4. Empirical psychiatry starts to get into problems here as soon as it forgets that the vessel metaphor of depression is just a metaphor, and develops rating scales in the erroneous belief that it is possible to measure depression.

Jackie

Jackie starts to hear voices. She is very upset by them because they say unpleasant things to her. She goes to see a psychiatrist. She talks to the psychiatrist who asks her a few questions: 'Do they speak about you in the third person? Do they pass a running commentary on your thoughts and actions?' 'Yes,' says Jackie, 'they talk about me, tell me I'm rubbish, that I'm useless, that everything I do is a waste of time.' At the end of the interview Jackie asks, 'Why do I hear voices?' The doctor tells her that the voices are a symptom of schizophrenia. They are caused by a disorder of the brain, an overactivity in dopamine systems. She says that this imbalance can be rectified by neuroleptic drugs, which reduce the overactivity in the brain's dopamine systems. If she takes the medication her voices will go away and she will feel better. Jackie listens carefully to the psychiatrist and decides to follow her advice. She goes home and takes the medication. A few weeks later the voices have more or less disappeared, and she is feeling better. She remains on medication and sees the psychiatrist every three months. After she has been taking the medication for a year or so she asks the psychiatrist if she can stop taking it. The doctor says it might not be a good idea because she would run the risk of having a relapse, and the voices might come back. Jackie isn't happy with this advice, so she decides to stop her medication, which she does suddenly. Two weeks later she is admitted to hospital because she isn't sleeping, is extremely tense and anxious, and the voices have returned. The psychiatrist tells her she has had a relapse of schizophrenia.

Jill

Jill starts to hear voices. She is very upset by them because they say unpleasant things to her. She goes to see a psychiatrist. She talks to the psychiatrist who asks her a few questions: 'Do they speak about you in the third person? Do they pass a running commentary on your thoughts and actions?' 'Yes,' says Jill, 'they talk about me, tell me I'm rubbish, that I'm useless, that everything I do is a waste of time.' The doctor listens carefully to what Jill says. At the end of the interview Jill asks, 'Why do I hear voices?' The doctor tells Jill she isn't sure; she needs to spend more time to get to know her, so they arrange to meet a week or so later. In the meantime she gives Jill a prescription for a small dose of neuroleptic medication, telling her it may help her to feel less distressed by the voices. The next time they meet, Jill is feeling a little better. The voices are still there but she isn't as upset by them. The psychiatrist has set an hour aside to listen to Jill's story.

During the course of this it emerges that although the voices started to trouble Jill only recently, this was because they started saying unpleasant things to her. In fact she had been hearing voices for many years since the age of six when something terrible had happened to her involving a family 'friend'. Jill told the doctor that the voices comforted her, telling her it wasn't her fault, and that she wasn't to blame for what had happened to her. The tone of the voices changed dramatically a few weeks before she saw the doctor. Her ex-boyfriend had attempted to rape her. She was devastated, and the next day her voices began to accuse her and to blame her for what had taken place. She began to feel a little easier as she told the doctor, even though the voices were still angry with her and scolded her for speaking about them. A few weeks later she reduced and then stopped the medication, and was seeing the psychiatrist regularly to talk about what had happened to her and her voices. She was keeping a journal and was halfway through writing out her life story. Although her voices hadn't completely gone away, she was coping with them much better and able to carry on with her life. After a year or so she was on no medication, and although she still occasionally heard voices she didn't find them troublesome or distressing. She was back at college studying for a degree in psychology.

The moral consequences of different narratives of psychosis

These two women were given quite different stories by their doctors. The story given to Jackie by her psychiatrist was that her voices were a symptom of schizophrenia, a brain disorder that required her to take medication. In contrast, Jill's psychiatrist didn't give her a story at all. Instead she agreed to make time available so she could hear Jill's story. She didn't make a diagnosis, although this didn't prevent her from suggesting to Jill that she might find a small dose of medication helpful. When they met again the doctor had set aside time to listen to Jill's account. She began by asking her some open-ended questions about her and her voices: 'Tell me about your life. Was there anything going on in your life when the voices began? How did you feel then? Tell me about your childhood. Did anything unpleasant ever happen to you? Can you remember how you felt at the time?'

Of course, we don't know what might have happened had Jill not been able to remember these events, and their relationship to the voices. Neither do we know what might have happened had her voices started and changed in the absence of traumatic events in her childhood and recent past. We do know, however, that many people who hear voices have experienced trauma (see Chapter 4). We also know from the work of Marius Romme and Sandra Escher (Romme *et al*, 2009; Romme & Escher, 2012) that having the opportunity to understand the meaning of voices in relation to one's life history is important in being able to live with or recover from the experience.

Equally, we do not know what might have happened had Jackie's psychiatrist responded to her and her experiences in the way that Jill's psychiatrist did. All we can say is that if Jackie had had similar events in her life, and had her voices borne a similar relationship with these events, then she might not have received a diagnosis of schizophrenia and may not have been given long-term neuroleptic drugs. But for this to have happened, Jackie's psychiatrist would have had to respond to Jackie in the same way that Jill's psychiatrist responded to Jill.

Even then it is possible that both psychiatrists might have chosen to disregard these parts of Jackie's story and Jill's story. They might not have regarded it as important, or they may not have wanted to engage with yet more suffering. They are, after all, ultimately in a position not only to ignore how Jackie and Jill interpret their voices and all the events in their lives that led up to this, but to impose their interpretations on these two women, to force them to accept medication against their wishes, and to justify this use of force by saying that they are mentally disordered. That's not how Jill's psychiatrist responded, and it's important to note that whereas Jackie was given a diagnosis of schizophrenia, Jill wasn't *told* that the reason she heard voices was because she had experienced trauma. She established this link for herself. It emerged as she was encouraged to talk about her experiences and her life.

What really matters, though, about this thought experiment, are the moral consequences of these two stories. What I mean by this is the way that these stories have remarkably different outcomes as far as the possibilities for action, or *agency*, of the two women are concerned. In other words if we experience psychosis, the type of stories that are presented to us, and whose strands we may pick up and weave into our lives, open up or close down future possibilities for us. Jackie was told that her voices are a symptom of schizophrenia, a disorder of the brain caused by overactivity of dopamine systems. This biomedical explanation of psychosis is based in non-intentional causality. Jackie's voices arose from circumstances and events in the natural word (in her brain) over which she had no control. Because her voices arose as a consequence of non-intentional causality there is no possibility of understanding the significance of her voices through her life story in terms of things that happened to her, especially things that happened as a result of other people's intentions and actions towards her. The abuse she experienced in the past is unimportant. This places her future entirely in the hands of the experts, doctors and psychiatrists who hold the knowledge and mastery, or so it seems, over the physically causal events in her brain. Thus in the story of how she copes with her voices, Jackie is relegated to a bit-part, a walk-on role in the clinic once every three months or so for a routine check-up. The real hero in this piece is her doctor. This is precisely how Arthur Frank describes the relationship between patient and doctor in the restitution narrative (Frank, 1995).

In contrast, by talking about her experiences with her psychiatrist, who listened carefully and opened up a space in the relationship for Jill to tell her story, Jill came to the conclusion that her voices originated in painful and traumatic events in her past. Her voices began at a point in her life when she had been sexually abused by a neighbour. Her doctor didn't tell her that this was the case. Instead she listened to Jill's story. We know from Chapter 4 that there is extensive evidence linking psychosis to trauma. Romme and Escher (1993a, 2006) have shown that between 70 to 80 per cent of people who hear voices relate their experiences to traumatic events in their lives, including sexual and physical abuse, bullying and emotional neglect, most of which occur in childhood.

In telling her story, Jill also drew on cultural narratives, stories that are important in all our lives, to make sense of the role played by the voices in her life. She told the doctor that when her voices began in her childhood, she believed their identities were kind fairies: 'I suppose they were a bit like the fairy godmother in Cinderella' she said. 'They reassured me; they told me that what had happened to me wasn't my fault.' Cinderella was her favourite story, and she made the link between the fairy godmother and her voices. Of course, not all versions of the Cinderella story have the fairy godmother as a character, but the version she was familiar with did. Even though the abuse came to an end after a few months, the voices persisted, reassuring her whenever she was treated unfairly. As she grew up she heard the voices less frequently until the rape. This, she told her doctor, was a particularly humiliating event for her. Until that moment she had been deeply in love with her violator, and had hoped that they might settle down together. After the event she was not only bitterly angry with him because of the way he betrayed her trust, but also she blamed herself for misjudging his character. The voices returned with a vengeance, and turned on her immediately she made this judgement about herself. They picked up the theme of betrayal and her self-blame, expressing critical comments about everything she did or said, reinforcing her own lack of faith in her ability to judge people, and trust them. She was overwhelmed. She couldn't speak. She had a chaos narrative.

The recent sexual attack reinvoked a sense of powerlessness, horror and anger that went all the way back to the age of six, and which her long-standing voices had protected her against. Through this insight, which was validated by her psychiatrist, not only did she have a different story about her voices, but also a story that had the potential to put her in a very different moral relationship with them. She was able to see that they had arisen in response to human actions and intentions, terrible things done to her by other people. In other words her voices arose out of intentional causality. This meant that she could understand the founding action (the terrible things that had happened to her as a child), her voices, and her struggle to cope with and make sense of her story, in moral terms. Something terrible had happened to her; we can see her struggle to understand and make sense of it all as a quest narrative and as an act of courage.

This is why narrative is so important in psychiatric practice. If we are able to help a person who experiences psychosis of distress to find the story that suits them best, possibilities for action open up for them. For some people the right story might just be 'schizophrenia', the metaphor of dopamine overactivity and neuroleptic medication, but for many, probably the majority, this is an unhelpful, disempowering narrative. Jill, through telling her story, through having her story witnessed, was able to understand her voices. In the next chapter I want to explore how narrative psychiatry can provide a framework for helping people from different cultural traditions who present with distress.

Recommended Reading

Frank, A. (1995) *The Wounded Storyteller: Body, illness and ethics*. Chicago: University of Chicago Press.

Greenhalgh, T. (1999) Narrative based medicine in an evidence based world. *British Medical Journal, 318*, 323–5.

Holmes, J. (2000) Narrative in psychiatry and psychotherapy: The evidence? *Journal of Medical Ethics: Medical Humanities, 26*, 92–6.

Lewis, B. (2011) *Narrative Psychiatry: How stories can shape clinical practice*. Baltimore, MD: Johns Hopkins University Press.

White, M. & Epston, D. (1990) *Narrative Means to Therapeutic Ends*. New York: W.W. Norton.

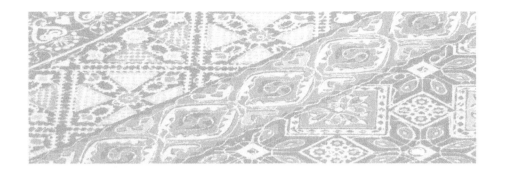

Section 4

Stories in and of
Clinical Practice

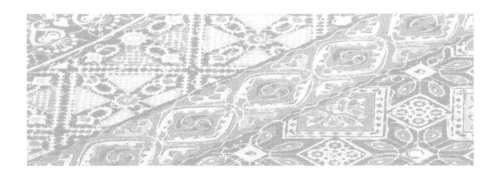

Two Stories of Loss and Sadness   8

It is said that depression is the most common mental disorder in community settings. According to the World Health Organization it affects 350 million people worldwide (WHO, 2012a). The *World Mental Health Survey* found that one in twenty people reported an episode of depression in the previous year (Marcus *et al*, 2012), and its treatment and management is a priority for the WHO's mhGAP (*Mental Health Gap Action Programme*), a global initiative aimed at pressurising the governments of all nations to invest more resources in the management and treatment of mental disorders. The priority is the provision of 'evidence-based' treatments such as antidepressants, brief structured psychological therapies, behavioural activation and relaxation training (WHO, 2012b). Depression, however, is not simply a matter of concern to those who experience sadness, their families, and mental health professionals. It has become an enormous economic problem, a burden to global capitalism demanding a global response. According to the World Bank (1993), it is the fourth most common cause of disability in the world, and is projected to become the second most common cause by 2020. One might be forgiven for believing that all that matters in relation to depression is its economic consequences through loss of productivity, and its economic burden through social welfare benefits for those who are afflicted and unable to work.

If you read the specialist literature on depression, clinical practice guidelines like those produced in England by NICE, or the WHO technical documents on depression in mhGAP, two things stand out. First, it assumes that depression is a disorder with a biological basis, although the precise nature of this remains unknown. It may be genetic, biochemical or endocrinological, but it is primarily biological. Psychological and social factors are important to a point, but a yet-to-be-established biological 'vulnerability' is seen as the most important factor.[1] The question that technological interpretations of sadness (i.e., the clinical entity

1. See, for example, National Collaborating Centre for Mental Health, 2003, especially page 20. Accessed on 13th February 2014 at http://www.nice.org.uk/nicemedia/pdf/cg023fullguideline. pdf

'depression') raises for narrative psychiatry is how such understandings relate to the human processes that take place with people who experience sadness of such intensity and duration that they find their way into the psychiatrist's outpatient clinic. This question becomes even more pertinent in a global context. European cultures have become increasingly diverse, and global programmes like those supported by WHO are putting non-Western countries under increasing pressure to deliver technological interventions for depression to their populations. Those most likely to benefit from this form of neo-colonialism, as Suman Fernando (2011) points out, are the global pharmaceutical companies. At the same time multiculturalism, another consequence of globalisation, is giving rise to a debate about whether members of diasporas should be assimilated within British culture, or whether they should be integrated. Setting aside political arguments about how society should respond to multiculturalism, the reality in the clinic is that diasporas are generating complex, hybrid identities, and this inevitably has implications for narrative psychiatry.

This chapter deals with two stories of sadness, or depression. They are semi-fictional accounts based in the experiences of a number of women I saw when I was a clinician. I want to use these stories to draw attention to the way that the meaning of the word 'depression', and the different understandings that come with it, are closely tied to our different traditions and beliefs. In effect, they are one aspect of the narrative identities we considered in the previous chapter. In turn, these different meanings have implications for how we might respond to someone with the experience. The subjects of these stories are identical as far as age, gender and the role of loss in triggering their sadness, but they differ in one crucial respect – they come from different cultures. One, Kath, is a working class woman from an Irish Catholic background. The other, Amina, is a Muslim woman originally from a small village in the Punjab in Pakistan. Through these stories I want to demonstrate an important feature of narrative psychiatry: its ability to engage with different narrative identities. At the same time I will show that there are limits to this ability.

If we see these stories simply as medical narratives or 'cases' we might be entitled to conclude that they are identical, and it follows that what happens to the two women, their treatment and management, will also be identical. However, attention to the stories reveals important differences in detail that require different responses in terms of the help and support that the women receive. Both make positive responses to the help they receive. They get 'better' or recover. They get over their sadness and are able to carry on with their lives, each in her own way.

Kath

The letter from Dr Wilson didn't say a great deal. I read it as I walked down to the reception area.

Dear Doctor

Re: Kathleen Harrison

I'd be grateful if you could see this 55-year-old secretary who is depressed. Her husband died suddenly of a heart attack eighteen months ago. She has had a course of Prozac and some counselling in the surgery, and although she seemed to do well initially, her depression has since relapsed. Her children have grown up and moved away, and she lives alone. Her general health is good.

Yours sincerely

Two women were sat reading magazines in the waiting area. I introduced myself and asked which one was Kath. One of them stood up, smiling.

'I'm her friend, Joan. Can I come in with her?'

'Is that okay with you?' I asked the other. Kath didn't say anything. She looked at me and nodded.

'Only we've known each other for years' Joan continued. 'We used to work together.'

Back in my office I began by outlining what would happen over the next forty minutes or so. 'Perhaps you could start by telling me how things have been going for you.' Kath gave me the following story.

She had been fine until about two years before, when Kevin, her husband, started to suffer with angina. Although at that stage he wasn't seriously ill, he had a lot of investigations in hospital, and was started on medication. Shortly after this she began to worry a lot about him.

'He seemed to get old very quickly' she said. 'One minute he was running around playing football in his early fifties, then the angina hit him really badly. It slowed him down. His colour changed. His face and his hair turned grey over the course of a few weeks. I began to worry about him, and started to have these attacks, panic attacks the doctor said. I couldn't breathe, and had this terrible thumping in my chest. I'd lie awake at night with this awful feeling hanging over me, like something dreadful was going to happen. I couldn't sleep, and I'd wake up each morning feeling absolutely worn out.' Her voice faded out as she remembered how she had felt. She dabbed her eyes with a handkerchief before continuing. 'Then he had a week off sick. His angina was getting worse, so the doctor signed him off and arranged an urgent appointment. I went to work that morning.' She looked through the window. Outside it was a hot August day, but she sat with hunched shoulders, as though trying to ward off the cold. 'It wasn't like this' she said, waving at the window, 'It was snowing heavily. Snow!' The word drained her, and her voice trailed off again. For a moment she looked as though she was trying hard to remember something; or perhaps I was wrong, maybe she was trying hard not to remember something. She shook her head slowly. 'The buses were late. At work they said I had to get to the hospital right away. I knew something bad had happened. I knew.' Her body shook as tears took over. I gave her a glass of water. Joan knelt beside her, an arm around her shoulders, doing her best to comfort her.

Kath continued. She told me that she had 'kept the lid on' her feelings at Kevin's funeral so she could be strong for her children, but during the weeks and months that followed she described herself as 'slipping into a pit' out of which she could not climb. She said she felt increasingly 'depressed' each day (her word), until about six months later she could no longer manage work. She felt exhausted and was still unable to sleep. She awoke earlier than usual, feeling unrefreshed. Her appetite was poor and she lost over five kilograms in weight. She also noticed that she had become very forgetful.

At this point Joan commented that she lost interest in her appearance and activities that she normally enjoyed, like reading, or going to the cinema. Her self-confidence was so low that she cancelled a week away with her eldest son and his new girlfriend. 'I just couldn't face meeting people, or going anywhere,' Kath added. In the end, Joan managed to persuade her to go to see her doctor.

'I was really worried about her' said Joan. 'She blamed herself for his death. I couldn't reason with her. She began to feel hopeless about life, saying she didn't know how she could carry on.'

'Did you think you might do something about it?' Kath's gaze was fixed on her lap, the fingers of her right hand fiddling with her wedding ring. She looked up at me. 'Did you have any plans?'

'No. I was brought up a Catholic ... I've not been to church since I was a girl. I suppose I miss it really, but I just couldn't go back to it, not after all the terrible things that have happened, the way it treats women, but I do miss it ...'

We moved on to get some details about her life. She was born into a working-class family, with two of her grandparents originally from Ireland. Her maternal grandmother came to the North of England to work in the mills, where she met her miner husband. Her paternal grandfather, originally from County Clare, had fought in the British Army in the Great War and settled in Lancashire afterwards. His only son (Kath's father) was also a soldier, but he was killed in a road traffic accident in the Big Freeze in early 1963 when Kath was six years old. She told me that she had never got over her father's death, and she still felt very close to him. One of her most treasured possessions was a button off his army tunic. Her childhood was otherwise uneventful, as was her comprehensive school education. She trained as a secretary, and apart from having time off when her children were babies she had always worked. Those were the days when working-class women lived close to their extended families, with grandmothers on hand to look after the children. Her eldest child, a son, worked as a teacher in Manchester. Another son worked as a mechanic. Her youngest child, her only daughter, was reading law at a university in the south of England. No one in the family had ever suffered from depression, or seen a psychiatrist.

'We've nearly finished now' I said, scribbling a few notes, 'but could you give me some idea why you think this has happened to you?'

Her eyes filled again.

'Shall I?' asked Joan. Kath nodded. 'She's ashamed because she believes she caused Kevin's death. I've tried to reason with her but it's impossible. All I can get from her is that she's a bad person because she believes she caused it. It's not true; they had a marvellous relationship.'

'Can you say a bit more about it, Kath?' But by now she was too upset so I changed tack.

'What do you think is the matter with you?' I asked.

She looked at Joan. 'Go on, tell him!'

'I think I'm depressed' she replied.

'Can you tell me what that means to you?'

She shook her head and cleared her throat. 'I don't know. I suppose it's an illness, like something wrong with the chemicals in my brain.' She told me about an article she'd read in a women's magazine, and a story line from *Coronation Street* about a young woman who'd suffered from postnatal depression.

'Do you have any idea what might help you to feel better?'

'I don't know. I don't think I'll ever really get over this.'

I wanted to ask her what it was that she thought she would never really get over, but it didn't feel right at the time. 'I'm sure you'll feel better soon. It seems to me that there's a lot you need to talk about, but it's obviously very difficult for you to do that the way you feel right now.'

'Perhaps I need more tablets' she volunteered. 'Maybe I didn't take them long enough last time. What do you think?'

I said I thought she was probably correct. She'd only taken fluoxetine for eight weeks or so, and although her family doctor had referred her for brief psychotherapy in the surgery, she hadn't found this helpful because she said the therapist was too young. 'We just weren't on the same wavelength' she added.

'Okay, how does this sound? I'll start you on some tablets today, very similar to the ones you had before, only they have more sedative properties so they'll help you to sleep better and make you feel less anxious during the day. It's called fluvoxamine. Your GP will continue them if you find them helpful. Then, when you're feeling a bit better, we'll arrange for you to have a course of cognitive therapy. Have you come across it?'

She looked at Joan. 'Is it the one you were telling me about?'

'Yes' replied Joan. 'I had it myself a few years ago. I found it really helpful to get on top of my OCD.' She smiled at Kath, then squeezed her hand.

There were no more questions, so I outlined the side effects of the medication, and wrote her a prescription before ending the interview. Six weeks later she was feeling better. The quality of her sleep had improved, and she was less anxious. Her appetite was better, and she was regaining weight. She had some side effects, but was prepared to put up with them because she believed the medication was helping. She had started to read again, although she hadn't managed to get back to work; neither had she been to the cinema with Joan, 'But we're going this weekend' she added. She was due to attend for her first session of cognitive therapy the following week.

We met on a couple of occasions following this, the last being a month or so after she had finished therapy. She was getting over her depression. She was taking pride in her appearance again, and moved with greater purpose and direction. She carried herself into the world with greater confidence, and no longer appeared overburdened as she had when she first came to see me. She had been back at work for a month or so. We discussed the medication, how long she should remain on it, and I stressed the importance of reducing the dose gradually and not stopping it suddenly.

'How did the therapy go?'

'Well' she replied. 'It helped me to get a sense of proportion on my problems, on my life. The psychologist was great. She made me feel an equal, and that we were working on my depression together. That made me feel so much better in itself.'

'Are you seeing her again?'

'No. She discharged me the last time we met, but she said I could get in touch with her if I felt I needed to.' She looked out of the window. Snow was falling heavily outside, a white blanket for Easter. There was something on her mind. 'You know it was on a day just like this that Kevin died. 'I remember slamming the front door shut and looking at the crocuses struggling to poke their heads through the ice and snow in the garden. I can't see crocuses in the snow without thinking of Kevin not being here. I got to the gate, leant on it; and looked back at my footsteps. I wanted to go back and cover them over, pretend I hadn't left the house, and that I was still inside with him.' She fell silent again, lost in the snow outside.

'Why was that?'

'It was the last time I ever saw him. It would have been our thirtieth anniversary that year. We'd had a blazing row that morning, a stupid thing really, over nothing at all, but I was too stubborn. I stormed out into the white without kissing him, or telling him I loved him, without even saying goodbye. It was my dad over again. Now do you understand?'

Amina

The letter from Dr Khan was typically brief and to the point. I read it as I walked down the corridor to meet the patient he was referring.

```
Dear Doctor

Re: Amina Begum

I'd be grateful if you could see this 55-year-old housewife
who is depressed. Her husband died suddenly of a heart
attack eighteen months ago. She has had a course of Prozac
and some counselling in the surgery, and although she seemed
to do well initially, her depression has since relapsed.
She lives with two of her children and their families, and
her general health is good.

Yours sincerely
```

Two South Asian women both wearing hijabs were sitting next to each other in reception. I introduced myself, and asked which one was Amina Begum. The younger of the two stood up.

'I'm Naima, her daughter. Can I come in with her?'

'Is that okay with you?' I asked the other, who frowned at me. Her daughter spoke to her in Urdu.

'Yes, that's fine,' she says. 'My mother speaks some English, but not enough to make herself understood.'

Back in the office I outlined what would happen over the course of the next forty minutes or so. 'Perhaps you could start by telling me how things have been for you.' Through her daughter, who acted as an interpreter, she gave me the following story.

Amina Begum had been well until about two years before, when her husband, Bashir, began to suffer with angina. At that stage he wasn't seriously ill, but he had a lot of investigations in hospital, and was started on medication. Shortly after this she began to worry a lot about him.

'He seemed to age very quickly' said Naima. 'One minute he was running around with his two grandsons teaching them to play cricket. He loved cricket. He used to play into his fifties. Then his heart problem hit him really hard and he suddenly looked very old.' Her mother nodded, and then fiddled with her hijab, trying to make it sit as she wanted on her head. She spoke again to Naima.

'My mother said that she couldn't breathe at night, and she had bad feelings in her chest.' She spoke to her mother again in Urdu. 'And she couldn't sleep. She used to wake up in the morning feeling worn out.' At this point Amina Begum began to cry. 'Then he had a week off sick because the chest pains were getting so bad. Dr Khan arranged an urgent appointment at the hospital. I was at college at the time, and my mother phoned my mobile, saying he had to go to hospital right away and that I'd better come up. It was the day before Eid. On the bus home I knew that something terrible had happened.' Her mother was gently patting the upper part of her chest with the palm of her left hand. 'Could she have a glass of water?' I poured her one as Naima knelt beside her mother, an arm around her shoulder trying to comfort her as she moaned quietly.

Her daughter continued the story crouched by her mother's side. The next day the funeral had to take place according to the Muslim tradition, even though it was Eid. In the six months or so that followed, Amina was clearly struggling with life. She complained of frequent headaches, and sensations in her chest 'like a sinking feeling'. She had no energy, felt extremely tired, and had become quite forgetful. Her sleep was poor, and she woke earlier than usual each morning, feeling unrefreshed. She found it increasingly difficult to keep on top of her housework. She complained frequently about her health, expressing the fear that she had a serious physical illness. She saw Dr Khan, requesting tests and investigations to find out what was wrong. He performed some blood tests the results of which were normal. The family knew that there was a serious problem when she appeared to be so unwell that she lost interest in her grandsons, waving them away as she spent all day in her bedroom. Her daughter said that Amina believed she was a bad person because she had let the family down. She also became increasingly anxious about money. Her husband had always handled the family's finances, and after his death she struggled to manage them. There were letters from the bank and utilities to deal with, and she hid them from the family so that routine matters became urgent problems that had to be resolved. This was why her daughter decided to take time off from her studies at university, where she was reading law, to help her mother sort the finances out, and to help her around the house.

'That just made things worse' said Naima. 'We all thought it would help her, but she just blamed herself all the more.'

At this point Amina began to weep as she mumbled in Urdu. 'She says she is a bad person' said Naima. 'She says she is worthless because we cannot rely on her to do the things that she should be doing for us. But it's not true.' She broke off and spoke to her mother quietly, trying to reassure her. 'It's just that it's so difficult for us to talk about what's happened. He was my mother's husband, but he was also my father. We all miss him terribly.'

'How does your mother see the future?'

They spoke again. 'It's difficult' replied Naima. 'She believes that she must have faith because she knows that's what everyone who matters to her expects. But she feels that she is lost in darkness and cannot see her way out.'

'Do you think she has lost faith completely?'

'No. She spends a lot of time reading from the Qur'an and that seems to give her some hope. She prays too, and that helps. But she is lonely. She has withdrawn from us and won't discuss anything, but then I think it's impossible for her to do that with her children.'

'Have you worried that she might be so hopeless that she would consider taking her own life?'

'No, not at all. That would be a terrible thing against our faith. I think she just accepts that this is the way life is for her now. She says this is what God intends for her.'

Through Naima I was able to get an account of her mother's early life. She was born in a small village in rural Punjab, about a hundred miles from Lahore. Her family had been farmers in the area for generations. Uncles on her father's side had fought for the British Army in World War Two and moved to England afterwards. Her early life was unremarkable, although she had suffered from tuberculosis as a child, from which she made a full recovery. At the age of eighteen she was introduced to her future husband, a second cousin who had been born and brought up in Birmingham. Naima said her mother had always laughed when she heard her husband speak. 'She had never heard Urdu spoken with a Brummie accent before' she said. A year later they married in Punjab and he returned to England. She joined him a year or so later, and in the next five years they had three children, two sons and Naima, the youngest. Her daughter described Amina as a very conscientious woman who took her responsibilities to her family, community and her faith very seriously. 'We were, we still are, her life' she said, 'and she was full of joy when her first grandchild was born a few years ago. She is close to my eldest brother's wife. She has given her a lot of support, at least until a few months ago.'

Naima's eldest brother (the father of her two nephews) worked as a teacher at a secondary school in Leeds, and her middle brother, who had just married in Pakistan, was working as a motor mechanic. Naima was halfway through a law degree.

'Shouldn't you be at lectures?' I asked.

'I've suspended my studies for the time being to help Mum get sorted out. I was worrying too much about her. I couldn't concentrate on my work. It's only temporary and I fully intend to go back when things are more settled. But it's for the best right now.'

'We've nearly finished.' I spent a few seconds scribbling some notes. 'Could you ask your mother why she thinks this has happened to her?'

Amina Begum's eyes filled with tears again, and she shook her head as they exchanged more words.

'It's impossible for her to talk about it with you, or with me for that matter' she replied. 'But I think she feels ashamed because she feels she has let us down. Her faith and her family are the two most important things in the world to her, but she feels she is not worthy of God's love because she can't do what she has always done for us.'

Whilst I listened I was going through my inner checklist to make sure I had covered everything. I had forgotten something important, but hesitated before speaking. 'Could you ask your mother if she feels depressed?' She spoke to her mother again. Whilst they were talking her mother occasionally pointed to different parts of her body, her head, her chest and her abdomen.

'It's difficult' said Naima. 'I think she probably has been feeling what you would call depressed, but it's not an easy word to translate. She says she has felt very sad, and has been crying a lot. She has also had many strange feelings in her body, a sort of sinking feeling in her stomach, like a heavy stone weighing her down is how she put it.'

I made some more notes, and then asked Naima to ask her mother how she thought I might be able to help her. They spoke again, for longer this time.

'It's very tricky. Although she feels she is a bad person, she also believes that this is the way her life will be from now on. It's what God has planned for her, and nothing can change that. She says she just has to accept that is the way things are, and carry on her life as best she can.' Her mother interrupted and they spoke again for a few seconds. 'She also says she is very worried that she has an illness, and that she might die. She knows you are a doctor so she wants you to do some tests to make sure that she isn't seriously ill.'

'I see. Do you think she would consider taking tablets to see if they might help her.'

'No. She didn't take the tablets Dr Khan gave her. She felt bad about it because she has a lot of respect for him, but she didn't think they would do anything for her.'

'And the therapy?'

Naima smiled. 'She went a couple of times to the surgery. They have a young Muslim psychologist who spoke Urdu, but to be frank with you, I think Mum spent most of the time offering her advice about the best flour for chapatis. I don't think there was much therapy.'

I was facing a familiar problem. The bilingual psychiatrist Ajit Shah has written about the practical difficulties he experiences carrying out clinical assessments of South Asian patients who speak no English. There is a real problem because of the absence of a matching vocabulary for signs and symptoms of psychiatric disorders based in the patient's language. There may be words corresponding to depression in Gujarati and Urdu but they do not have the precise clinical connotations carried by the English word. As a result he (Shah, 1999) struggles to ask questions about symptoms based on Western diagnostic systems. Amina Begum's distress was every bit as real and incapacitating as Kath's, but the word 'depression' was anchored not only to meanings that were strange to her, but also to consequences and actions that were even stranger: therapy and drugs. As is the case when you are flummoxed, honesty is the best course of action, so I outlined my dilemma to Naima. 'What do you think would help your mother?'

She smiled again. She only needed to be asked. 'Two things would make a big difference. She feels really guilty that I have had to take time away from my studies to help her out. My middle brother has recently married, but his wife is stuck over in Pakistan. We want her over because she can help us all, and that means I could get back to my studies. That would help my mother feel less guilty about me. We have tried to persuade the authorities to grant her a visa, but they are dragging their heels. Dr Khan wrote a letter of support, but our solicitor says they would be more likely to pay attention to a consultant's letter.'

'No problem' I replied, 'and the second thing?'

'My mother is very lonely. She gets a lot of comfort reading the Qur'an, but I think she really needs other women like her to share this with. I don't suppose you know of a group of Muslim women she could meet with?'

'I don't, I'm afraid, but I know someone who does.'

I wrote the letter, organised a blood screen, and later that day spoke to a community development worker who worked in a community mental health project for Asian women. Yes, she knew of a group of Muslim women, mostly about Amina's age, who had experienced sadness. Some had been to see their GPs with 'depression' before finding their way to the group. She arranged to speak to mother and daughter, then try to get Amina involved with the group. Several weeks later I saw Amina and her daughter in the clinic.

'How are things?' I asked.

'She is gradually getting over it' came the reply. 'She goes to the group once a week, and I think she finds it very helpful. She has made new friends there. They talk about their families, their children, and they also read from the Qur'an and pray.' They were still waiting to hear from the immigration authorities, but the family's solicitor was more hopeful that the daughter-in-law would be soon granted a visa.

'You know, my father's death came at a very difficult time for us all' said Naima. 'He was buried on the morning of *Eid-ul-Fitr*, the end of Ramadan. We should all have been celebrating as a family, but instead we were thrown into sadness and were unable to. But it was difficult most of all for my mother. She loved Eid, going to the market, preparing special food, doing Mehndi [painting of hands, feet or body with henna] with me and my cousins. But she couldn't do any of these things for us. Now do you understand?'

Meaning, Language and Culture

When we talk about our lives, we share stories about ourselves with others. Those we speak to are usually from the same cultural background. They share certain expectations, referents and meanings about the stories we tell, and how those stories are to be understood. They are already primed with values, beliefs, traditions and stories that help them to understand how we feel. This is also true of psychiatrists engaged in the daily practice of clinical psychiatry, working with people who experience distress and madness. When we use language to narrate our stories we engage in a shared, communal activity. The languages we use are embedded in cultural and historical traditions that shape the plots and metaphors that enable us to interpret and understand our experiences. At this point I want to examine these stories to see how the two women's cultural backgrounds shape the meanings of their stories, and the responses their stories require. In doing this it is not my intention to reify culture, or to see it in a deterministic way. I am not trying to impose particular features of a culture upon individuals, stripping them of their uniqueness and difference. That said, it is worth remembering that these stories are based in real people's lives. The stories only relate to the individuals whose lives they refer to. They should not be taken as generalisations true for all women from a particular group, or who have a particular cultural identity

Superficially the stories are similar. The women are the same age, at the same point in their lives, and both have recently lost their husbands. They have children of identical ages and genders. They present with broadly similar experiences of distress, at least as far as the physical manifestations of this are concerned. Both appear to have improved some months after the initial consultation. The clinician who listens to these stories is privileged to be able to interpret them in a variety of ways. This act of interpretation changes these patients' stories into the clinician's story. If the clinician interprets the story according to the logic of EBM, the resulting narrative is one of clinical depression requiring treatment with medication and CBT. A more nuanced reading reveals the complexity of the situation, with the result that the clinician holds two different stories about these women.

First, they present to the clinic in different ways. Kath, whose children have grown up and left home, attends with her friend Joan. This gives a clue to an important aspect of Kath's identity as a person, a clue that emerges in the first sentence of the GP's letter, where he describes her as a 'secretary'. This, together with the fact that she comes to the clinic accompanied by a friend, a former workmate, suggests that a significant part of her identity is invested in relationships and activities outside her immediate family. In contrast, Amina, described by her GP as a 'housewife', attends the clinic with her daughter, suggesting that her identity is tied to family relationships. Little information is available at interview either from Amina or her daughter to form a view about the extent of her friendships or activities outside the family, other than Naima making the point that in her view her mother is lonely. Of course, one reason for this may have been an expectation on my part that the relationships of a Muslim Asian woman in her mid-fifties would in any case largely revolve around her family, with the result that I didn't bother to ask. This of course could be seen as a stereotype, but in this particular woman's case, this is how her life was. In any case, the differences between the two women are confirmed as their stories emerge. The role of faith and religion is another important difference between the two. Kath describes how she has lost her faith since a Catholic childhood, but I sensed a wistfulness about this, because she made it clear that she misses it. Nevertheless it plays no part in her life, and certainly has no role to play for her in understanding her sadness and loss. In contrast, faith is a really important part of Amina's life. She believes that the reason she feels the way she does is because it is the will of God. The circumstances of Bashir's death are also closely related to an important religious festival, one that would normally draw her together with her family.

Kath describes how she felt after Kevin's death in terms of loss of self-confidence and loss of pleasure and enjoyment. This curtailed her social activities, going to the cinema with Joan, going away for a week with her son and his new girlfriend. We might conclude from this that before Kevin's death, Kath's activities and relationships outside the home, for example her work, meant a great deal to her. They are important aspects of her narrative identity. Her subsequent loss of confidence and inability to enjoy these activities became an important feature of the story she gives about her distress. Most significant is her use of the word 'depression' to describe how she makes sense of what has happened to her. She not only makes clear that this is how she understands herself, but also she is quite clear about its meaning. For Kath, depression means having a problem with the chemicals in her brain. She warrants this view of her problems with reference to information and stories that feature prominently in popular culture, magazine articles and a soap opera story line.

The way that Amina talks about her experiences is quite different. The emphasis in her story is less upon loss of pleasure and self-confidence, but rather her belief that she is a bad person because she has let her family down. We can understand this if we remember the importance for her of her role as a mother within the family, and the obligations she experiences as a result of this to her children and other members of her family. She sees herself as a bad person because she became unable to fulfil these obligations. She believed that she had let her family down. This can be seen in her response to her daughter's taking time away from her studies to support her, which, paradoxically, made things worse for her. This is because it emphasised the extent to which she was no longer able to support her family, and required help herself, most notably with practical tasks like running the family finances, something she had never had to do when Bashir was alive. This doesn't mean that family relationships are unimportant for Kath, just that they did not feature in the same way in her identity as they did in Amina's.

In addition, the word 'depression' is problematic for Amina and her daughter (at least in her role as interpreter with her mother). This can be seen in the difficulty that Naima has in translating the word into Urdu. A word corresponding to 'depression' may exist in some South Asian languages, but it does not convey the sense of clinical depression or disorder that Kath accepted in relation to her experiences. Yes, Naima agrees that her mother has probably been feeling depressed, but she immediately qualifies this by adding the non-clinical word, 'sad'. In addition, there is a strong sense that the way Amina feels is tied to her view that she is letting her family down. In turn she understands her sadness through her faith. It is God's doing. God took her husband away from her, and there can be no questioning God's intentions. She must accept that this is the way her life will be.

Kath's understanding of the word 'depression' is close to that of most mental health professionals. Depression is a change located inside the self and affecting the self. These changes occur either through chemical abnormalities in brain function, or through dysfunctional thinking processes (cognitions). The sort of self that is affected by such disturbances is quite different from the way that Amina sees her self. At first glance it may appear that Kath's story about her depression conforms closely to the view of non-intentional causality that we considered in Chapter 7. Events happened in her life over which she had no control (Kevin's death). Her depression arose through events over which she also had no control (a chemical imbalance). Only at the end of her story does the plot reveal that things are not quite as simple as they seem. They had had an argument, and she 'stormed out into the white', angry with him. She didn't say goodbye, didn't kiss him, didn't tell him she loved him. Under ordinary circumstances she might not have done any of these things on leaving for work in the morning. She might have said casually 'see you later' or words to that effect. However, given what happened after she left the house and the emotional tone of her departure, it assumed enormous significance for her. That moment in time, the full significance of the scene, the cold, the spring flowers struggling to emerge through the ice, her footprints fresh in the snow stretching back to the front door which she had just slammed shut; all were seared into her memory, an anchor point tied to her last contact with Kevin, feeling hurt and angry, not saying goodbye. Crocuses, a symbol of renewal, regeneration and hope, had for Kath become emblematic of her loss, and more. It was only in our last meeting that she was able to face up to the mode of her departure and acknowledge its significance for her. In our first meeting it must have been too painful for her to acknowledge. Perhaps she felt ashamed about it. She had stormed out presumably to save face, but with unforeseen consequences. Of course she may have thought to herself later, that at the time she was unaware that less than a couple of hours later he would be dead. Then again it is quite possible that as part of her depression she would blame herself for Kevin's death. Indeed, this was the case. A clinical interpretation of such a statement would see it as an example of distorted cognition, a cardinal feature of depression to be remedied by CBT. Although it is conceivable that the stress of their argument might have been sufficient to compromise his cardiac function (given that he was suffering from severe angina) with the result that he had a cardiac arrest, this seems unlikely. In contrast, a narrative approach would see such a belief as an attempt to make sense of his death, one based in intentional causality: we had a row; I stormed out; it stressed him out and he died. His loss thus becomes tied to acts of commission and omission on her part. She becomes a moral agent in what takes place, albeit not in a virtuous sense, but she nevertheless assumes a more active role in events. If it is the nature of being human in Kath's culture to search for human agency when something goes seriously wrong, then in Amina's culture it is to ascribe suffering to the will of God.

Kath might also have thought to herself that had she said goodbye, she would have felt differently after his death. It might not have been quite so painful for her. This, it seems to me, is why her remembering seeing her footprints in the snow is such a poignant feature of her story. The footprints symbolise her walking away, leaving him behind, her separation from him in time and space. When she spoke about seeing the footprints behind her she did so with a deliberateness that made me feel that the prints were vividly present to her. She looked at the floor as she described them, and she did so slowly and deliberately as though feeling her weight press down into the snow. It felt to me that she wasn't seeing the carpet in my office, but the snow on her path with her prints freshly made. She wanted to cover them over or undo them, but of course she couldn't. Her footprints marked out not only the fact of their separation and his loss, but also the mode of it, the intensity of feeling associated with it.

Then again, there is one element in her story that we haven't considered, and which might entitle her to believe that even if she had kissed him goodbye it wouldn't have changed her response to his death. This part of her story tied loss and death to the winter snow, and the death of her father in 1963. There is an extensive sociological literature on the importance of childhood experiences of parental loss and separation in adult depression. The work of George Brown and Tirril Harris established this link convincingly in a series of well-executed studies.[2] Sadly, this work seems largely to have been forgotten about (possibly for the reasons described by John Read; see Chapter 4, this volume). This work on early experiences of loss fits well with narrative understandings of depression in terms of a *leitmotif* that runs throughout a person's life. It is important work that is well worth revisiting. It is arguable that the death of her father when she was six had profound implications for her view of relationships and her expectations of them. No matter how much she loved someone, the capricious nature of the world meant that she could never take love for granted. We are always on the cusp of having love snatched away from us. For Kath the white transition from winter to spring marked the loss of her father, and that of Kevin. Stasis in the snow, frozen crocuses, hope submerged.

This relationship, between loss and depression or sadness, has figured prominently in Western culture for hundreds of years. Freud famously wrote about it in *Mourning and Melancholia*. Brown and Harris saw depression as a response to the social and psychological circumstances of loss and loneliness in people's lives. They write as follows:

> The immediate response to loss of an important source of positive value is likely to be a sense of hopelessness, accompanied by a gamut of feelings, ranging from distress, depression, and shame to anger. Feelings of hopelessness will not always be restricted to the provoking incident – large or small. It may lead to thoughts about the hopelessness of one's life in general.

---

2. See, for example, Brown *et al* (1977). Although their work demonstrates the link between depression in adult women and the loss before age eleven of their mothers, they also show links between more severe forms of depression (i.e., 'psychotic' depression) and bereavement losses.

> It is such *generalization* of hopelessness that we believe forms the central
> core of depressive disorder. (Brown & Harris, 1978: 235)

They were writing about depression as a clinical disorder from the perspective of social science researchers in the West. The Sri Lankan anthropologist Gananath Obeyesekere points out that to a Buddhist such a statement sounds odd. Hopelessness is not simply a feature of an individual's life. Buddhists see it as an inevitable consequence of life that originates in the nature of the world. Life is sorrow brought about by attachment and desire for others. He (Obeyesekere, 1985) argues that Western interpretations of sadness in people from non-Western cultures as depressive illness are not shared by people in those cultures. The difficulty in part arises because the methods of science (in this case epidemiology) require that we define and investigate concepts like depression outside the specific cultural contexts in which they are used. He questions the idea that it is possible for us to use a word that has specific meaning in English on the assumption that they convey precisely the same meaning in another language. Kleinman (1991) makes the same point:[3]

> A word, after all, is a sign that signifies a meaningful phenomenon. That
> phenomenon ... exists in the world mediated by a cultural apparatus of
> language, values, taxonomy, notions of relevance, and rules for interpretation.
> (Kleinman, 1991: 11)

Obeyesekere also points out that holy days are fundamentally important to all faith traditions. They mark a break from the routine existence that most of us endure. They draw us into communion with those we love, our families, and our communities. They also open up a window for us on worlds that we mostly live in ignorance of, or at least of which we are unaware. This is the world of priests, sadhus, imams and other holy men and women. This is true of Eid, Easter and other great religious festivals. Amina's husband died suddenly on the morning of Eid, marking the end of Ramadan, one of the most important Muslim festivals. Under normal circumstances this would be a very busy time for Amina. She would buy in provisions to prepare special dishes to celebrate the end of fasting. Cities and towns that have large Muslim communities often feature special markets to celebrate *Chaand Raat* (Urdu – the Night of the Moon), with music, entertainment and stalls selling special sweets and food.

This is a time that brings families together, but for Amina and her family this Eid was blighted. Instead of gaining pleasure from sharing in the family's celebration of the event, celebrations that to a large extent depended upon her hard work in preparing the home and food, they were thrown together in grief.

---

3. And elsewhere, Tim Thornton, Ajit Shah and I used the idea of language games, drawn from the later philosophy of Ludwig Wittgenstein, to make the same point (Thomas *et al*, 2009).

Bashir had been ill for some time, and in the last week of Ramadan his condition deteriorated. This was a time when she would have been busily preparing for Eid, a time not unlike the week leading up to Christmas for those in the Christian tradition. Her husband was dying at home, and Amina spent this time caring for him as best she could, fearing what was about to happen. There was no time for preparation. Celebration was far from her mind, and it was at this point, with her loyalties torn between her husband and her family, that she began to speak about having let them down and being a bad person. Her family reassured her, saying that her most important task was to care for her husband. Before she went to college that morning, her daughter told her that there would always be Eids in the future; that it didn't matter if they missed one.

Although, like Kath, the loss is closely related to the experience of profound sadness, the way in which this developed (or if you prefer, the plot) is quite different for Amina because it is a story told through a different narrative identity. Amina's sense of who she is has little to do with autonomy and personal agency as is the case for Kath. It is set out in terms of her relationships to her family, her faith and her community. This has implications for the way she sees herself in relation to the events that unfolded in her life. If the ideal self in Western cultures is an autonomous one that prizes personal agency, this is not an important feature in South Asian cultures. Sastry and Ross (1998) found that personal control featured much less prominently in people of South Asian heritage, and that it also played a less prominent role in psychological distress.

As I read this chapter in the process of editing and rewriting, I am aware that something is missing. I am struck by another contrast between Kath's story and Amina's story, one of my making. This is a contrast between *my* telling of Kath's story and *my* telling of Amina's story. In her book *Doctors' Stories*, Hunter (1991) describes the 'narrative incommensurability' of doctors' and patients' accounts of illness. She writes as follows:

> The patient's account of illness and the medical version of that account are fundamentally, irreducibly different narratives, and this difference is essential to the work of medical care. Sick people who seek a physician's advice and help are in quest of exactly this difference, for, physicians are believed not only to know more about the body but also see its disorders clearly and without shame. Yet because it is scarcely acknowledged by either patient or physician, the difference between their accounts of the patient's malady can warp understanding between them. (Hunter, 1991: 123)

She is of course writing about narratives in clinical medicine, but precisely the same warping of understanding can occur if psychiatrists re-tell patients' stories solely from within the framework of evidence-based medicine. The story I have told about Kath, even though superficially this is told within an evidence-based framework, is so much more richly embroidered than the story I have told about Amina. Earlier in this chapter I made the point that when we tell other people stories about our lives, we do so to people who are not only close to us emotionally, but also close to us culturally. I am much closer to Kath's culture than I am to Amina's. My background is British working class, with some Irish roots (albeit in my case, Protestant not Catholic), and my wife comes from a British working-class background with strong Irish Catholic roots. In contrast, although I have many Muslim friends (mostly male), especially Muslims of Pakistani heritage, and I have visited Pakistan, I am not a Muslim and I do not speak Urdu. Consequently a gulf exists between Amina and me. This is unavoidable, but its inevitability makes it all the more important that I acknowledge it, that I am aware of it, and that I try to take steps to bridge it.

My story about Kath is what the anthropologist Geertz (1975) would call a 'thick' description, one that engages with the complexities and ambiguities of Kath's own story at many levels, even though in the clinic Kath only wanted technological interventions from within the framework of evidence-based medicine. In contrast my account of Amina's story is, I believe, much 'thinner'. If I am to respond to Amina's distress justly and fairly I need to find a way of enabling her story to be told that engages with the complexity of intentions and meanings that her story deserves. Our ability as clinicians to engage with and understand the stories our patients recount depends to some extent upon our familiarity with the patient's culture. But the nature of this familiarity takes us much deeper than the familiarity we might gain through training in cultural competency, which is generally restricted to issues of custom, diet and tradition. Narrative practice in my opinion requires a much deeper embodied familiarity with culture, one that is capable of recognising and engaging with the emotional significance of events in people's lives, in the context of a specific cultural tradition. We can best grasp this if we have grown up in the same culture as the patient. Like Kath I understood deeply the significance of the winter of 1962–1963, even though I hadn't lost a parent in it. I was capable of grasping the significance of snow, ice and crocuses. Of course, this cultural closeness is an ideal situation rarely encountered in the clinic. However, the growing diversity of our society means the practice of narrative psychiatry requires that we draw on resources, individuals and groups, in communities that share the specific cultural origins of our patients. This is why, as we will see in Chapter 13, community development is such a valuable resource in mental health practice. It was for this reason that Pat Bracken and I turned to community development when we worked in Bradford. It is not possible here to set out in detail the origins and background of community development, but I will end this chapter with a brief reference to a group set up by the community development project Sharing Voices Bradford (see http://sharingvoices.org.uk/about-us.html) and from which I drew inspiration in writing about Amina's story.

Hamdard (from an Urdu word meaning companion in pain or one who supports) is a group exactly like the one that Amina attended. It was set up by a Muslim woman who had experienced family and marital problems in her life.

With the help of a Muslim female community-development worker, who also supported her in her personal life, she set up the group for other Muslim women. Over the nine months of the Sainsbury Centre evaluation (Seebohm *et al*, 2005), the group, which had its own constitution and funding, was regularly attended by an average of ten women drawn from different communities including Mirpuri, Kashmiri, Pataan, Punjabi and a white English Muslim. All the women experienced distress related to family or relationship problems. Most had consulted their family doctors and been prescribed medication. Some had used mental health services, including hospital admissions. None had been offered or used psychotherapy. The women described how they valued the opportunity to come together as Muslims to understand their experiences in terms of their faith. Reading and discussing the Qur'an featured prominently in their activities, as did preparing food together and craft activities. The fact that they were Muslims but from different cultural traditions drew them closer together, enhancing their solidarity and mutual understanding. Three women moved on to work or training over this period, and its founder is now a qualified social worker. The words of one of its members, Shazia, could have been spoken by Amina:

> Through these friendships I've discovered my identity as a Muslim woman and by establishing my prayers I feel I've become a lot more focused. The 'real' me is now more strong, clear and content with who I am. (Seebohm *et al*, 2005: 49)

Recommended Reading

Brown, G. & Harris, T. (1978) *The Social Origins of Depression: A study of psychiatric disorder in women*. New York: The Free Press.

Obeyesekere, G. (1985) Depression, Buddhism, and the work of culture in Sri Lanka. Chapter 4 in (Eds. A. Kleinman & B. Good) *Culture and Depression* (pp. 134–52). Berkeley and Los Angeles: University of California Press.

Shah, A.K. (1999) Difficulties experienced by a Gujarati psychiatrist in interviewing elderly Gujaratis in Gujarati. *International Journal of Geriatric Psychiatry, 14*, 1072–4.

Thomas, P., Shah, A. & Thornton, T. (2009) Language, games and interpretation: A Wittgensteinian thought experiment. *Medical Humanities, 35*, 13–18.

Danni's Story: Voices and Trauma in a Secure Unit

9

Danni was a twenty-two-year-old woman who was referred by a consultant forensic psychiatrist. She was admitted to a regional secure unit (RSU) four months earlier after she had been assessed in a women's prison. She had been convicted of attacking a stranger on a bus with a knife. He wasn't seriously injured, but required surgery. A liaison psychiatric nurse assessed her when she was on remand in a local prison. The forensic psychiatrist recommended that she should be transferred to the RSU under his care on Section 37 of the Mental Health Act, a six-month treatment order for people convicted of an offence who are believed to require treatment for a mental disorder. The referral letter indicated that she assaulted the stranger when she was '... hearing verbal auditory hallucinations ...'. The voices commented on her thoughts and actions, gave her instructions, and occasionally ordered her to do things. She also experienced visual disturbances '... a shadowy figure that passes through her body ...' and profound mood changes, with sudden and intense episodes of anger, which she believed were caused by external influences. The letter described these as '... made affects, or passivity experiences ...' (positive symptoms of schizophrenia). She also cut herself, inflicting deep incisions down to the muscle layer on her arms.

The diagnosis was schizophrenia, and although they considered the possibility that she had borderline personality disorder, the intensity and duration of her psychotic experiences made schizophrenia more likely. On the RSU she appeared tense and preoccupied. She often whispered to herself, and cut herself on two or three occasions, but there were no violent incidents. They started treatment with a depot neuroleptic (Clopixol, 400mg every two weeks), and carbamazepine, a mood stabiliser widely used to control impulsive behaviour. Her consultant was only too aware of the problems experienced by women detained in forensic hospitals, and was keen to move her into a less restrictive environment, and then back into the community. A few days later I drove over to the RSU to see her.

She thumped into the office, her arms tightly clasped in front of her, cradling a mug of tea beneath her chin, and banged herself down in the chair. Tea slopped out of the cup onto the floor. She ignored my extended hand, and sat head bowed staring at the surface of the dark brown liquid. Three five-pointed stars were tattooed on the inside of her left wrist. She wore a black t-shirt underneath an amorphous woolly cardigan, which she left unbuttoned, blue jeans the knees of which gaped like a toothless mouth, and a pair of trainers, which were on their last legs. Her shaved head sat on a pair of woolly boulders for shoulders. Both forearms were heavily bandaged, and there were old and healing scars visible on the exposed skin above and below the bandages.

'Hello, Danni, my name's Phil. I'm the consultant psychiatrist who has been asked to see you.'

She twirled a stud piercing the skin just beneath her lower lip. She lifted her head momentarily to glare at me wordlessly, and then resumed her contemplation of the surface of her tea. I was shocked at how young she appeared. She seemed barely old enough to be out of school.

'What? You mean get me out of this place?'

'Yes.'

'Where to?'

'To the ward where my patients are admitted.'

'That place?'

'Yes. That place.'

'The loony bin.' She stopped twirling the stud to sip her tea. Then she looked at me again, this time with suspicion and incredulity. She was sizing me up.

'Really?'

'Yes. Your consultant feels you don't need to be here. What do you think?'

'Bloody 'ell, too right.' Her eyes narrowed. 'You're not winding me up are you?'

'No. Can you tell me what you want to happen?'

'I want out of this place, out of hospital. I want my own place, and I want back to college. I was in my second year at university before this happened.'

'What were you studying?'

'Physics.'

'Wow! I really struggled with physics at school.' She shot another glance at me, this time without suspicion.

'I want to teach it.'

'That's great', I replied. 'So, how come you ended up here?' She told me about the assault, her voices and the arrest. 'When did your voices start?'

'About a year ago.'

'OK. Had you ever heard voices before?' She fell silent and twirled the stud vigorously. 'Only, in my experience, it's often the case that people hear voices for a long time before they ever end up seeing someone like me.' The twirling increased, stretching and distorting her lower lip. Then I realised she was whispering under her breath. 'Danni, I don't care what the voice is saying to you right now ...'

'How do you know?' She looked at me quizzically.

'Because I've seen it before, many times, and I guess the voices are giving you grief just now. All I want to do is to help you to do the things you've just told me that you want, a place of your own, college. But if I'm to do that, it's important we trust each other enough to be completely open with each other. And for you that starts right now by telling me about the voices.'

After a few seconds the twirling stopped. She finished her tea and wiped her mouth on the back of her bandaged right arm, then continued to stare at the empty mug in silence.

'Please Danni, I want to help you.' There was a barely perceptible nodding of her head. She took a deep breath before ridding herself of it through puffed out cheeks.

'I was five when it started. It came on at school. I thought everyone heard it. Then I realised it was only me. I asked my best friend. "Julie," I said, "Can you hear that voice?" And do you know what she said?' I shook my head. 'She said you're a loony, you. Only loonies hear voices. You'll end up in the loony bin. So that was it. I never told anyone again, never. I kept it to myself. But it was alright. I learned to live with it, and then for a few years it went away. But it came back again when I was fourteen at secondary school. It wouldn't go away this time and I found it really difficult to cope with. That's when I started cutting. Then last year it got right out of control.'

'Why do you think that was?'

'I was raped. I'd been to the pub with my girlfriend, and we were walking back home together. We kissed goodnight, but this gang of blokes was following us. They started hurling abuse so I clobbered one of them. They grabbed hold of me and beat me, so I told my girlfriend to run for it. They carried me into the park and raped me.' While she was telling me this she suddenly became animated, then when she finished she lapsed back into a frozen silence.

We sat for a minute or two, both deep in thought. I reflected on what she had said. It had taken much courage to tell me this on our first meeting, and I knew there would be more to come. Her courage and honesty convinced me that we could work together.

'OK, Danni, it must have been really difficult for you to tell me this, and I want to thank you for being so honest with me. When do you want to come over?'

'You mean you'll take me on?'

'Of course.'

'Fuckin' 'ell.' Her eyes widened behind her glasses. 'So, when?'

'When do you want?'

'Right now. I want out of here as soon as possible.'

I phoned the ward to confirm that the bed I'd provisionally booked was still available. 'When you come over, the first thing I'd like to do is to introduce you to Karen, the social worker I work with. Then I'll ask you to write your life story for me. When you've done that, and we've been through it together, I want to go through an interview with you about your voices. How does that sound?'

'Scary.'

'Do you think you can go through with it?'

'I have to. I don't have any choice if I want my life back.'

We shook hands and I left.

She was transferred over that evening. A few days later I saw her on the ward and introduced her to Karen, who had a background in Transactional Analysis.[1] We had worked together several times with people who heard voices, and we had had preliminary discussions about using it to help Danni in her relationship with her voices. TA provides a really useful way of helping someone to understand current difficulties in relationships in terms of past relationships, including problematic relationships with voices. We hoped that this would help Danni to see her relationship with the voices in developmental terms.

Medication was another priority. She had been on neuroleptics for several months, and said she'd gained no benefit from them. If anything the Clopixol was making things worse. She still heard voices, but the medication made her feel tired, and sapped her 'resistance' as she put it. She had gained weight, and this badly affected her self-esteem. The voices picked up on this, accusing her of being 'fat' and 'ugly'. On the other hand she believed that the carbamazepine had helped her feel calmer. It reduced her tension, making it easier for her to resist the urge to harm herself. We agreed she would stay on the carbamazepine whilst we reduced and stopped the Clopixol over the next three to six months. We also agreed that she could ask for diazepam if the voices were very troublesome, or if she occasionally needed help to sleep. She had found this helpful on the RSU. The point was to put as much control as possible into her hands, rather than take it away from her.

She agreed to write her life story, and to share this with Karen and me. I usually encourage someone to write their life story prior to working with them on their voices.[2] This is helpful for two reasons. It provides an important context against which a voice interview[3] takes place. More important, though, is that writing a first-person narrative about the self and its vicissitudes can help to strengthen the sense the person has of an autobiographical self. After a few days she presented me with several pages of neatly written text in which she set out the story of her life as follows.

---

1. Transactional Analysis (TA) is a form of psychotherapy developed by the Canadian-born psychiatrist Eric Berne (1964). This is a theory of personality structure and interpersonal behaviour that examines human relationships at three levels: Parent, Adult and Child. It provides a way of understanding how difficulties in relationships in the present originate in problems experienced in childhood. It is one component in voice dialogue work described by Dirk Corstens and colleagues (Corstens *et al*, 2012).

2. Davies *et al*, 1999; Leudar & Thomas, 2000, see Chapter 7, Working with Voices, pp. 129–47.

3. This was originally developed in 1987 by Marius Romme and Sandra Escher as a research interview for use with voice hearers, but it was then modified to help voice hearers to explore their experiences. The interview (Romme & Escher, 2000) is neutral in regard to theories about voices, and covers many different aspects of the experience. These include voice characteristics, personal history of voice hearing, triggers for voices, voice content, personal understanding of the experience, and the impact the voices have on the person's life. It ends with questions about childhood experiences, treatment history and social networks.

I was born in 1985 on a council estate in Leeds. I have two half-brothers age sixteen and thirteen, and a half-sister age ten. My dad worked on the railways, but when I was three years old he left us for another woman. He was fed up with Mum's drinking. This started when she was carrying me, and it got worse after I was born. Throughout my early years she had a serious problem through drink. She was often in trouble with the police for shoplifting, being drunk, or getting into fights. She had a real paddy, Mum, especially after a few. Most weekends I'd be left with her sister while she went off on the bottle. She'd end up in casualty because she was drunk and fallen and injured herself, or had been in a fight. I had to grow up very quickly, learn how to look after myself. For all her problems, she still loved us; I just know she did, and I love her to bits. I'd do anything for her.

When I was about four, social services got involved. They arranged foster placements for me with this family in Bramley whenever Mum was bad with the booze. That's where the trouble really started. The social worker had this little blue car and she used to take me over there in it. My heart sank whenever I saw it outside our house. I'd stay in Bramley for a week or two, however long it would take for Mum to sort herself out. This must have happened several times from when I was four to when I was six years old. They had a teenage son, and very quickly I learnt to avoid him; only I couldn't. He started touching me, and getting me to touch him, and it progressed from there. He'd threaten me, tell me I was this and that, and that he'd tell everyone I was a dirty little cow, and worse. As time went by and the abuse got worse, I'd refuse to go, but they'd drag me over.

When I was six Mum met this new bloke. I don't know how she managed, but she got her boozing under control, and for a while things settled down. Alan, my step-dad, is a lovely bloke. He had a really positive influence on Mum. My brothers were born, then our kid sister, and all seemed fine. I began to do well at school and started to make friends. But when I went to comprehensive things went downhill. I was put in the top stream, and my mates started to bully me. I think they were jealous because I was doing well. They played tricks on me, snide things, like trip me up so I'd fall in the mud, fill my school bag with water and ruin my homework, calling me all sorts. I suffered really badly with nerves and was physically sick in the morning, so Mum kept us off school. Then, when I was thirteen, I became aware that the way I felt wasn't just to do with what was happening at school. There was something else, something inside that didn't feel right. I started to realise there was something different about me. The other girls were dating lads and going crazy about boy bands and suchlike, and I was wondering what all the fuss was. I tried it once, dated this lad, but it left me cold.

It became clear when this new girl joined our class. She was black and so beautiful, tall and athletic, with skin that shone, and twinkly eyes, and high cheekbones like a supermodel. It was more than a crush; I fell in love with her. But she was straight, and never once looked at me. All the lads were crazy about her. I never told anyone, and was terrified that people would find out. No one ever admitted to being gay in them days, least not on a council estate in Leeds. I had this burning feeling deep inside, so much so that whenever anyone said anything about gays or such like, I believed they were talking about me. It was awful. That's when the voice started again, saying folk knew I was gay. I started to feel really tense, and it was then I found that cutting made me feel better.

Looking back I can see that wasn't a good way of coping, but I had no one to talk with. It was partly because I shut myself off from friends and schoolmates that I started to work hard. I found that really helpful. I'd get lost in physics and maths so much so I'd forget about my problems. I love calculus and equations, and I'd spend hours puzzling over them in my bedroom, trying to see links between different laws, like thermodynamics and electromagnetism. And of course the more I did that the better I got at it so the teachers were impressed and encouraging. I did really well at GCSEs, and went on to pure and applied maths and physics at sixth form college. The teachers wanted me to apply to Oxford, but that's not me. I'm not posh, or anything like that. So I did A-levels, got good grades, and was accepted at Leeds to do physics. I didn't want to move way. At sixth form college I'd met other gay people, and came out. Mum and Dad were brilliant about it. I got involved in the gay scene, and had lots of gay friends in the city, but I didn't want to have to start over again in a new city, which is what would have happened had I gone down south. I also wanted to be at hand for my mum, and my kid brothers and sister. I'd worry too much about what might happen if I was far away, especially for my kid sister. She's beautiful and I love her to bits. I feel for her.

After A-levels I had a year out and travelled about Europe, and came back to start my degree. I lived at home and at the end of my first year I met my first real girlfriend, Vickie. She's studying english. We hadn't been going out long; it was the start of the second year, and we'd been out for a few drinks. On the way home this gang of blokes followed us, calling us when we kissed goodnight. I turned around and told them to lay off, but they wouldn't, so I clobbered one of them. They were shocked; they weren't expecting someone like me to give the lad a good braying. They were right angry and surrounded me, beating and kicking. The one I'd laid out got up and said he'd teach me a lesson. I shouted at Vickie, told her to get out of it, which she did. Then they held me down while he raped me. I can't remember what happened after that. I was told an Asian taxi driver found me in the middle of the road, and took me to casualty. The nurse said she'd phone the police to report it, but I couldn't face up to going over it again so she gave me a phone number and told me to speak to them when I felt better.

When I got home that morning the voice started flooding the room with abuse. It was the same one I'd heard before. I couldn't sleep, or think. It went on and on, blaming me for what happened, telling me the police wouldn't believe me if I did report it, so the next day I stayed in bed, and the day after, and so it went on. I wouldn't speak to Mum or Dad. I started cutting myself badly again, and I felt so bad about that, I stopped going to lectures. At the end of that term I dropped out altogether. A few weeks later I was waiting for the bus to town to sign on, and the voices were really bad. Two lads were stood next to me in the queue, and the voice kept saying that one of them was the lad who raped me, so I turned on him and laid him out. His mate ran off and called the police. They arrested me and put me on bail. Then the same happened a couple of weeks later. Every time I went out I believed this lad was following me, and the voice taunted me, saying he was behind me and he was going to do it again. I started carrying a blade for my own *protection. I'd end up threatening someone, or hitting them, and I was arrested several times over the course of the next few weeks. Sometimes when I was out I'd see this shadowy figure to one side. Then it would move in front of me when I was walking so I'd bump into it, but at the last moment it walked straight through me and I'd feel all iced-up inside. I never saw his face. In the end I was on this bus back home from town and it was crowded. The only free seat was the one next to me, and this bloke sat in it. The voice kept saying it was him and he was going to do it again when I got off the bus. I was absolutely terrified, so I stabbed him in the arm. I can't remember much about it, but that's what the police said from the witnesses who saw what happened. All I remember is the bus screeching to a halt, and this bloke screaming at me with blood dripping down his arm onto the floor. They called the police, who slammed me up in the Bridewell, and that's how I ended up in here.*

I read Danni's story, and with her permission shared it with Karen, before meeting up to discuss the voice interview. It took nearly two hours over two sessions to go through the interview with Danni and Karen. With her permission I recorded the interview, and then summarised it. I asked Danni to check the first draft for accuracy and to prompt for further responses, and used the corrected version to summarise the interview and generate the voice construct as set out in Chapter 12. The summary of Danni's experiences of voice hearing at that stage was as follows.

Voice Interview – summary

Originally, Danni heard a single voice. When it first started she was shocked and distressed by it. It was very loud, and completely took over her mind. She heard it in her head and ears at the same time. On occasions it came from the shape or shadow of a person she could see. When it first started she couldn't say anything to it, but over the years this changed and now she could communicate with it either by speaking out aloud, or whispering, or less frequently by speaking to it in her mind. Recently she had discovered that speaking to it aloud was the most powerful way of addressing the voice.

The voice started when she was nearly five years old. Its onset was related to the abuse she experienced at the hands of the teenage son of her foster parents. At first it was that of a stranger, but over the course of several months it changed, becoming the voice of her abuser threatening her, 'I'll murder you if you tell anyone', 'I'll cut your throat', 'No one believes you because you're evil', 'You're a dirty little slut' – all things that her abuser said to her.

By the time she was seven years old her life was more settled, and the voice had largely disappeared. However, when she was thirteen or fourteen and in turmoil over her sexual identity, the voice reappeared. This time it made derogatory comments about her appearance and sexuality. It picked up on her anxieties about herself, especially over her relationship with her peers. She was extremely sensitive about how others saw her. The voice commented on this, fuelling her insecurities. At that time she found two ways of coping, negatively through self-harm, and positively through her work, and gradually the frequency and intensity of the voice diminished. It had been infrequent until the rape, but immediately following this shattering experience it returned with renewed intensity, and overwhelmed her. It blamed her for what had happened, accusing her of inviting the attacker on. It told her it was her fault, and she deserved it; it was no more than she was worth.

But on this occasion the original voice was joined by several new voices, all male, but not as loud as the first voice. These new voices repeated everything the original voice said in chorus with it. Over the following weeks when she dropped out of college and cut herself off from family and friends, the voices increased in frequency and volume. Nothing she could do eased them, and they became much worse if she went out, which she had to do to sign on and get her benefits. When she knifed the stranger on the bus, she was fairly certain this wasn't because the voice told her to. She was overwhelmed by voices and fear, and she couldn't remember exactly what happened when she stabbed him, other than that she was convinced he was her attacker, and that he was about to strike again. The rape and the voices' response to this resonated powerfully with the events early in her life when she was abused, coerced and had no control over what was happening to her body.

After the attack she heard the voices more or less continually. They were particularly likely to come on in social situations, for example at mealtimes and social breaks in prison and the RSU, commenting on her thoughts, actions and appearance, always disparagingly. They commented that other people were looking or staring at her, and as a result she ended up confronting the person concerned, occasionally getting into fights. This was particularly likely if she felt emotionally vulnerable or anxious. The voices continued to call her unpleasant names, and at times she believed they could take over her thoughts and actions, making her think and do things against her control. Her fear about the voices and their impact on her life resulted in her avoiding all contact with other patients on the RSU. She became a recluse.

Although the voices seemed all-powerful, the psychologist on the RSU encouraged her to talk back to them, questioning their motives and challenging the negative things they said about her. She found this helpful and achieved modest success in challenging the voices. The work with the psychologist also identified agitation as an important trigger for the voices and increasing the risk of cutting herself. She understood the link between the voices and self-harm. Reducing the extent of her social interactions helped to reduce the agitation, and she managed this by returning to her room and listening to music. She could also reduce her tension by working on mathematical equations and puzzles, 'anything without people and without words' as she said.

Karen went through the summary with Danni, and a few days later we all met to review progress and plan the work ahead. Shortly after the voice interview Danni told us that she had begun to hear a new voice. It woke her up the night before when she dreaming. At first she couldn't remember what the dream was about, but she was certain that the voice had figured in it, and it had been present ever since. It was an older woman's voice, a 'cold, uncaring voice' that told her to cut herself. The strange thing was that she hadn't felt tense, and hadn't cut herself for two weeks; neither did she act on the new voice's instructions. The voice was dismissive of Danni, making her feel small and insignificant, but unlike the other voices it wasn't abusive or threatening. For example, earlier that day she had been going through some course work in mathematics, which she continued to do to keep in touch with her work, and to cope with her distress. As soon as she opened the notebook the voice said, 'I don't know why you're doing that. It's a waste of time. You know it is.' She argued back, but this took a lot out of her. The voice argued back, and she ended up feeling drained. It had, however, said some positive things about her: 'She's all right is our Danni', and 'You'll be OK, girl, I know you will. You're stronger than you think.'

The new voice had no name and hadn't told her who it was. It didn't sound like anyone she knew, because it was too 'posh', but there was something vaguely familiar about it. It reminded her of someone. We had moved on to discuss further reductions in her medication when she suddenly interrupted me.

'The dream. I remember it.' She bounced up and down on her chair, gesticulating with her hands, her eyes sparkling behind her lenses. I hadn't seen her as animated as this. 'It was all jumbled up, but it was about when I was a kid. Remember I told you about the little blue motor? Well I was getting into it, but this time I was an adult, and this posh voice was saying "You'll be all right, Danni. I know you will." But when I looked out of the window it was Mum speaking. Then I thought that can't be right, she doesn't speak like that. Then the car drove off, but there was no driver, and the voice said, "Go on, Danni, you can do it, you can drive it yourself. You're a big girl now." So I took the steering wheel and drove off out into the country miles from anywhere, right out into the wilds. It started to get dark, and the voice said you can stop here if you want, so I stopped and got out. It was calm and peaceful, and the air pure and clear. The sun set, and a gentle breeze wrapped itself around my body. I looked around and saw that I was on a vast beach, but the sea was miles away. The world was empty, no birds, animals or other people, just me and this space stretching on forever. The sky was black and enormous, and the stars were so clear that I could reach out and touch them. Over in the east the sky lightened as a dull moon rose out of the ocean, like a heavy dark blood clot turning the water purple and red. Then the voice said, "You can cut yourself if you want to. That's all that's left for you", meaning the blood sea, the moon and the emptiness. "Everything else is a waste of time." And that's how it ended.' Her voice faded away, as she stared into the middle distance.

'You were talking about your mum yesterday', said Karen. 'It seems that the dream and the voice have something to do with her.'

'Aye', replied Danni, after a silence.

'What do you make of it?'

'Not sure.' She was twirling the stud again, and whispering under her breath.

'Do you mind if I tell Phil what we talked about yesterday?' asked Karen.

She eyed me up suspiciously, her sizing-me-up expression. She shook her head. 'No. Not now, not yet. Later perhaps.' She stretched and yawned heavily. 'I'm bloody knackered. Can we leave it there?'

I was intrigued by what they might have spoken about, but it was important that Karen didn't compromise Danni's trust. Over the coming weeks, she had regular sessions with Karen, and we met regularly to review progress. Danni was coping well with the reduction in the Clopixol, and was generally less tense. At her request she was spending more time at home with her family, and had two or three uneventful overnight stays at home. She said she wanted to be sure that everyone was happy at home, that there were no problems. Karen arranged for Danni to visit a project that offered women with mental health problems supported accommodation, and then agreed to referral in preparation for discharge. Things were moving ahead smoothly when Karen and I met up to discuss progress.

'One of the really important issues that's emerged is the difficulty she has with her family.'

'In what way?' I asked.

'She loves them, especially her brothers and sister, but it's almost that she loves them too much.'

'How?'

'Take her brothers and sister. She's very protective of them, but it feels out of proportion. I suspect there's a part of Danni that's stuck as a four-year-old, so that in caring for them she's also caring for herself. That's why ever since she's been in here she has to go home to check that they are OK, that nothing has happened to them.'

'Isn't it just because she's close to them?'

'No. It's not as simple as that. She's gone home feeling like shit warmed up, pretending that everything is well with her when it's not. I strongly suspect her mum has absolutely no idea what she's been through. I'm certain she's told her nothing. All she says is that she's a bit depressed.'

'That makes sense, at least as far as the voices are concerned. I can see how her relationship with the male voice is so problematic because it originated in an impossibly one-sided relationship. What I can't fathom is the significance of the female voice and how that ties in with her relationship with her mother.'

'The problem, I think, is Danni's need to preserve the idea that her mother wasn't to blame for anything that happened in her childhood. That's why she hasn't told her mother anything. It's partly because her abuser coerced her not only sexually, but also into believing that it was her fault. Blame the victim. As long as she can pretend it's all her fault, then she doesn't have to face up to the possibility that these awful things would never have happened to her had her mum not had the problems she had after Danni's birth. We've been through this repeatedly. She sees the sense of it intellectually, but hasn't grasped its emotional significance.'

This felt right. Danni loved her mother deeply, but only through idealising her at the cost of continuing to blame herself for her misfortunes. This meant denying her angry feelings – towards her abuser and towards her mother – by splitting herself off from them, or dissociating from them. The problem was that her anger was so powerful it demanded expression, which it did through the voices and ultimately her self-harm. Key elements of her relationship with her voices reflected a psychological reality that she had faced since the age of four: her powerlessness in the face of an abusive male figure, and her complex ambivalent relationship with her mother. This found expression through the cold and rejecting female voice that expressed ambivalent concern for her. It was clear that Danni was making progress in understanding her voices, although there was still some way to go.

Karen and I saw Danni a few days later, just before Karen was due to take a week's leave. Danni said that she felt she could live alongside the voices. They were still there much of the time, but she was able to turn her mind to other things. They were having much less of an emotional impact upon her life. We agreed that she should spend more time at home on leave, and that we would tail her medication off.

'What about your section?' I asked her towards the end of our interview.

'What do you mean?'

'Well it runs out in six weeks, and if you are happy with the treatment plan, tailing off the medication, continuing the work with Karen, spending more time at home, then there seems to be little point in keeping you on it.'

She frowned, then stared at Karen.

'Can I tell him what we discussed yesterday?' said Karen.

'Go on.'

'We talked about this because I guessed you'd probably raise it today. If I understand Danni correctly she feels safer for the time being on the section. She sees that she's made a lot of progress. She can think things through for herself more clearly, and that makes living and coping with the voices a lot easier. But she's terrified if something were to happen she might lose control and that would undo all the progress she's made. She'd prefer to stay on it just for the moment.'

'Yeah. It's a safety net', added Danni.

We agreed that for the time being she would stay on the section.

That night she went home for a night's leave, but failed to return to the ward the next morning. Her mother phoned, very upset, saying that Danni had arrived home and then suddenly ran off later in the evening and not returned. The police returned her to the ward later that morning, badly hung over. They said that she had got drunk at a pub on the estate, and then stopped outside a neighbour's house, shouted abuse at him, and smashed several downstairs windows. When I saw her the following Monday she refused to talk. She was in 'overwhelm' mode, shoulders hunched, stud twirling, no eye contact and whispering furiously to herself. It was clear that something had happened, and that she was troubled by it. I also had a strong feeling she was angry with me, or to be more accurate, with us. Karen, of course, was on annual leave and so Danni wouldn't be able to see her for another week. There were other things besides that. I wondered if I had reduced her medication too quickly. She hadn't slept well for a few days following the last reduction, and the nursing staff reported that she had been requesting more diazepam because she was feeling more tense. She had made very good progress in reducing the neuroleptic medication, but it was possible that the most recent reduction coupled with the emotionally demanding work on her voices had been too much, triggering off severe anxiety, making it more difficult for her to cope with the voices.

The next day I saw her on my way home. This time she was prepared to talk. She told me her mother had phoned and she'd had to go home to see her. She didn't want to tell me what they had spoken about. She did say, however, that the female voice had told her that the man who had abused her was living on their estate, just around the corner from her mother's house. That was why she went round and smashed his windows. She now recognised that he wasn't there, and she was deeply embarrassed by her actions. She resolved to be much more circumspect before doing anything on the basis of what her voices said. She was shocked by what had happened, especially the contribution made by alcohol to her loss of control. 'It made me realise how alike my mum and I are,' she said, adding cryptically, 'in more ways than one.' She said she had to be much more careful in her use of alcohol. She had also been feeling more tense since the last reduction in her medication, and we agreed it would be sensible to increase the dose slightly for a couple of weeks before reducing the dose in smaller steps.

The next week Karen was back and we saw Danni together. She told Karen what had happened the week before, and that since then she had been sleeping better. Both voices had been less frequent, and not particularly troublesome. She felt calmer and hadn't harmed herself. She was also buoyed by news from Karen that the supported accommodation project had agreed to offer Danni a place on discharge. She was working hard on her relationship with her mother with Karen. Moving away from home and achieving greater independence was an essential part of this process. I was still in the dark about what had happened between her and her mother, but that didn't matter. The main thing was that Danni was moving in directions that she wanted – a place of her own and, ultimately, back to college. We arranged a period of trial leave to the supported accommodation, following which, if all went well, she would be discharged.

The trial passed without incident, and she was discharged. Her new bedsit was a short walk from my community office, and over the following months I visited her regularly. Karen usually accompanied me, and sometimes her support worker. Danni continued to make good progress. She stopped neuroleptics, although she remained on carbamazepine, which we were gradually reducing. She was in regular contact with her family, and was back in touch with her girlfriend. She was also working as a volunteer at a women's refuge two-half days a week.

'How are the voices now?' I had arranged to see her to review her care plan. She was about to stop carbamazepine, and was soon to restart the second year of her degree course.

'OK. They don't cause me any trouble. I still hear them, the male voice less often, but if it does come on I challenge it, and it shuts up.'

'And the woman's voice?'

'I hear that more often than the other one, but it's changed.'

'In what way?'

'Well it used to be cold and off-hand, but not anymore. It's more friendly and helpful. It even supports me, tells me I'm doing OK. Most of all it tells me the other voice has no right to speak to me the way it does. It tells it to shut up and leave me alone.'

'Good', I nodded. 'So are you coping better with them now?'

'Definitely. I guess I'll always hear them, but they don't upset me anymore. I understand why they're there, how they came about. They're a part of me, of my life and my past. I can accept that now.'

'How are things at home?'

'Good. I babysit once a week for Mum and Dad, and have lots of fun especially with my younger sister. She reminds me so much of me when I was that age.' She paused for a moment. A doubt crossed her face. She looked at me, then Karen. 'Can I tell him?'

'It's up to you', replied Karen.

'Only I want to.' Her gaze returned to me. She stared at me. I was being sized up again. 'You remember when I went AWOL and smashed the neighbour's windows?'

'Yes.'

'The reason I left was because Mum phoned. She wanted me to go round. She said it in a way that I just knew I had to go. I had to find out what it was. I got home, and she made a brew and we sat down at the kitchen table. She was crying. I'd never seen her that way before, really upset, wailing and sobbing. She said she'd wanted to tell me what she was about to tell me for years, but she was so ashamed about it she couldn't. She knew all along about my problems. She'd suspected the abuse at the foster parents because I was so reluctant to go there. She knew all about the self-harm, and the voices even though I'd never told her. "But how?" I asked. "How could you know all that?" Because she'd been through it herself, she said. An uncle had abused her when she was a schoolgirl, and it affected her in much the same way that it affected me. She'd recognised the signs for years because of her own experience. But do you know what really set it all off? She said that although she got over it as she grew up, the moment she discovered she was pregnant with me it all came back. She was overwhelmed by memories of what had happened to her as a girl. That's when she started drinking really heavy and lost control.'

'Did she say why it happened then?' I asked.

'Because she was terrified the same would happen to me. She had this thing about history repeating itself. Well when she said that, something just clicked inside me and the woman's voice started yelling at me saying that my abuser had moved into a maisonette on the other side of the estate, and he'd do to me kid sister what he'd done to me. I was terrified for her, for Mum and for me. I ran off and got pissed, then went round and smashed what I thought were his windows. You know the rest.'

I nodded and we sat in silence for a moment or two. This time there was no stud-twirling, no boulder shoulders, just silence, and the shadow of a smile flitting across her lips.

'I see now', I said. The smile broadened. 'What is it?'

'I saw Mum the other day and we talked about it for the first time. You know, *really* talked about it. She said she'd always loved me so much, and she'd dreaded that what had happened would ruin my life, like it almost ruined hers. I said to her, "Well it has happened to me, but it's not your fault, and it hasn't ruined my life. I feel stronger for what happened." And we hugged each other, and wiped each other's faces dry, and no more words were necessary.'

Brian's Story: Young, Black and Mad 10

On my first day as a consultant I walked onto the inpatient unit and was confronted by something that defied explanation. Ten of the twelve men whose care I had taken over that morning were black. I was shocked and puzzled. When I interviewed them, and went through their notes, I became even more troubled. It continues to trouble me even today. In my psychiatric training in Edinburgh I acquired practical skills in mental state assessment, formulation (a narrative summary of the origins of the person's problems) and diagnosis. My teachers were amongst the foremost authorities on psychiatric diagnosis. I became a lecturer in the Department of Psychiatry in Edinburgh University, and worked with one of them, the late Professor Bob Kendell. We carried out a research project to investigate the use of language analysis in the diagnosis of schizophrenia (Fraser *et al*, 1986). Under Bob Kendell's supervision I interviewed and assessed over a hundred people using the Present State Examination[1] to make research diagnoses. I was, to cut to the point, experienced in a rigorous approach to psychiatric diagnosis for clinical and research purposes, and knew how to make a diagnosis of schizophrenia.

What troubles me is that very few of the young black men who came under my care that day in September 1983, and since then, appeared to have experiences that made it possible to say without doubt that they had a diagnosis of schizophrenia. They were all very distressed and disturbed; most were very disorganised and had unusual ideas and beliefs or probably heard voices; many had not been functioning effectively in the world outside but very few appeared to experience either specific forms of verbal auditory hallucinations (and I use this expression here deliberately because of its diagnostic significance in relation to schizophrenia), or specific delusions of the sort that made it possible for me to say beyond doubt that the diagnosis was schizophrenia. When I tried to

---

1. The Present State Examination was a standardised interview widely used in psychiatric research in the 1970s and 1980s. It was often used with a computer program to yield research diagnoses.

interview them, most remained silent, some laughed strangely to themselves; less frequently they might whisper incoherently. But they wouldn't talk to me, tell me what was on their minds, share their fears and hopes, or say what life was like for them. They wouldn't speak about their families, or what had happened in their lives that resulted in them coming into hospital. For reasons I didn't understand I felt I was being forced into a form of veterinary psychiatric practice. The young men I wanted to help wouldn't engage in the most fundamentally human activity, the use of language to talk about themselves. Why? What was going on here? This experience stands in conflict with the evidence we considered in Chapter 5, that schizophrenia is more common in black people in this country. The purpose of this chapter is to try to understand why this is. It tries to find a way through this conflict. I also want to show that if we are to find a way forward we cannot do so unless we work with the community.

There are some other points I need to raise before I launch into the story. Thirty years ago it was considered good practice to observe anyone recently admitted to hospital for a few days in order to get to know them. There was no rush to start newly admitted patients on drugs. That has changed. The imperative now is to treat as quickly as possible. This is partly fuelled by the idea that early intervention reduces the duration of untreated psychosis (DUP), which has a 'toxic' effect on the brain making it more likely that psychosis will become chronic. There are also economic pressures to reduce length of admission, the same pressures that have reduced staffing levels on most acute admission wards. Little surprise then that doctors often feel rushed into starting patients on treatment, usually by nurses anxious about how they can cope with people whose behaviour is perceived as difficult and challenging.

As time passed, and I struggled to understand this troubling situation, something else became clear. Many of the staff I worked with, nurses on the wards, community nurses, social workers, police and others, were deeply troubled by these young men, although few admitted it. They found them intimidating. Some feared them because they saw them as potentially violent. Most of these young men didn't find their way into hospital the way most people did. They were admitted via the police out of hours, and this may have contributed to a view that they might be difficult to manage. Many were taken by the police to hospital because they were behaving oddly on the streets. Many were seen and assessed in police stations or local prisons where they had been held on remand after committing some trivial offence.

There is a final point that particularly troubled me. It seemed that many were admitted from nowhere, to where they returned on discharge. They were unlike their white or Asian peers, who were frequently visited by their families, anxious mothers and fathers, brothers and sisters who wanted to know what was happening, what treatment would be offered, what the prognosis was, and so on. It seemed to me as though these young black men dwelt in a forgotten land. Many had lost contact with their families, who were rarely to be seen visiting them in hospital. It is of course possible that this was merely an artefact of the way services were organised when I first became a consultant. Although from the start of my career I worked from a community base, the Victorian asylums dominated care for most, and even though I worked closely with community mental health teams, and held clinics in local health centres, there was no significant contact with local communities. At first there was no way of engaging with these communities, with the families of these young black men, their peers, girlfriends, and youth workers – those who really knew what life was like for a black person living on the streets of our cities and towns. This was why I became involved in working with people from Manchester's black community to help set up what was then the Manchester African Caribbean Mental Health Project; and later on, in Bradford, I became involved with Pat Bracken and others who set up the community development project, Sharing Voices Bradford.

This preamble sets the scene for a fictional account of a young African-Caribbean man who could have been any one of the hundreds I encountered as a consultant. It points to the importance of working not just in, but with, communities. In the story that follows we will see how a community development worker played a key role in filling in the void, helping to bring voices into the silence that surrounds the admission of young black men to hospital.[2] It is important to remember that from 2005 to 2010 the Department of Health in England and Wales ran a five-year strategy, 'Delivering Race Equality'. This resulted in the employment of over 500 community development workers in key strategic areas aimed at tackling the discrimination experienced by people from black and minority ethnic (BME) communities. The policy was established as part of the government's response to the recommendations following the death of David Bennett, a Rastafari, in a private secure unit (NSC NHS Strategic Health Authority, 2003). That policy has now ended and nothing has replaced it at a time of austerity when issues of race and social justice no longer appear important.[3] Although the story I am about to relate is fictional, it is broadly based in my own experiences of work undertaken by community development workers in mental health services.

---

2. The focus here is on young black men, because numerically they are the group most over-represented in statistics for compulsory admission and the diagnosis of schizophrenia. The same is true, however, of black women, albeit to a lesser extent. The same is also true for black people of African heritage, men and women.

3. A point made poignantly by Doreen Lawrence, the mother of murdered teenager Stephen Lawrence. See http://www.guardian.co.uk/uk/2012/dec/18/stephen-lawrence-mother-race-discrimination, accessed on 14th May 2013.

At first I thought the room was empty. The curtains were drawn and what little light there was struggled through a heavy blue pall. My nose and eyes stung.

'Brian. Wake up! You've been told not to smoke in your room.' The nurse tugged the edge of the duvet.

As my eyes accustomed to the gloom I could just make out a shape beneath the duvet. The bed was chaos; a sheet abandoned on the floor, and a confetti of orange peel, torn-up Rizla papers, cigarette ash and sinuous strands of cigarette tobacco littered the mattress.

'Brian, the doctor's here to see you. Wake up!'

Beneath the tobacco I noticed a deeper, heavier smell; that of poverty, of a life lived in boarded-up houses, and spent scavenging wheelie bins for cast-off food. I approached the bed and gently lifted the duvet. I caught a glance of tight curls and ringlets, tousled and matted, covering a black face, skin that glowed in the faint light, a blackness that defied the dark, refusing to be engulfed by it. I lifted the duvet a little higher to reveal an arm, then a grey t-shirt that might once have been yellow.

'Brian, my name's Doctor Thomas. I'm your consultant. Can we speak, please?' Nothing broke the silence. Without warning a slim hand appeared from beneath the duvet, and drew the edge firmly back over the head, before withdrawing noiselessly under cover. The movement was calm and precise, unhurried and graceful.

'I'm sorry to disturb you, Brian, but it's important we talk. I need to understand how you ended up in here. Can you tell me?' Beneath the duvet the body tensed, and then a muffled response which I couldn't make out. 'I'm sorry, but I didn't catch that.'

'Leave me alone.'

'Just five minutes?'

'Leave me alone.'

'OK. I'll see how you are later on.'

Back in the office his notes contained only a short report from the duty psychiatrist. Brian had been arrested for shoplifting outside a local supermarket, and had allegedly resisted arrest, assaulting two police officers in the process. When he was taken to the police station to be charged there were concerns about his wellbeing, so the police requested a psychiatric assessment. The duty psychiatrist's report said that Brian appeared very disorganised in his thinking, appeared to be hallucinating, and his self-care was extremely poor. All this strongly suggested that he was suffering from mental disorder, and that he required assessment in a psychiatric hospital. He was admitted the next day on Section Two of the Mental Health Act, a twenty-eight-day assessment order.

The charge nurse told me that since admission Brian had refused to cooperate. He had kept himself in his room with the curtains drawn, smoking continuously. He refused to answer questions, and ignored food that staff offered him. He only drank water that he ran for himself from the tap. On several occasions nurses had heard him shouting in his room, but when asked why, he denied that anything was amiss and then refused to speak about it. On the basis of this they concluded that he was hearing voices. 'It sounds like he's saying "Where are you Scooby?", or Booby, or something like that. But he won't tell us about it,' said the nurse.

'Has he had visitors?'

'None', replied the charge nurse, checking through the nurses' notes.

'Phone calls?'

'Nothing.'

'And medication?'

'He was written up for the usual if required, but so far he hasn't caused any problems so he's not had any.'

In the team meeting later that morning the junior doctor presented Brian's case as follows.

> Brian is a twenty-year-old, single, unemployed African-Caribbean man who had been sleeping rough before admission. As far as we can establish he was born and brought up in England; he has a local accent. He was admitted under Section Two of the Mental Health Act after he had been arrested for shoplifting and assault. This is his first admission to psychiatric hospital, although he has been in and out of Youth Offender Institutions since the age of fifteen for repeated offences of theft, shoplifting, criminal damage, assault, and possession of drugs (cannabis). He refused to cooperate at interview, so it was not possible to obtain background information, his family and personal history. He also refused to cooperate with mental state assessment and physical examination. At interview he presented as a tall, slim man whose self-care was very poor. He established no eye contact, and spent most of the time at interview sat on the floor in a corner of the room whispering to himself. It was difficult to hear what he was saying, but it seems likely this was in response to auditory hallucinations. It's also likely that the content of these experiences is persecutory. For example he whispered 'They are going to kill me, Scooby', but he wouldn't elaborate. He also had strange mannerisms. He shook his hands as if shaking water off them, and had unusual facial grimaces. He'd bare his teeth, then cover them with his lips, and rapidly alternate these movements for several seconds. His mood was incongruous and labile. For example, when he said, 'They are going to poison you', he smiled and laughed. Then he suddenly became angry, hitting the wall with his fist.

The junior doctor ended by summarising the possible diagnoses: schizophrenia, an affective psychosis (mood disorder), drug-induced psychosis, or organic psychosis. It was clear to me that this was not only speculation, but irrelevant speculation. In truth we had no idea what was going on. Our hands were tied because he wouldn't speak with us to tell us what had been happening to him, how he saw the world, what sense he made of it.

'That's why on balance paranoid schizophrenia is the most likely diagnosis', said the junior doctor. 'After all, we know that young black men are much more likely than other groups to develop the condition.'

'I agree,' said the charge nurse 'and I don't think we should wait for the situation to deteriorate.'

'He spoke to me yesterday for the first and only time', said his named nurse. 'Something about Scooby. I said, "Do you mean Scooby Doo, the cartoon dog?" and he said yes. He gave this strange little smile, like a grimace, and said the voice told him they'd kill him like they killed Scooby.'

'Would he say any more about it?' I asked.

'No, that was it. Then he started to cry and got angry.'

'Sounds to me like a schizophrenic illness', said the junior doctor chewing a paper clip while he scribbled in the notes.

The charge nurse agreed. 'The sooner we start treatment the sooner he'll get better and out of hospital. I'm also worried that he's on a short fuse and that things could get out of hand. We've a responsibility to the other patients and staff.'

I listened carefully to the different points of view and sensed unvoiced thoughts and fears between the spoken words. 'The difficulty is that we are discussing treating him in complete ignorance of his background, the events that led to him being here, and with no clear understanding. We need more information. We need to talk with his family.'

The charge nurse shook his head. There was no clear consensus. The charge nurse and junior doctor wanted him on medication. The social worker, Brian's named nurse and I were less sure. Everyone agreed that we had to find out more about him. In the end we decided to hold off medication whilst we tried to find out more about him. I arranged to visit his mother at home, and to discuss Brian with Trevor, a community development worker at a local black mental health project.

The next day I was knocking on the door of a maisonette in a leafy cul-de-sac on a large estate just off one of the main thoroughfares into the city. The small front garden was well tended, with a neat lawn, small rose shrubs about to bloom, and a battered mountain bike chained to a drain pipe. I knocked again and could hear movement inside. The door opened a few inches on a security chain and a woman peered out.

'Yes?'

'It's the doctor. I phoned yesterday. Are you Claudia?'

'Yes.' She frowned, her knuckles white as she gripped the door.

'Can I come in and talk with you about Brian?'

'Is he in trouble again? Oh dear God.'

'No, not in that way, but I do need to talk about him with you if that's OK?'

'Yes of course. I'm sorry.' She undid the chain and opened the door. I followed her through to the living room and sat on the sofa facing her. 'So, are you a detective, a plain-clothes man? Oh Lord, what's he been up to now? Which prison is he in? Is he OK? I do want to see him.' Her questions panicked out.

'Let's start from the beginning. He's been in hospital since earlier this week. He's all right, but we need to talk about what's happened to him.'

'Hospital? What's the matter with him? Has he had an accident?'

'No. He came from prison.'

'So you *are* a policeman.' She gasped.

This was something I was sadly accustomed to. I shall never forget the first time a mother mistook me for a police officer. I was taken aback, but now I was prepared. 'No. I'm his consultant. He's in a psychiatric hospital.' She burst into tears. I waited while she composed herself, wiping her face with her hands, before giving her the scant details we had about her son. 'We are desperate to know what happened to him. That's why I'm here. I need to ask you lots of questions, and doubtless you have many for me.'

'This is bad, real bad.' Her breath still stuttered out in staccato bursts. 'This is awful. It's happening over again.'

'How do you mean?'

'Lynton, Brian's dad. He's in a secure mental hospital. They locked him away there years ago. It happened when Brian was two. He never got out since. I still see him once a month, but it's a long trip, doctor. Two trains, two buses and a long walk. I have to go alone, cos Brian has nothing to do with his dad.' She rummaged around in a cupboard for some tissues, wiped her eyes again, and blew her nose loudly. 'There, that's better. Now, what do you want to know?'

'Just tell me in your own words about Brian's life.'

She told me that he was born in Nottingham in 1989, the same city his mother was born and brought up in. Her parents were from Jamaica, and Lynton, Brian's father, was from Barbados. When Brian was two years old there was a lot of tension in the city between different gangs involved in drug dealing. Lynton wasn't involved in it, but he became caught up in a riot as a bystander, and was arrested. Something happened to him in the cells, and she thinks he might have been beaten up. Whatever it was affected his mind, and he suddenly developed strange ideas and began to hear voices. He ended up in hospital and had never been the same since. She started to cry again. 'I'm sorry, but this is so terrible. The same is happening to Brian. I can feel it.' I stood up and put a hand on her shoulder.

'No. That's why I'm here. If we work together we can stop that happening.' She offered to make some tea and when she returned she continued telling me about Brian's life. When he was four Claudia moved up to Manchester. She needed to get away from the unhappiness in Nottingham, and Lynton had been transferred to a secure unit in the north of England. Her sister had moved to Manchester a few years earlier so it made sense for her to move. At school she said that Brian's teachers always saw him as a problem. He was a daydreamer, shy, and not an easy child to get on with. He started to get into trouble for disobedience, and was frequently excluded from class. At the age of nine he was accused of fighting with other kids and he hit a teacher. They expelled him. Shortly after this he began to get into trouble with the police.

'You know,' she said, breaking off for a moment, 'he is like his dad. Lynton used to get mad about being picked on. "It's not right," he used to say. "It's unfair the way people pick on you because you're black." I think Brian felt the same. One of his teachers said he had the biggest chip on his shoulder she'd ever seen.'

By the age of ten he was regularly in trouble for shoplifting, with frequent court appearances for theft (sweets, chocolates and cigarettes at first, then alcohol), criminal damage (usually cars, especially police cars) and assault. Three years later came his first arrest for possession of drugs (cannabis), and he was hanging around with what she described as a bad crowd.

'He wasn't really close to them. He was on the fringe. I'd say he was quite lonely really. He wasn't a ringleader. I don't know if it was because he was easily led, or whether it was being a black kid he just had to have one over authority.'

'Has he ever worked?'

'No. When he was fourteen he dropped out of school, and then he was sentenced to six months in a young offenders' institution. Over the next three years he must have been inside at least three times. It was after his last spell that I noticed a change in him. I'm certain that something had happened when he was inside but he wouldn't talk about it. He was eighteen, and when he came home he was very quiet. He didn't go out and wasn't interested in seeing his old friends. At first I thought it was a good sign. He even spoke about wanting to go to college and getting a job, but nothing came of it. Instead he spent all his time in his room, very withdrawn, not wanting to see anyone, not even his sisters or Auntie. He was smoking lots of cannabis, and listening to loud music, playing video games. He'd be awake most of the night then sleep all day. I could hear him talking to himself when he was awake, then shouting out. I knew he wasn't right. I couldn't speak to anyone about it, not even in church. People were scared of it, scared and frightened. My friend Geraldine's son is a youth worker. One day after church I plucked up courage and spoke to him. He agreed to come and talk to Brian, to see if he could persuade him to come along to the club, but he wouldn't talk with him.'

'When was that?'

'A few months back. He wouldn't even go with him to sort out his benefits. He was claiming nothing, not helping with the upkeep of the house. I'm a single parent with three children. I work in town, but it's not easy. The girls help out as best they can, but we're all so worried about Brian.'

'Did you see his GP?'

'Yes, a month before he disappeared, but she said that unless Brian came to see her by himself there was nothing she could do. I tried to persuade him, but he wouldn't. Oh please, what's the matter with him doctor?'

'I'm honestly not sure', I replied, shaking my head. 'It's obvious he's a very troubled young man, but he won't talk to us.'

'Aren't there tests you can do to find out what's wrong with him?'

'I'm afraid not. Psychiatry isn't like other branches of medicine. There are no physical tests to help us make a diagnosis. We rely heavily on what the patient and family tell us.'

'Do you think he's schizophrenic?'

'It's very difficult to say for a number of reasons. He won't tell us how he feels. There are aspects of his behaviour that make the diagnosis a possibility, but that's not enough. We need to know why he behaves that way, what's on his mind, is he hearing voices and so on. We also need to know what has been happening to him, in prison the last time, outside the supermarket, all those years at school when he was in trouble. We need to know what all that's about.'

There was a commotion at the front door, and two teenage girls ran in, breathless and laughing. Claudia introduced me to her daughters. 'I didn't realise it was that time', she said, checking her watch.

'I'd best be off', I replied. 'Here's my phone number. Get in touch if you're worried or want to talk some more, and thanks for your time. It's been really helpful.'

On my way home the phone rang. It was the duty doctor to say that they had had to transfer Brian to the secure ward. He'd hit another patient, then refused to accept medication, so they had to restrain him to force an injection of Clopixol, a neuroleptic drug widely used in the rapid tranquilisation of aggressive patients. I went to see him first thing next morning.

He was snoring heavily on his bed, watched over by a nurse. I checked his drug chart. He had also been started on regular medication, a long-acting injection. I read the duty doctor's account of events the previous evening. Brian had asked the nursing staff if he could go out into the courtyard for some fresh air. This wasn't part of his management plan so his request had been refused. A few minutes later he was seen arguing with another patient who was using the public phone. Brian wanted to use it. He returned a couple of minutes later to find the phone still in use, so he tried to grab it off the other man. A scuffle followed, and the two were separated. Brian was escorted back to his room, but the other patient followed him down the corridor, shouting at him. Brian turned suddenly and hit the other patient in the jaw, knocking him to the ground, and breaking a tooth. The nursing staff intervened again, restraining him, and calling the duty doctor who wrote him up for the medication, before arranging his transfer to the secure ward. The nursing staff confirmed this account, saying that if they had more staff things might have turned out differently. I was less certain. The situation was deeply frustrating, and getting out of control.

That afternoon I met with Trevor, a community development worker with a black mental health project. We met every fortnight to talk about individuals we were both involved in, and wider matters concerning the relationship between the city's black community and the services. I summarised Brian's predicament, saying that although it was clear that he had problems, it was far from clear that psychiatry was the best way of helping him. Whatever Brian thought about his situation, and we still had no idea how he saw it, he didn't see psychiatry as offering a solution. On the other hand we had a duty to help him out because of our relationship with the criminal justice system, but it wasn't working out.

'He just won't talk with us', I added. 'I can understand a young black lad not wanting to talk with a middle-aged white bloke who has the power to lock him away and fill him up with powerful drugs, but he won't talk with any of our black staff.'

Trevor was very familiar with the problem. 'My guess is he probably doesn't see them as black', he said.

'How do you mean?'

'They've sold out to the White Man. He probably sees them as Uncle Toms.'

'OK, I take your point, but it doesn't solve his problems, or ours for that matter.'

'Look, I'm free next Monday afternoon. Do you want me to see him?'

'Would you?' In the past Trevor had been really helpful in engaging young men like Brian. 'I really want to try to understand what's been going on with him. I can't put my finger on it, but there's something about Brian, the way he conducts himself, his bearing.'

'We've just opened up a new studio in the basement, loads of kit for music-making. If I can get him down here there's a chance he might open up. But I must see him alone, not with you or any of your staff. If he gets wind that I'm in league with you then forget it.'

'Of course', I replied. 'But depending on how things go, I really do want to talk with him at some point, find out what makes him tick.'

'We'll see.'

Over the next three weeks Trevor took Brian out on escorted leave to the project. There were no further incidents on the ward, although tensions were high when it was time for him to receive medication. I had extremely mixed feelings about this. Brian appeared to be changing. The nursing staff and the junior doctor believed this was because his psychosis was beginning to respond to neuroleptic medication. I had serious doubts that this was so, but there was little to be gained by confronting them with my doubts when they believed that the medication was helping. I had to agree that Brian appeared calmer, but although there were no more outbursts, he remained very suspicious and unwilling to talk to the staff about himself. He simply refused to open up to them. Staff believed this was because he probably still heard voices and had paranoid delusions. In support of this they reported that he continued to talk to himself, and that his emotional responses were odd and incongruous.

Time passed and a difficult decision loomed: his section was about to expire. We had to decide whether or not to place Brian on a Section Three, a treatment order, to continue giving him medication against his wishes over the next three months. He had also appealed against his section, and this was due to be heard the following day. It was quite likely that his appeal would be successful, in which case he would be taken off his section, and be free to leave hospital. My view was that medication wasn't 'treating' an underlying psychosis; rather it was simply blunting his responses to things that were going on in his social environment. It was sedating him to some extent, but it was making him indifferent to events that previously would have distressed him, and made him very upset. Latterly he had appeared to be warmer, and even smiled on one occasion to his named nurse, just about the only member of staff he trusted. I formed the view that this slight thaw in his relationship with us was to do with something other than medication.

This was confirmed at a team meeting on the inpatient unit attended by Trevor, who described Brian as a very disaffected young man, but no more disaffected than countless thousands of others who had to put up with racial abuse, harassment and attacks every day of their lives. He didn't go into detail, but I knew from what he said that Trevor was beginning to make progress. Brian had been to the project on four occasions, and was engaging with it. According to Trevor he had initially hung around on the periphery, but once he went into the studio he began to come out of himself. He had keyboard skills, but had never used a computer and sequencer before; however, he quickly picked it up. In doing so he began to make new friends and was developing a closer relationship to Trevor.

'My view is that it's difficult to make the case to extend his section', I said as the discussion drew to an end. 'It's quite clear he is going to win his appeal.'

'Well shouldn't we take him off it?' said the junior doctor. 'All we have to do is put his aftercare package together.' There was broad agreement with this.

'I'm not so sure', I replied. 'Yes, he probably will win and be taken off his section, but I suspect that it may be better for it to happen that way, rather than it being something we do. It feels right, under the circumstances, that he successfully challenges the power that we have over him.'

'That's not exactly good practice', said the social worker.

'That's true if you consider it narrowly from the perspective of the guidance we have in the operation of the Mental Health Act. But consider this: most of his experiences of white people in authority over him have been experiences of disempowerment.'

'Right!' said Trevor who had been following the discussion closely. 'There are too many people like Brian locked up by the system for no good reason other than no one really knows what to do with them. Let him have his say.'

I kept him on his section, and two days later I presented myself at his appeal. It was quite amicable. His solicitor politely grilled me. Was he suffering from a mental disorder? (Yes, he probably was.) Is he still suffering from mental disorder? (Difficult to say because he still refuses to talk to us.) Is he a risk to himself or others? (He may have been when he was admitted. He was very vulnerable when he was on remand. He certainly posed a threat to some people in hospital.) Is he currently a risk to himself or to others, or is he likely to pose such a risk in the future? (Difficult to say, but there had been no recent incidents, and the way things were moving at this stage suggested that risk was not an issue.) The nursing staff and his social worker reported that he was improving, and Trevor reported positively on Brian's progress at the project. He was taken off his section, and later that day returned home to his mother and sisters.

A few weeks later Trevor phoned me and asked if I would come over because someone wanted to talk with me. The project was housed in a curious brick blockhouse on the fringes of what had been an industrial estate. Outside the building I could sense more than hear a booming base line, which rattled the windows. The main entrance was on the first floor reached by a metal staircase painted rainbow colours, starting in red at the bottom, transitioning to violet by the time you reached the top. I plunged into the cool dark, and dimly made out a jostling throng. It took a few moments for my eyes to adjust, but the small reception area was bustling with young people, African-Caribbean, African, South

Asian, and from many different faiths: there were kufi caps, hijabs, veils, turbans. The walls were covered by photos and posters including Bob Marley, Ghandi, Rosa Parks, Martin Luther King, and Mary Seacole. Trevor greeted me and led me up to a quiet room on the second floor before disappearing off downstairs again. He returned a few seconds later with Brian. It was some time since we'd last met and at first I didn't recognise him. He was slimmer, and had regained the fluidity of movement and agility that I sensed only briefly when he was first admitted. For the first time he now looked at me, not just looked at me, but took me in and weighed me up. He took my hand.

'What are *you* doing here?' he asked.

'He's here at my invite', said Trevor. 'Remember?'

'Yeah', Brian nodded and smiled.

'Well? You said you wanted him to know ...'

'What, now?'

'As good as any time. I'd be drawing my pension if it were up to you.'

We sat down and fell into an awkward silence.

'You're looking very well, Brian. How are you keeping?'

He smiled, this time anxiously, and sucked his teeth.

'Well tell him!' said Trevor.

'You begin. It was your idea.'

'My idea? Bullshit. *You* said.' By now they were both smiling.

'Would someone please tell me what's going on?' I pleaded.

They looked at each other. 'Let me start then', said Trevor. 'There are things both Brian and I think it's important you know. We've spent a lot of time discussing this, and the time's right.'

'About what happened to you before you were admitted?'

'Yeah, and in hospital.'

'Go on.'

'OK. You remember the time I was locked up?'

'Yes.'

'I hit that white guy, right.'

'Yes.'

'We'd had a row. He was hogging the phone and I wanted to talk with Mum. They wouldn't let me into the courtyard, and thought maybe if she spoke to them or if she came down she could take me there. All I wanted was some fresh air, feel the rain on my face. I hated being cooped up. Anyhow, this guy just kept hogging the phone so I couldn't use it. In the end I tried to grab it off him and we scuffled. The nurses broke it up but he followed me as they marched me back to my room, shouting at me, right, shouting abuse. "You fucking stinking nigger! You black bastard." I just saw red and went for him. And do you know what happened? He gets away with it. Me? I get jumped on, stuck full of drugs, and carted off to the locked ward. All because I'm the black guy who stands up for himself, and ain't gonna take no shit from no one.'

'I understand', I replied, far from convincingly.

'Do you, Doc? Do you really? I don't think so. It's the same all through if you're black. At school as a kid, I mean the teachers, man, they're not racist!' He smiled. 'But believe me, if you've got colour, people believe you're more into fighting than reading. And because you've got some muscle then they think, OK, we'll stick a book in front of him and then we'll pull him up. Like my English teacher, right? I was nine and he said "Don't end up like those other black boys." So I said to him, "What do you mean, man, I *am* black." And he said again, "Just don't turn out like those other black kids." What did he take me for? I saw red and hit him.'

I remembered my visit to his mother's house, her telling me about his expulsion at the age of nine. Trevor was stretched back in his chair, listening carefully. 'Tell him about the police.'

'Where do I start? OK. I was playing football with some mates, mostly black, a couple of Asians. One of the Asian guys called me a nigger, so a minute later I went in on him and tackled him real hard. We ended up fighting. The next thing the police van turns up, lights and siren, and they let this Asian guy go. But this white lad who's been watching shouts out "Fuck the pigs", and they arrested me for it, dumped me in the van and slapped me up. If you're black you're always getting shit off other kids, right? White and Asian particularly. But it's the police; they really have it in for you. I wouldn't stand for it.' He paused as something flitted across his face, obscuring the light in his eyes, a shadow, a memory. He hung his head briefly and it vanished, then the defiance returned. 'My old man wouldn't stand for it either, not from anyone. My mum told me about him, about the way he'd been taught by his mum to hold his head up. He used to say to my mum it makes no difference what happened to us all in the past, but today we hold our heads up, and never take no shit from anyone.'

'Only I'm sure she never used that word', said Trevor.

'Yeah. But she said never, I was never to hang my head. I kept complaining to the teachers about all the shit they used to hand out, and all they could say was that I had a chip on my shoulder.' He paused for a moment, drumming his fingers on the table in front of him.

Trevor leaned forward and patted him on the knee. 'You're doing fine, kid. Tell him about prison.'

'When I was eighteen?'

'Yeah.'

'Last time I was in I met up with this guy I used to hang around with. Scooby was his nickname. He sang scat real good, like Ella, and he mixed scat and rap so everyone called him Scooby Doo. We used to play football, listen to music, but I hadn't seen him for years. Anyway there was this screw; we called him the Screaming Skull 'cos he was thin and grey like a corpse, with black rims around his eyes. He hated us black kids. He used to call us all sorts. "You fucking niggers," he'd say, "why don't you all crawl back to the jungle?" So one day he says to

Scooby "Fuck off back home!" "OK," says Scoob, "give me £1.50." "Why?" asks the Skull. "'Cos that's what a single to Moss Side costs," replies Scooby. We're all laughing, but the Skull loses his cool and jumps Scooby, pushes him to the floor, boot in, and screaming at him. This other screw just stands there laughing.' He closed his eyes for a moment. 'Real bad, blood all over the place and the bastard goes on laying into him, while I'm watching; I'm frozen. By now Scoob's almost unconscious and moaning, whimpering like a whipped puppy, so the Skull drags him over to the stairs, presses the alarm, and when the others arrive he tells them he slipped at the top and fell down the stairs. They cart Scoob off, and the Skull comes up to me and says, "You, nigger, are next if you don't behave." I heard later on that Scoob was in a coma for several days, and that he is paralysed, lost the use of his right side, and worst of all, he can't speak or sing. No more scat, man.'

The club was silent when I left. The kids had gone. I groped my way down the dimly lit stairs to the reception area. I paused and waited for Trevor.

'You know we all thought he was hearing the voice of a cartoon dog telling him he was going to be killed.'

'Does it make sense now?'

'It does,' I replied, 'thanks to you.'

I pushed the door open and was dazzled by the light. I missed the first step down and almost fell headlong down, but felt a strong hand grab my outstretched arm. Trevor stopped me from falling.

'Steady. I keep saying to the management committee we must do something about these steps, but they keep saying we just don't have the money.'

I paused to get my breath back, and turned to face him. 'I'm really shocked.'

'Why?'

'Nowhere in his notes was there any mention of the racial abuse he experienced.'

'They probably didn't think it important. They probably didn't even notice it.'

'But it's disgraceful, terrible.'

'It's institutional racism. Have you never read Stokely Carmichael? Listen, like many of us, Brian has a story in his family that goes way back. That's why it's so important we keep holding our heads held high.'

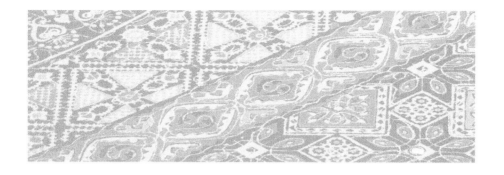

Section 5

Communities, Solidarity and Meaning

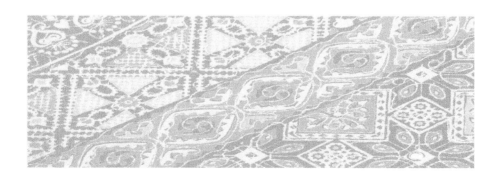

Resisting Psychiatry: The Rise of the Service User/Survivor Movement

11

> Mental health services are not relevant or helpful in the way I surf
> my waves of madness: less a life jacket, more a circling shark.
>
> (Andy Smith, in Stastny & Lehmann, 2007: 51)

Perhaps the most notable feature of the second half of the twentieth century, more immediate and striking for many of us than the moon landing, was the rise to prominence of movements of liberation. In America, black people challenged the oppression they had experienced at the hands of white people through the civil rights movement. Northern Ireland witnessed a similar phenomenon, only here it was Catholics who challenged oppression by the Protestant majority. Elsewhere in Africa, South Asia and the Caribbean, people who for centuries had been encouraged to think of themselves as the colonial subjects of distant foreign powers, struggled for freedom and independence. The women's movement and feminism challenged and rejected male authority and paternalism in all its guises. Disabled people, gay people, lesbians and transgendered people questioned and challenged the marginal position assigned to them by the non-disabled, patriarchal and heterosexual majority. The last will be first and the first will be last.

Liberation of course refers to the act of setting free, but this meaning misses something that is really important about these movements. It implies that liberation is something that is granted, or handed over, to those who are liberated. This overlooks a political reality, that the freedom of a group of people, whose identities share some common, defining features, has been limited and constrained by another group who do not share these features. These constraints vary considerably in how they operate, the mechanisms that sustain them, and the sites at which they operate (societies, communities, groups, families and individuals). However, a central feature of these constraints is that their power to limit the freedom of the oppressed group operates through a set of deeply ingrained assumptions shared by both oppressed and oppressors. These assumptions are so deeply held that, historically, they have been taken for granted by all. They are based on a set of beliefs that the oppressed are in some way inferior, or weaker, or undesirable, or irrational.[1] The power of the oppressors to define the lives and subjectivities of the oppressed in these negative terms is the focus of liberatory movements. Think, for example, of Black Power, Gay Pride and Women's Liberation. The rise of the service user and survivor movement over the last thirty years can be understood within this tradition.

Liberation is not something that can be granted by the oppressors, as the word implies. Movements of liberation begin with resistance, the struggle of oppressed minorities (or in some cases, majorities, as is so for countries which previously were 'colonies') against those who oppress them. In turn these various movements have changed all of us, as can be seen in the *Universal Declaration of Human Rights* and the equalities legislation that has been adopted across Europe. Yet the rights of mad people have yet to be fully confirmed within this framework, although significant progress is being made here, most notable through the Center for the Human Rights of Users and Survivors of Psychiatry.[2]

It is important to be clear that this chapter does not represent an attempt to write a history of the survivor movement. Those who write, and especially those who write history, do so from a position of power and privilege. The act of writing means continually having to make decisions about what to include and what to leave out. History in particular has a propensity to paper over cracks and fissures, to elide difference, and thus to silence. I am acutely aware that the 'history' of the survivor movement is one in which many voices have been and still are silenced. For this reason the main focus in this chapter is on the implications of the rise of the survivor movement in the UK for critical psychiatry and mental health practice today. That said, I apologise in advance if my account of the movement is seen to be partial, or fails to acknowledge the important and significant contributions of particular groups and individuals.

The service user/survivor movement is changing the society we live in. It is inconceivable that critical psychiatry would exist in the form it does without a movement that created the word 'postpsychiatry' (Campbell, 1996).

In this chapter I want to explore the rise to prominence of the service user/survivor (SU/S) movement over the last thirty years. I will frame this with a short introduction through Michel Foucault's later ideas about the nature of power. This will help us to understand how the SU/S movement is creating new possibilities for people who use mental health services. Foucault's work is helpful in this respect, because it provides a way of understanding why the resistance of service users and survivors to psychiatric power is so important. The main purpose of this chapter is to set out some of the significant aspects of the work of the SU/S movement.

---

1. For example, Chapter 5 explored in some detail the role played by scientific theories of racial difference in racism and the oppression of black people by white.

2. See http://www.chrusp.org. Tina Minkowitz has written extensively about this work on her *Mad in America* blog (Minkowitz, 2013).

Understanding the different levels at which power operates is important here. At one level, psychiatrists are empowered to deprive people of their freedom, and impose physical treatments upon them. The rationale for this is the belief that they suffer from mental disorder and require treatment. We have already seen that here are many difficulties with this, not least the evidence from Chapter 2, that there is no established scientific or medical basis for mental disorder. In addition to this we saw in Chapter 3 that psychiatric interventions are very limited in terms of their effectiveness, and potentially very harmful.

Despite this, psychiatric power is a peculiarly coercive form of power, for if the person disagrees with the psychiatrist's opinion about the nature of his or her problems they are likely to be described as 'lacking insight'. This then is used as evidence that the person is psychotic and thus mentally disordered. There is no way out of this catch-22. Furthermore, the interventions meted out by psychiatrists are experienced by many as harmful, degrading and highly oppressive. This is why one of the most important developments in the field of mental health in recent years has been the rise of the SU/S movement. Not all people who use mental health services see themselves as survivors of psychiatry, but the fact that many do is important and cannot be ignored. There are no activist groups who identify themselves as survivors of cardiology or gastroenterology, in much the same way as there are no groups of clinicians who identify themselves as critical cardiologists or critical gastroenterologists.

Foucault on Power

The French philosopher and historian Michel Foucault is best known for his work on the origins of psychiatry and modern medicine. In the *History of Madness* (1961/2006a), Foucault described and wrote about the power of psychiatry to silence the voices of mad people:

> There is no common language: or rather, it no longer exists; the constitution of madness as mental illness, at the end of the eighteenth century, bears witness to a rupture in dialogue, gives the separation as already enacted, and expels from the memory all those imperfect words, of no fixed syntax, spoken falteringly, in which the exchange between madness and reason was carried out. The language of psychiatry, which is a monologue by reason about madness, could only have come into existence in such a silence. (Foucault, 1961/2006a: xxviii)

Towards the end of his life he wrote at length about the nature of power in ways that are helpful in understanding the importance of the SU/S movement as a focus of resistance against the power of psychiatry to silence. His analysis of power indicates that it isn't simply a negative phenomenon; it can have positive as well as negative properties. Power can of course be used to subjugate and oppress, but it can also serve to liberate. Indeed, power and liberty are closely intertwined. His later work (Foucault, 1982) helps us to think through how resistance to power by those who are subject to it is liberatory:

> ... it consists of using this resistance as a chemical catalyst so as to bring to light power relations, locate their position, find out their point of applications and the methods used. Rather than analyzing power from the point of view of its internal rationality, it consists of analyzing power relations through the *antagonism of strategies*. (Foucault, 1982: 210–11; emphasis added)

The second half of the twentieth century witnessed the rise of a number of antagonistic strategies, or contemporary 'oppositions', such as feminist opposition to the power of men, of the civil rights movement, and the voices of mental health service survivors opposed to psychiatry. Foucault argues that it is not possible to dismiss these social movements simply as mere rejection of authority. They share a number of features in common:

1. They extend beyond national boundaries, and are unrelated to specific political systems or economies.
2. The aim of such struggles is primarily directed at the analysis of power.
3. They are 'immediate' struggles in the sense that those engaged in them are those who are most directly affected by the source of their oppression.

These features characterise the SU/S movement. It is an international movement – witness the existence of the World Network of Users and Survivors of Psychiatry (http://www.wnusp.net) and the European Network of (ex)-Users and Survivors of Psychiatry (http://www.enusp.org). The resistance of survivors and service users to the power of psychiatry is evidenced through their writing, especially their personal narratives. There are powerful anthologies of survival and resistance against psychiatry to be found in Read and Reynolds (1996), Stastny and Lehmann (2007), Romme *et al* (2009), and Reynolds *et al* (2009). Foucault writes:

> In such struggles people criticize instances of power which are the closest to them, those which exercise their action on individuals. They do not look for the 'chief enemy', but for the immediate enemy. Nor do they expect to find a solution to their problem at a future date (that is, liberations, revolutions, end of class struggle). In comparison with a theoretical scale of explanations or a revolutionary order which polarizes the historian, they are *anarchistic struggles*. (Foucault, 2006b: 211, emphasis added)

His use of the word *anarchistic* is significant especially in relation to the struggles of survivors. It implies a rejection of established ways of ordering and structuring human, social and political relationships. This is a resistance that defies *this* explanatory language, or *that* model of distress. It seeks only the ability and the right to speak in its own terms about madness in its struggle with the rationalising power of psychiatry.

Another important aspect of resistance is that it asserts the right of individuals to be different by emphasising the value of everything that makes them truly different from others, be it skin colour, gender, sexuality or (ir)rationality. These struggles resist any attempt to separate and detach the individual from his or her community of difference, and to tie that individual or her to his or her own identity. Foucault points out that these struggles also stand in opposition to power linked to professional expertise (or 'knowledge, competence and qualification', *ibid*: 212), such as psychiatry. In addition they represent a struggle against mystification and the imposition of secretive representations on people. Mary O'Hagan's powerful record of her experiences in an acute psychiatric inpatient unit is an excellent example of this. She juxtaposes her account of her experiences of an admission to an acute psychiatric ward with the medical entries made in her notes concurrently by her psychiatrist. We find a stark contrast between her intensely felt personal experiences of psychosis, especially the agony and isolation she endured, and the detached, remote and objectifying attitude of her psychiatrist towards her. In the extract below, her account is in italics and her psychiatrist's in non-italic font:

> *Today I want to die. Everything was hurting. My body was screaming. I saw the doctor. I said nothing. Now I feel terrible. Nothing seems good and nothing seems possible.*
> *I am stuck in this twilight mood*
> *where I go down*
> *like the setting sun*
> *into a lonely black hole*
> *where there is room for only one.*
>
> Flat, lacking motivation, sleep and appetite good. Discussed aetiology. Cont LiCarb 250mg qid. Levels next time. (O'Hagan, 1996: 46)

Finally, Foucault proposes that these struggles are fundamentally concerned with the question of subjectivity, and who has the right to determine how we identify and understand ourselves as human beings:

> ... all these present struggles revolve around the question: Who are we? They are a refusal of these abstractions, of economic and ideological state violence which ignore who we are individually, and also a refusal of a scientific or administrative inquisition which determines who one is. (Foucault, 2006b: 212)

Many in the SU/S movement, for example the Hearing Voices Network, resist and reject the language of psychopathology, which originates in and bolsters its scientific expertise and authority. In challenging the power of psychiatry in this way it opens up what Blackman (2001) calls an 'ethical space' for different understandings of the experience.

The Rise of the Service User/Survivor Movement

There is an immediate problem in speaking about a multi-voiced and multi-faceted movement like the SU/S movement: that of terminology. A number of terms have been used to describe the broad alliance of individuals and groups who at some time or another in their lives have used mental health services. These include service users, survivors, clients, consumers, ex-patients, and experts by experience (which comes from the Dutch word *ervaringsdeskundigen*). There are also differences between Europe and the USA. The expression used in the UK, the service user/survivor movement, is taken from *On Our Own Terms*, a research study undertaken by a group of prominent service users/survivors, published by the Sainsbury Centre for Mental Health (Wallcraft *et al*, 2003). The project steering committee agreed the following definition of the term, which most of those who responded to the survey agreed with:

> The 'service user/survivor movement' is a term used to describe the existence of numerous individuals who speak out for their own rights and those of others, and local groups and national organisations set up to provide mutual support or to promote the rights of current and former mental health service users to have a voice.
>
> Group members and individuals may call themselves 'survivors', 'service users', 'clients', 'ex-patients' or other similar terms.
>
> The term 'movement' implies that these individuals, groups and organisations share some common goals and are moving in a similar direction. (Wallcraft *et al*, 2003: 3)

It is probably more accurate to refer to 'movements', because service user/survivor movements are multi-voiced and heterogeneous, but for the sake of simplicity of style, I shall continue to use the singular.

The prominent activist Peter Campbell (1989, 2009) who, along with many others, has played an important part in the emergence of the SU/S movement over the last thirty years, has written about its growth from the 1970s to the present day. His view is that the critiques of Laing, Cooper and others had little impact upon psychiatric practice. He argues that the anti-psychiatry movement failed to engage survivor activists, and had at best a marginal impact on the growth of the movement. This may be true if you consider anti-psychiatry narrowly in terms of its leading protagonists and activities. If considered from that perspective it was a movement dominated by critical professionals and academics, and had little to say about service user empowerment or involvement, self-advocacy or self-organisation. In contrast, the SU/S movement in England drew inspiration from the struggles of other marginalised and oppressed groups to have their human rights recognised, especially from the survivor movements in the Netherlands. In the early days, many activists hoped that the era of community care would open up a more equal, democratic and participatory relationship between service users and professionals, but in 1989 the reality was different:

> As a result of 'open door' policies and chemotherapy, users now believe they are part of the community; indeed, they have no general reason to doubt that they are. Yet in reality although they are invited to the party they are forced to sit out on most of the dances. (Campbell, 1989: 208)

The situation did change, however, and others have argued that many of those involved in the very early days of the survivor movement in England were inspired by the work of Laing and Cooper (1964) in particular, as well as sharing a political alignment with the latter in Marxism. The work of Laing and Cooper challenged and questioned the assumptions and practices of traditional psychiatry, and many radical activists along with a small number of mental health professionals, especially nurses and social workers, were inspired to work more closely with people who were using psychiatric services. Helen Spandler's book *Asylum to Action* (2006) has described how the influence of Laing and Cooper, and those involved in the therapeutic community movement, was focused through the work of the Paddington Day Hospital, where in 1972 the first meeting of the Mental Patients Union (MPU) took place. Andrew Roberts,[3] another significant figure in survivor history, has recently described his own involvement in the early days of the MPU (Roberts, 2008). This, arguably one of the earliest contemporary survivor groups, was followed by a succession of grass-roots organisations such as the Community Organisation for Psychiatric Emergencies (COPE) which was inspired by the work of Laing and Cooper (Andy Smith & Eleanor Dace, personal communication, December 2013).

An important event in the origins of the SU/S movement took place at MIND's national conference in 1985 under the title *From Patients to People*. For some it was an event of symbolic significance because survivors and service users gave plenary talks and workshops; they dominated the proceedings. It took place just as the idea of self-advocacy was beginning to take hold, and the opportunities afforded by the conference, especially the publicity it attracted, made it possible for service users to see themselves and be seen by others as self-

---

3. There is a valuable resource devoted to service user and survivor history, the website maintained by Andrew Roberts: http://studymore.org.uk/mpu.htm accessed on 13th September 2013.

advocates and activists. This shift in self and public perception is important in resisting oppression. Another important outcome of the event was the formation of Survivors Speak Out, which became an important focus for SU/S activism nationally over the next fifteen years. At the same time Channel 4 broadcast *We're Not Mad, We're Angry*[4] in 1986, the first television documentary in which survivors and service users had a degree of editorial control. This film, which includes interviews with white and black service users, is deeply critical of the biomedical model in psychiatry. Sadly, its message is as relevant today as it was thirty years ago.

The SU/S movement really started to expand from the mid-1980s on. According to Peter Campbell, in those early days mental health workers played a part in supporting the movement. Most self-advocacy groups in the mid-1980s were alliances between service users and supportive mental health professionals. He regards these alliances as essential in fostering the growth and development of self-advocacy, and argues that professionals were encouraged to work in alliance with the early SU/S movements by the crisis of legitimacy facing psychiatry as it moved out of the asylum into the community. It was extremely difficult to challenge the theories and practice of psychiatry as long as it remained within its institutional base. Once it moved into the community, the relevance of psychiatry, especially the medical model, increasingly came under challenge.

It must be stressed that the SU/S movement has always encompassed a wide range of perspectives, from those who simply want mainstream mental health services to offer greater choice and better quality, to abolitionists who want to replace statutory services with survivor-led alternatives (Campbell, 1989, 2009). It is now the case that service users are routinely involved in the planning, commissioning and monitoring of mental health services. I'll return to this later. Despite the different perspectives, the SU/S movement shares a common belief in the '... essential competence of people with mental health problems ...' (Campbell, 2009: 48).

> What is clear is that a significant number of service user activists have not confined themselves to issues to do with the quality (or existence) of services but have inserted themselves into discussion about the nature of madness/ mental illness itself. (Campbell, 2009: 50)

This is precisely what Foucault has in mind when he talks about analysing power relationships through antagonistic strategies. The SU/S movement challenges the power of psychiatrists to speak authoritatively about the lives and experiences of service users and survivors. This presents psychiatrists with a challenge, that of adopting a more nuanced, self-aware and self-critical perspective on their theories and practice. It is this more than anything that made it possible, indeed,

---

4. The documentary can be seen on YouTube. Accessed on 25th August 2013 at http://www.youtube.com/watch?v=qD36m1mveoY

necessary, for a movement like critical psychiatry to exist.

We can begin to grasp the impact the movement has had on the wider field of mental health if we consider the main findings of the study *On Our Own Terms* (Wallcraft *et al*, 2003). It set out to describe the SU/S movement in England, with a particular focus on the extent of involvement and representation of black people. It also examined the extent to which the movement was involved with mainstream services, and in what capacity. It used a variety of methods including a postal questionnaire survey of groups (318 responses) and face-to-face interviews, focus groups and observational research of 25 groups. It also convened a national focus group for black service users and survivors, and visited seventeen local user-led projects.

A key finding was the role of individuals in the movement in providing mutual help and support at times of crisis for those who chose to move out of traditional services in the quest for recovery. This is achieved through peer-led alternatives, such as self-management, crisis support,[5] recovery and social action based on reintegration. In addition, nearly three-quarters of local groups were involved in consultation or decision-making bodies, usually concerned with the implementation of the National Service Framework (NSF), although the quality of this input and the extent to which it represented genuine involvement, as opposed to tokenism, varied considerably. Local groups were also involved in the education and training of mental health professionals in local services.

The survey highlights three problems facing the movement. First, it remains largely a white movement. Although there is a growing black SU/S movement, this was (and still is) struggling for resources and recognition. Much work remains necessary to enable the movement to reflect the diversity of British society. Second, many groups, especially those from BME communities, struggled to find funds to support their work. In particular there was a problem with the security of funding. This problem is even greater following the recession and the cuts in funding for third-sector organisations. Third, although there was broad agreement across the groups about the importance of being treated as an individual, and dissatisfaction with mainstream services, there were some

---

5. The first inkling I had of the extent and importance of informal crisis support occurred nearly twenty years ago shortly after I moved to Bradford. I held an informal drop-in once a month at Bradford MIND to offer advice to members about medication and other problems relating to treatment. Two people approached me, asking whether they could discuss a friend who had been admitted to hospital under my care in early January. The individual concerned had opened his flat over the period of Christmas and New Year celebrations to service users and survivors who were facing the holiday period in crisis, and who did not wish to be admitted to hospital. At one point he had twelve people sleeping on his floor. He found the emotional pressure of this so great that it had a negative impact on his own wellbeing, and was admitted to hospital in the first week of January. Had it not been for his efforts, a substantial number of the people he had helped out would probably have been admitted to hospital. His own admission was in part related to the stress he experienced in offering support, but also because he had no money after feeding up to nine or ten other people.

unresolved controversies. These concerned the role of compulsory treatment in mental health care, the role played by biomedical and social models, the relationship with the disability rights movement, and the role of pharmaceutical company funding of the SU/S movement. The most striking thing to emerge from the survey, however, was the growth and development of SU/S-led groups through organisations like the Hearing Voices Network (HVN) and UK Advocacy Network (UKAN).

It is important to recognise that people who experience states of madness and distress find many ways of coping with their experiences without resorting to professional help. A comprehensive account of these non-professional systems of help and support can be found in *Alternatives Beyond Psychiatry* (Stastny & Lehmann, 2007). This anthology includes contributions from fourteen people who describe the things they have found helpful in coping outside mental health services. They have either enabled the contributors to move out of mental health services, or helped them to avoid having contact with services. The strategies described include the use of peer-support networks and self-help (ten people); engagement in creative activities including films, music and gardening (six people); engagement in silence or retreating from the world, or social activism (four people each); exercise, relationships with pets and animals, fasting and diet (three people each); meditation and sleeping (two people each); and massage, personalised budgets or advance directives[6] (one person each).

The following quotes from *Alternatives Beyond Psychiatry* give some idea as to how these strategies are helpful.

> When you are experiencing internal chaos, the exercise of control and the act of creation in editing a piece [film], no matter the outcome, can be healing. (Sarah Carr, *ibid*: 55)

> Institutionalised societal silence on [male violence, child abuse, rape, assault] makes me mad ... Fighting back, finding my voice and refusing to shut up are my remedy to despair. (Merinda Epstein, *ibid*: 58)

> What I learned is that silence is my best friend. Silence is what I found at the heart of my being. Silence is where all my thoughts come from and where they all return to. This silence, not my sometimes crazy mind, is who I am. And in this silence, which was always and already forever inside me, I finally found peace after overlooking it for so many years. (David Webb, *ibid*: 70)

> There is no science to remaining mentally well, as opposed to the supposed science of being mentally ill. It is an art form. (Tina Coldham, *ibid*: 71)

------

6. Advance directives, or advance statements (see also p. 269) are plans drawn up by a person who has full capacity setting out the sort of help and care they want to receive in future, should they lack capacity through psychosis or severe distress.

Service-User-led Research

The growing influence of the SU/S movements can be discerned in academic research in psychiatry and mental health, which increasingly includes the perspectives of people who have first-hand experience of madness and distress. This is exemplified by the work of academics including Professor Peter Beresford at Brunel University and Professor Diana Rose, Co-director of the Service User Research Enterprise (SURE) in the Institute of Psychiatry (Rose, 2001).[7] But at the same time there is another strand of SU/S research that is carried out entirely by service users and survivors. This work, usually led by independent survivor researchers like Alison Faulkner or Jayasree Kalathil, and supported by NGOs like the Mental Health Foundation or the Sainsbury Centre, is designed, carried out and written up entirely by service users and survivors (see, for example, Faulkner & Layzell, 2000; Mental Health Foundation, 1997). Service users and survivors set the research questions, which originate in their own experiences, and train other service users in basic qualitative research methods, enabling their peers to undertake the research.

A key feature of this work is that it deals exclusively with the concerns of service users and survivors. It is designed and undertaken in such a way as to maximise the likelihood that people whose experiences and opinions are inaccessible to most other forms of research will be included. Given the difficulties that the SU/S movements have in reflecting the views of people from black communities, I will describe a recent study by Jayasree Kalathil and colleagues (2011) which examined how black British women who have used mental health services understood 'recovery'. Much of the evidence on the impact of social adversity on the mental health of black people in Chapter 5 originated in studies of black men. This is an area that has been much less well studied from the perspective of women, despite the fact that they are equally disadvantaged by social adversity. The purpose of Jayasree Kalathil's carefully designed and executed study, which used depth interviews with twenty-seven women, was to explore their experiences with particular reference to their identities as black people.

They recruited African, Caribbean and South Asian women who had recovered (defined in their own terms) from distress, through user and survivor networks, organisations working with women, faith groups, newsletters and on-line forums. They identified twenty-four women, eight from each community. Participants gave a narrative interview using a semi-structured interview schedule that enables the person to tell her story whilst at the same time providing a framework for subsequent analysis.

Not surprisingly the women understood recovery in terms of their understandings of their distress. This included a variety of narratives that drew on socio-cultural and family factors, as well as personal experience and biomedical

7. An overview of the range and extent of SU/S research can be found in Sweeney et al (2009).

factors. Culture, gender and the spiritual aspects of personal identity were all important in how they made sense of and recovered from their distress.[8] Recovery in this sense meant engaging with a sense of self, overcoming negative social experiences, and forging a:

> ... shared sense of identity and social justice through collective action, and having access to 'recovery spaces' where specific socio-cultural aspects of distress could be safely addressed. (Kalathil et al, 2011: 9)

Some people related their distress to oppressive experiences originating in family relationships, including domestic violence and sexual abuse, as well as bereavement and obligations in fulfilling family roles. The meaning of recovery here depended on the extent to which women were able to manage their difficulties and regain control over their lives. For some women, faith and spirituality were particularly important in helping them achieve this. It may come as a surprise to discover that psychiatrists had a role to play in the recovery of some women. However, the extent to which a biomedical framework was helpful in facilitating recovery depended on the quality of the therapeutic relationship,[9] especially the extent to which the doctor used a shared decision-making approach. Most women who found a biomedical framework helpful made a clear distinction between the limited role of medication in symptom control and genuine recovery, which involved being free of medication. Only a small number of women found the concept of recovery used by mental health services consistent with their personal understandings of the term, and '... some wanted to distance themselves from the term because they saw it as professional-led, pressurising and meaningless' (ibid: 10).

Service User and Survivor Involvement in Services

The emphasis so far in this chapter has been on the activities of service users and survivors outside services, but the rise of the movement has resulted in major changes and improvements in mental health services. It is now a matter of routine that service users (and carers) are involved in the organisation, delivery and monitoring of services locally, and at a national level they are involved in the development of mental health policy. There is evidence that service user involvement has beneficial effects on outcomes. Simpson and House (2002) carried out a systematic review of randomised controlled trials ($n = 5$), and other comparative studies ($n = 7$) of service user involvement in the delivery and

---

8. This evidence supports the arguments in Chapter 7 on the importance of narrative identity in recovery.

9. This is entirely consistent with the analysis of the evidence from EBM studies of the effectiveness of psychiatric interventions presented in Chapter 3.

evaluation of mental health services. Half of the studies concerned service users who were involved in case management. They found that service user involvement in care was associated with higher levels of patient satisfaction with care and fewer hospitalisations. In addition, mental health professionals who had been trained by service users had more positive attitudes towards the people whose care they were involved with. Another systematic review by Mike Crawford and colleagues identified over forty papers on service user involvement. Most described changes to services that were attributable to patient involvement, including attempts to improve the accessibility of services and the production of information leaflets. Changes in the attitudes of organisations to involving patients and positive responses from patients who took part in initiatives were also reported. They concluded that patient involvement has contributed to changes in services in a range of settings (Crawford *et al*, 2002). Involving service users in care not only is feasible, but also has beneficial effects on the outcome of care (Bowles *et al*, 2002).

Despite this, many SU/S are suspicious and wary of being involved with services. In part this is because they feel strongly that they are not really listened to, and that their presence is little more than tokenism. These views are confirmed by my personal experiences of talking to service users and mental health professionals. Many mental health nurses have spoken to me about the input they receive from SU/S during their degree courses. Many see this as challenging but invaluable because it forces them to think carefully and critically about their practice. However, once they return to ward environments the attitudes of some senior staff across disciplines, together with work pressures, make it difficult if not impossible to work in a reflective manner.

What does this mean in practice? How might the role of the service user involved in services work out? To take one example based in our experience in Bradford, Peter Relton and I have described the role of the service-user development worker (SUDW) in the Bradford Home Treatment Service, which was set up by Pat Bracken, Valerie Rhodes and Peter Relton in the mid-1990s (Relton & Thomas, 2002). The service, which opened in 1996, offered a 24-hours-a-day, seven-days-a-week alternative to acute inpatient care for an inner-city community. The service-user development worker (Peter Relton) was one of the first appointments to the team. The aim of the post, which was open only to someone who had used mental health services, was to provide a user perspective at the heart of the team in an attempt to address the issue of power between people who used the service and mental health professionals, especially the psychiatrists. The SUDW was involved in the short-listing, interviewing and selection of all team members as the service was set up. Once the service was operating, the worker attended all team and review meetings, and provided information and training for the team on service user- and survivor-led research. He also made an active contribution to local and national SU/S activities, and in particular acted as a bridge between the team and informal SU/S support networks locally, many of which were organised around Bradford Mind and Bradford and Airedale Mental

Health Advocacy Group, both of which were led and run by service users and survivors. He also visited individuals using the service at home if they wanted to get involved in political activism with other survivors, or explore opportunities for volunteering.

One of the most important aspects of Peter Relton's work was to challenge and support the team in developing and maintaining a non-medical philosophy. This helped to keep the focus of team discussion away from diagnosis and treatment to the struggle to engage more fully with people's narratives in order to understand and make sense of their experiences. His contributions also helped to move team discussions about risk to a more nuanced engagement with the complexities of human predicaments. In particular, discussions about the use of the Mental Health Act to remove individuals from the community into hospital became more participative, and were more likely to engage the service user and his or her immediate family or carers. This made these decisions more complex and difficult, but paradoxically this was more satisfying because it increased the team's engagement with the ethical complexities of mental health work.

Another strand of work that provides support for service user and carer input to team decision making is Bill Fulford's work on values-based practice (Woodbridge & Fulford, 2004). This draws attention to the potential conflicts that can arise in multi-disciplinary teamwork, from the various models and understandings that different actors use in mental health work. The values attached to these models have an important influence on shared decision making (Colombo *et al*, 2003). The involvement of service users and carers in team discussions helps to draw out the conflicting values between the participants' explanatory models, and helps to retain a focus on the interests and concerns of service users and families. For this reason the first element of shared decision making as set out by the Care Services Improvement Agency and National Institute for Mental Health in England (CSIP/NIMHE, 2008) is the involvement of service users and carers in assessments:

> It is well recognised that service users and carers should be actively involved in how their problems are treated so that they can work together in a shared process with practitioners to develop independence and self-management skills. (CSIP/NIMHE, 2008: 6)

Service-user development workers function well in services that they have been involved in setting up, but they face real problems if they are simply parachuted into existing services in the expectation that unaided they will be able to bring about fundamental changes in teams' values and attitudes. Bradford's Assertive Outreach team was set up in the same way as Home Treatment, with the service-user development worker as the first member appointed to the team. The team's values and philosophy were explicitly non-medical, in the sense that we did not use diagnoses (other than for strictly administrative purposes); we worked hard to engage with the social, community and cultural contexts in which our patients lived, and we strove to minimise the use and harmful effects of medication. My experience of working with that team was that the service-user development worker's role was essential in keeping us focused on those values and ways of working. Her presence meant that without knowing it, we became involved in our patients' stories. It was both a challenging and a richly rewarding way of working.

Recommended Reading

Campbell, P. (1996) Challenging loss of power. In J. Read & J. Reynolds (Eds.) *Speaking Our Minds: An anthology* (pp. 56–62). London: Macmillan/Open University.

Campbell, P. (2009) The service user/survivor movement. In J. Reynolds, R. Muston, T. Heller, J. Leach, M. McCormick, J. Wallcraft & M. Walsh (Eds.) *Mental Health Still Matters* (pp. 46–52). Basingstoke/Milton Keynes: Palgrave Macmillan/Open University.

Faulkner, A. & Layzell, S. (2000) *Strategies for Living: A report of user-led research into people's strategies for living with mental distress*. London: Mental Health Foundation.

Foucault, M. (1982) Afterword. In H. Dreyfus & P. Rabinow (Eds.) *Michel Foucault: Beyond structuralism and hermeneutics* (pp. 208–6). New York: Harvester Wheatsheaf.

Kalathil, J., Collier, B., Bhakta, R., Daniel, O., Joseph, D. & Trivedi, P. (2011) *Recovery and Resilience: African, African-Caribbean and South Asian women's narratives of recovery from mental distress*. London: Mental Health Foundation.

Mental Health Foundation (1997) *Knowing Our Own Minds: A survey of how people in emotional distress take control of their lives*. London: Mental Health Foundation.

Stastny, P. & Lehmann, P. (2007) *Alternatives Beyond Psychiatry*. Berlin/Eugene, OR/Shrewsbury: Peter Lehmann Publishing.

Wallcraft, J., Read, J. & Sweeney, A. (2003) *On Our Own Terms: Users and survivors of mental health services working together for support and change*. London: Sainsbury Centre for Mental Health.

New (and Old) Paths to Meaning and Healing in Psychosis 12

In the last chapter we saw that the rise of the service user/survivor movement could be seen as part of a growing concern with human rights in the second half of the twentieth century. The foundation of the movement was an act of resistance and self-determination in which mental health professionals played only a marginal role. That began to change once the movement became established. The possibility of alliances between the movement and professionals began to open up. The most influential and successful example of this is to be found in the work of the Hearing Voices Network. It has drawn attention to the fundamentally meaningful nature of the experiences of psychosis, something that mainstream psychiatry had avoided or denied for many years. In doing so it encouraged and reinvigorated those of us who drew inspiration from the early work of R.D. Laing. There is an important tradition in psychiatry that maintains that psychosis is potentially understandable, which extends back through Laing to the work of Harry Stack Sullivan in the early part of the twentieth century. This tradition was largely influenced by psychoanalytic and psychodynamic thought, as can be seen, for example, in the work of Freda Fromm-Reichmann in the US, Brian Martindale and Alison Summers in the UK NHS, and the work of Loren Mosher and Soteria House.

In this chapter I want to examine these two strands of work. Despite their origins in different traditions, they share a number of important features. They both recognise the meaningful nature of psychosis; and they have both contributed to collaborative work between people who experience psychosis, and mental health professionals and others. This is giving rise to new ways of working between voice hearers and professionals, and new theories about psychosis. Both traditions sit comfortably alongside the use of narrative in mental health practice described in Chapter 7. They share a common belief that the experiences of psychosis are meaningful, and that self-defined recovery is achievable without or with medication. In Hearing Voices groups, people share their experiences and stories through peer support. They encourage each other to reflect on the possible personal meanings of their experiences – an important part of the process towards healing or recovery. Soteria offered a safe space for people with chaos narratives to develop trusting relationships that made it possible for them to start the process of putting words to their experiences. It is important to note that although neither approach is opposed to the use of neuroleptic drugs, both stress that whether or not these drugs should be taken is a matter of choice for the individual.

The two approaches occupy quite different positions in relation to mental health practice today. The work of the HVN is now international in its scope – groups are found across the world. There are important alliances and links between HVN and mental health professionals, although as we will see, these links are not without their dangers. In contrast, there are only a few Soteria houses scattered across the USA and Europe. Despite this, there are groups actively campaigning for the development and provision of Soteria houses, or models of community support that have much in common with Soteria, and the Scandinavian work grounded in psychodynamic and psychoanalytic approaches to psychosis is becoming increasingly influential across the world, see also the work of ISPS, p. 244 for link. The City of New York has just announced major plans to reconfigure its acute psychiatric services along the lines of the Parachute Project, which will be described at the end of this chapter (New York City Department of Health and Mental Hygiene, 2013). This is a major breakthrough.

The Hearing Voices Network

Just as the service user/survivor movement (SU/S) was unfurling its wings in England, events were taking place in the Netherlands that were to open up radical new possibilities for social action, and new ways of helping and supporting people who hear voices. The striking feature about this development, a feature that came to symbolise the movement it founded, was that it involved a psychiatric patient appearing on a Dutch television programme with her psychiatrist. This marked the beginning of what was to become the Hearing Voices movement. The account given by psychiatrist Marius Romme and journalist Sandra Escher (1993b) is valuable and worth reporting in some detail because from it emerges the kernel of the work of the Hearing Voices Network (HVN) today. These elements are peer support and self-advocacy, the provision of non-medical systems of support for people who would otherwise be diagnosed with psychoses, and in particular the establishment of new alliances between service users and survivors and mental health professionals (including psychiatrists). These alliances are becoming increasingly important in research into the experience of hearing voices, and the development of new ways of helping people with the experience. One result of this is that the work of the HVN has brought people who hear voices – people who within a psychiatric context would be diagnosed with 'schizophrenia' – into collaboration with clinicians and researchers.

Marius Romme was struggling to help his patient. She had spent lengthy periods in psychiatric hospital, received a diagnosis of schizophrenia, and different neuroleptic drugs, none of which had helped to stop or reduce her voices. The drugs tired her out and reduced her alertness, although they did reduce her anxiety. Her voices were having an increasingly powerful hold over her life, and she was becoming increasingly lonely and isolated as a result. She felt hopeless and defeated, and began to speak about ending her life. Romme and Escher noted that the only positive aspect of the conversations between patient and psychiatrist at that time concerned her theory about why she heard voices. She had read Julian Jaynes' (1976) book, *The Origins of Consciousness in the Breakdown of the Bicameral Mind*, which argues that the experience of hearing voices was an important and 'normal' stage in the origins of consciousness. Romme was impressed by her ability to talk concerning her ideas about her experiences and, worried with regard to her isolation, believed it would be helpful for her if she could have contact with other people who heard voices. Together, they organised a series of meetings with other voice hearers, which Romme attended:

> As I sat there listening to their conversations, I was struck by the eagerness with which they recognized one another's experiences. Initially, I found it difficult to follow these conversations: to my ears, the contents were bizarre and extraordinary, and yet this was all freely discussed *as though it constituted a real world, of and unto itself.* (Romme & Escher, 1993b: 11, emphasis added)

Although it was clear that they gained benefit from meeting together and talking about their experiences, Romme and Escher were struck by the voice hearers' powerlessness in relation to their voices. None appeared able to cope with their experiences or challenge their voices. For this reason they devised a way of bringing voice hearers into contact with people who heard voices but could cope with them, people who didn't experience this terrible powerlessness. Romme and his patient appeared on a popular Dutch television programme to discuss hearing voices, and to encourage people to phone in after the broadcast. About 700 people did so, 450 of whom heard voices. Roughly two-thirds said they couldn't cope with the experience, whereas the remainder said they could. They sent out a questionnaire and received responses from 173, roughly a third of whom were 'copers' and two-thirds 'non-copers'. Those who were able to cope with their experiences generally heard voices that were friendly and positive, whereas the voices of those unable to cope were negative and aggressive. In addition, copers were better able to listen selectively to their voices and to set limits for them (e.g., to set aside a specific time to attend to their voices). Not surprisingly, copers felt stronger than their voices.

Romme and Escher drew an important conclusion from the results of the survey. People who were able to cope with their voices not only had more positive relationships with their voices, but also with their social environments. They were, for example, more likely to discuss their experiences with others. In contrast, non-copers rarely did this:

> We may therefore view the experience of voices not solely as a *discrete individual psychological experience, but as an interactional phenomenon reflecting the nature of the individual's relationship to his or her own environment,* and indeed vice versa. In other words, *it is not only a psychological but also a social phenomenon.* (Romme & Escher, 1993b: 16, emphasis added)

This is a profound insight, and it is important to grasp its significance. At one level it challenges deeply held philosophical assumptions about the nature of self and subjectivity, particularly dualistic divisions between the mental world and the social world, or what is referred to by some philosophers as epistemological dualism (the split between the mental world of the knowing subject and known-about world).[1] In addition, Marius Romme and Sandra Escher's insight reveals the influence of Romme's training and background in Dutch social psychiatry, and particularly the work of his teacher and mentor, Arie Querido (1966). Querido was an influential social psychiatrist who worked in Amsterdam in the mid-twentieth century, where in 1934 he set up an early version of home treatment. His understanding of psychosis and distress was based in his ideas about social homeostasis, that our wellbeing is dependent upon a balance and adjustment between competing social factors and pressures. Understanding the significance of this social perspective on the experience of hearing voices is the key to understanding why the hearing voices movement has become so influential, and has formed such an important element of self-help and peer support over the last twenty-five years. It also helps us to understand why it has been so influential with critical psychiatrists, clinical psychologists and other mental health professionals. This is because Romme and Escher's work places the social and narrative contexts that we explored in Chapters 4 and 5 at the heart of our attempts to understand experiences like voices and unusual beliefs. It represents a major break with the psychopathological tradition in psychiatry that sees the experiences of psychosis as meaningless.

Following the postal questionnaire, Romme and Escher organised a conference for people who heard voices. This was held in a non-medical setting, and the main speakers were all people who heard voices and who had responded to the questionnaire. This conference was in effect the first Hearing Voices Congress.

The community development worker Paul Baker has described the arrival of HVN in Britain (Baker, 1993). Marius Romme and Sandra Escher came to England to speak at public meetings in Manchester, Liverpool and Sheffield in 1989. This was followed by a national meeting in London, with groups subsequently established in London and Manchester. In 1992 the first attempt to involve professionals and academics in dialogue with the blossoming HVN took place in Liverpool, with contributions from the research clinical psychologist Richard Bentall, and others.

---

1. I examined some aspects of the philosophical consequence of this in Chapter 9 of *The Dialectics of Schizophrenia* (Thomas, 1997), as did Pat Bracken and I in Chapter 4 of *Postpsychiatry* (Bracken & Thomas, 2005).

Alec Jenner, at that time Professor of Psychiatry at the University of Sheffield, was also influential in supporting the work of Marius Romme and Sandra Escher in England. By 1993 the membership of HVN in Britain had reached 350, with groups in major cities in England, as well as in Scotland and Wales.

Since then the work of HVN has extended to most parts of the country, and indeed across the world. There are now over 180 groups in England, Scotland and Wales, and specialist groups for members of BME communities, people in prisons and secure settings, women and young people who hear voices. The principles behind HVN have now extended to people with other experiences that psychiatry would identify as 'pathological', such as strange and unusual beliefs. The work of Peter Bullimore in Sheffield and the Paranoia Network has been described by Tamasin Knight (2006), herself a survivor of mental health services, medically qualified and trained in psychiatry and public health, and Rufus May, a clinical psychologist and survivor of mental health services (2007). HVN today is almost entirely survivor led, from the national body, right down to the management and facilitation of local groups. Three of its trustees, Jacqui Dillon, Peter Bullimore and Rachel Waddingham are prominent survivors of psychiatry, with successful careers in survivor and professional training and development. Jacqui Dillon and another prominent survivor of psychiatry and doctoral research student in the University of Leeds, Eleanor Longden, have provided an overview of the contemporary work of HVN (Dillon & Longden, 2012).

They point out that a fundamental assumption of the work of HVN is that the experience of hearing voices is meaningful, and that meaning is tied to aspects of the person's life story. Coping with and recovering from the experience is possible not by suppressing it with neuroleptics, but by bringing people who have the experience together. Through sharing their stories and experiences it becomes possible for them to change their relationships with their voices. This becomes clear on reading some of the fifty stories presented by Romme *et al* (2009). If voice hearers are able to share their experiences in HVN groups they become less lonely and isolated, have the opportunity to explore different ways of coping with the experience, and can begin the process of trying to understand the experience. Dillon and Longden set out three main aims for the network:

1. To raise awareness of voice hearing, visions, tactile sensations and other sensory experiences.
2. To give men, women and children who have these, experience an opportunity to talk freely about this together.
3. To support anyone with these experiences seeking to understand, learn and grow from them in their own way. (Dillon & Longden, 2012: 130)

These aims – developed by trustees of HVN as part of the process of securing charitable status – are supported by research evidence that shows that voices are meaningfully linked to voice hearers' narratives. Dirk Corstens and Eleanor

Longden (2013) examined data taken from the constructs (a detailed summary description of the experience based in the Maastricht Interview; Romme & Escher, 2000) of 100 clinical voice hearers, most of whom (80%) had clinical diagnoses of schizophrenia. Nearly 90 per cent of the sample reported at least one adverse childhood experience, such as family conflict, neglect and bullying, or reported different forms of abuse. In 94 per cent of cases it was possible to understand the underlying emotional conflicts represented by voices, such as low self-esteem, anger, shame or guilt related to early experiences of adversity. In 78 per cent of cases it was also possible to identify the person(s) from the voice hearer's life represented by the voices. Voices are meaningful when understood within the context of the person's life narrative. In addition, there is also evidence that people who have the opportunity to discuss and explore their voices on their own terms, using their own language and explanatory systems, are better able to cope with them. In contrast, avoiding voices, refusing to talk about them, or denying voice hearers an opportunity to explore the experience make it more difficult for the person to cope (Escher, 1993; Veiga-Martinez et al, 2008). Understanding the meaning of voices is for many people an important part of recovery (see, e.g., Romme et al, 2009; Davies et al, 1999).

This raises an important problem. The education of most mental health professionals does not equip them to engage with voices in ways that are helpful and constructive for voice hearers. The experience is seen as a symptom of psychosis, schizophrenia, that requires treatment with neuroleptic medication. Indeed, many psychiatrists appear to believe that it is bad practice to engage voices hearers in discussion about their voices, or other experiences of madness.[2] In general, the training of psychiatrists and mental health professionals leaves them with a very limited repertoire for helping people who hear voices. Most are unaware of the wider range of coping mechanisms available to people who attend HVN groups. Fortunately this is changing. Romme and Escher's work on voice constructs, based on the Maastricht Interview (Romme & Escher, 2000) sets out a positive way for clinicians to engage with voice hearers' experiences, a resource frequently used by voice hearers who are involved in training mental health workers. Service users and survivors now play an important role in the re-education and training of mental health professionals (see, e.g., the work of Jacqui Dillon: http://www.jacquidillon.org/work/, and Peter Bullimore: http://www.nationalparanoianetwork.org/index.php?).

------

2. Evidence for this is to be found in McCabe et al's (2002) study of routine outpatient consultations of thirty-two patients (diagnoses of schizophrenia or schizoaffective disorder) with seven psychiatrists. They found that patients actively tried to discuss the content of their psychotic experiences, asking direct questions and repeating the questions again at the end of the consultation because they hadn't been answered. Psychiatrists' responses were characterised by hesitancies, or replying with a question rather than an answer. Sometimes they smiled or laughed in responses, indicating that they were embarrassed. They were either reluctant or unable to discuss their patients' experiences with them.

Hearing Voices Network groups are user led, although professional allies can be involved in advisory roles, or occasionally as co-facilitators with voice hearers. The user-led nature of the groups is essential to ensure that members are free to explore their experiences within their own frames of reference, and to learn from each other. Sharing informal narratives of recovery and transformation offers great hope to those starting the search for meaning. They also have an important social action function by empowering members to spread the ethos of acceptance of voices into wider society. This promotes the civil rights of people who hear voices, challenging stigma and promoting citizenship (May & Longden, 2010). This work operates locally, nationally and internationally, as can be seen in Eleanor Longden's highly successful TED (Technology, Education, Design) talk about her personal story of voice hearing[3] (Longden, 2013). The international work of the movement is now coordinated by Intervoice, with groups across the globe in over twenty countries, including two in Palestine (see http://www.intervoiceonline.org/about-intervoice/national-networks-2). In November 2013 at the World Hearing Voices Congress in Australia, the Melbourne Hearing Voices Declaration set out a commitment to building support for the hearing voices approach within mental health systems (http://www.prahranmission.org.au/declaration).

The work of Romme and Escher has important implications for the efforts of mental health professionals to help people who hear voices and have strange beliefs. There are four important lessons to be gained from their work. The first is the openness and receptiveness that characterises Romme and Escher's approach. It is not possible to work in the way they do without first of all setting to one side professional expertise, scientific models and paradigms. Only then is it possible to engage with voice hearers' understandings, no matter how unformed or inchoate they may be. This openness in part originated in their honesty in recognising the limitations and failings of conventional psychiatry to help many people who hear voices. It also originated in their compassionate curiosity about suffering human beings, something that lies at the heart of all good medical practice. In addition they demonstrate a genuine acceptance of the reality of the experience as far as the individual voice hearer was concerned.

Second, their work reveals a degree of humility in recognising the limits of psychiatry. The possibility that there might be people in society who hear voices, but who were able to live and cope with them without recourse to psychiatric help, was a truly remarkable insight for a psychiatrist to have thirty years ago. It contradicts a widely held assumption in psychiatry, that psychiatric disorders and psychopathology are universals applicable to all people at all times. It took vision and courage to think otherwise; to imagine that there might be people who hear voices and hold strange beliefs, but who do not see themselves as psychiatric patients. Once Marius Romme and his patient appeared on television and the

---

3. Accessed on 20th September 2013 at http://www.ted.com/talks/eleanor_longden_the_voices_in_my_head.html

public responses indicated that about a third of voice hearers had never seen a psychiatrist, then radical new possibilities became available for voice hearers within psychiatry.

Third, Romme and Escher's work started out as a public alliance between psychiatric patient and psychiatrist. Once it gained momentum, and voice hearers discovered the liberatory possibilities of sharing their experiences and stories through peer support, as well as new positive identities as voice hearers, Romme and Escher stepped back and let voice hearers take control of the movement for themselves. Peer support and self-advocacy are the most important elements of HVN groups. Community development workers and mental health professionals have a valuable role to play in helping to start groups up and supporting their work from a distance, but there their role ends. The idea of 'professionally led' HVN groups is a contradiction in terms, and raises the dangers of colonisation.

Finally, their work draws attention to the reality of voices from the voice hearer's perspective. To the person who hears voices, the experience is a real phenomenon. If we are to accept the reality of voices it is necessary first to set aside our own assumptions, beliefs and understandings about the nature of experience. Only then is it possible to approach the experience of voice hearing from an atheoretical position. This gives rise to a completely different type of information about voices, which then become understandable through the person's life history, just as we say in the case of Danni in Chapter 9.

Soteria

The work of HVN has an important message: that recovery from psychosis is not only possible without recourse to psychiatric expertise and knowledge, but that for many people psychiatry constitutes a barrier to recovery. This approach is embedded in trusting human relationships, of friendship, understanding and mutuality. If you like, it is an example of the human non-specific factors we considered in Chapter 3. This makes it extremely difficult to demonstrate its effectiveness through the scientific methods of evidence-based medicine. The closest we get to 'evidence' are the stories of recovery found on Hearing Voices Network and Intervoice websites, or in anthologies such as Romme et al (2009). In contrast, the effectiveness of Soteria has been evaluated.

Soteria was the name given by the American psychiatrist, Loren Mosher[4] to a residential facility which opened in San Jose, California, in 1971. It comes from the Greek word for 'deliverance' or 'salvation'. It was set up to help people who

---

4. Loren Mosher sadly died in 2004, shortly after visiting England, where he spoke about Soteria in London, Birmingham and Bradford. His lectures inspired those who attended to set up Soteria Network UK (http://www.soterianetwork.org.uk), dedicated to supporting local groups who are trying to set up Soteria-inspired facilities. At the time of writing there are groups in Bradford, Brighton, Derby and Manchester.

had received a diagnosis of schizophrenia to move towards recovery without, or with the minimal use of, neuroleptic medication. However, when he set the project up, Loren Mosher was Chief of the National Institute for Mental Health's Center for Studies of Schizophrenia, and Soteria doubled up as a research project aimed at investigating the effectiveness of the approach.

The House

The original Soteria House was in a multicultural working-class district of San Jose, California. It had twelve rooms, and accommodated up to six residents, two full-time staff members, volunteers and helpers. It was furnished to provide a comfortable 'domestic' ambience. The intention was to have a roughly equal mix of residents in crisis, and other residents who were sufficiently advanced on the path to recovery to act as helpers. Staff were non-professional (with the exception of part-time input from a house psychiatrist), and were selected for their ability to contribute to a safe, supportive, warm and relaxed environment. Everyone, staff and residents, shared domestic duties.

Staff were selected on the basis of having no preconceived views about the 'causes' of psychosis. Mosher attached considerable importance to selecting people with the personal qualities that he and his colleagues considered necessary for working with people who were acutely psychotic. Their experience indicated that having a professional background in this area of work was not necessary:

> One reason we recommend that degree and relevant experience not be sole selection criteria for work in community mental health programs is the wish to avoid, as much as feasible, staff who have been taught tightly organized, over-explanatory theories of the etiology or treatment of disturbed and disturbing behavior. We believe it is easier to interact with individual mad persons from an interpersonal phenomenologic[5] stance (i.e., open, accepting, without preconceptions) if previous learning does not have to be unlearned. (Mosher & Burti, 1994: 169–70)

This statement resonates strongly with the values that lie beneath the work of Romme and Escher, especially the importance they attach to locking theories and models away in the cupboard when working with voice hearers. The personal attributes of staff are more important than professional background and expertise. These attributes include a strong sense of self, the ability to tolerate uncertainty, open-mindedness and non-judgementalness, practicality, empathy, hopefulness, humour, humility, and an ability to think contextually (Mosher & Burti, 1994: 169).

When the house was first set up, there were three rules. Violence to self and others was prohibited. Visitors were allowed only with the prior permission of

---

5. Elsewhere I have described the main features of Mosher's interpersonal phenomenology, and compared it with the scientific-objective method in psychiatry (Thomas, 2013).

the residents. No street drugs were permitted in the house, and although alcohol was permitted, it was occasionally banned if someone in the house was abusing it. There was no rule prohibiting sexual relationships between residents, but an 'incest taboo' prohibiting sexual relations between staff and residents was introduced shortly after the house opened. This followed the admission of a young female resident who was vulnerable, disorganised, and sexually disinhibited with staff.

Loren Mosher's view of psychosis

Mosher *et al* (2004) set out a view of psychosis that helps us to understand how a therapeutic milieu aimed at helping people to recover should function. In this view, an acute psychosis ('schizophrenia') is an altered state of consciousness in response to a crisis. This is associated with a sense of loss of self brought about by fragmentation of the personality:

> As modalities of experience blend with one another, inner being becomes difficult to distinguish from outer, ambivalence reigns, and the disturbed person's terror is reinforced by others in his/her environment, who feel their own sanity challenged by the events taking place. Mystical experiences are common in this state beyond reason. (Mosher *et al*, 2004: 11)

Mystical experiences were regarded as metaphorically comprehensible, a task made easier by the 1970's Californian *Zeitgeist*. Indeed they make an analogy between the role of staff working with people in psychosis and that of a 'trip guide', someone who accompanies a person experimenting with LSD, but who doesn't necessarily take the drug themselves.

From this emerges the possibility of growth and reintegration. Staff were encouraged to engage with residents' feelings, beliefs and experiences, and to see in them the potential for psychological growth and reconstitution. This was facilitated by a strong view that the experiences of psychosis were simply extreme expressions of what are fundamentally human experiences. This view was further reinforced by staff values that respected individuality, tolerance, equality, and which resisted any pressure that people should conform. If we see the experiences of a psychotic person as symptoms of a disease, there is the risk that we negate the person. If their experiences are assumed to be meaningless, we place them beyond the ability of others to engage with them. This relegates the person to the status of a non-person. Instead,

> Soteria saw the individual experiencing a 'schizophrenic' reaction as someone to *be with* – tolerated, interacted with, indeed appreciated. (*ibid*: 12)

The emergence of a psychosis also affects the social environment, family, friends, work, in which that individual is embedded, so it was important to work with this social environment, not in a way that attributed blame, but in a way that fostered recovery within the person's social environment.

Soteria and medication

Loren Mosher famously resigned from the American Psychiatric Association (APA), claiming that its acronym more accurately reflected its metamorphosis into the American Psychopharmacological Association (Mosher, 1998), but it is wrong to assume that he was completely opposed to the use of medication in psychosis. He objected to the disingenuousness of a system whose spurious theories benefited the pharmaceutical industry, whilst claiming scientific validity. But he was a pragmatist and he recognised that some people benefited from medication, so he used neuroleptics and benzodiazepines sparingly and judiciously. The overriding considerations in his use of medication, however, were first that it had to be with the full consent of the person, and then his view that the medium- and long-term use of neuroleptic drugs could impede recovery.

The basis for this view was his conviction that twenty years of research (from the late 1950s on) had yielded no evidence that neuroleptics cured schizophrenia (see Chapter 3), whereas it was well-established that they caused extremely distressing, sometimes irreversible, toxic effects. For the first six weeks in Soteria all residents were as far as possible drug-free in order to give interpersonal phenomenology a chance to work. During this period medication was used only to reduce otherwise uncontrollable violence or self-destructive impulses, or to damp down unremitting psychological distress that had not responded to interpersonal phenomenology. It was also used if residents specifically requested it. During the first five years of operation, fewer than 10 per cent of residents received continuous medication. Mosher also occasionally used benzodiazepines for the short-term management of severe anxiety and sleep disturbances. There is evidence that these drugs are as effective as neuroleptics in the short-term management of schizophrenia (Wolkowitz & Pickar, 1991).

Interpersonal phenomenology and being with

Like most young doctors Loren Mosher struggled early in his career to come to terms with the existential problems raised by his first encounters with the reality of death. He describes his powerlessness to do anything to help his dying patients, other than trying to understand their experiences of it – something his medical education had ill-prepared him for (Mosher, 1999). So he turned to existential phenomenology in an attempt to grapple with the dilemmas posed by his awareness of mortality. He discovered Rollo May et al's *Existence* (1958) and this led him to the work of a number of existential/phenomenological writers, including Allers (1961), Boss (1963), Husserl (1967), Sartre (1958), and Tillich (1952). In an era of theory-driven rationalism he was attracted by their open-minded, non-categorising approach to the problems of suffering. He spent a year at the Tavistock Clinic (1966–1967) to undergo psychoanalytic training, and visited R.D. Laing at Kingsley Hall. Laing (1960, 1967) was of course the pre-eminent authority on existentialism and madness, and it was here that Mosher began to think about how a community-based social milieu could facilitate the reintegration of psychologically disintegrated individuals, whilst minimising the harm of institutional care and psychiatric drugs.

Although Laing's influence is apparent in his work, it is important to state that Mosher was not an 'antipsychiatrist' (a term that in any case Laing rejected; see Beveridge, 2011, especially p. 317). Mosher was sceptical of models of 'schizophrenia' because he believed they stood in the way of a phenomenological view of psychosis (Aderhold *et al*, 2007). He regarded psychosis as a way of coping with traumatic events that caused the person to retreat from reality. He saw the experiences of psychosis – terror, irrationality and mystical experiences – as extremes of ordinary human responses.

In his early career he worked with Sullivanian analysts at Harvard. Harry Stack Sullivan pioneered psychoanalytic work with people suffering from schizophrenia (Sullivan, 1931). He was also one of the first to recognise the value of employing people with no specialist mental health background in working with psychotic people. Freda Fromm-Reichmann (1948) was another important influence. She was another pioneer of psychoanalysis in schizophrenia, famously depicted in the novel *I Never Promised You a Rose Garden*, written by survivor Joanne Greenberg under the pen name of Hannah Green. The influence of the object-relations school of psychoanalysis is also apparent in his work, especially that of Ronald Fairbairn, the Edinburgh psychoanalyst who was primarily interested in the relationships *between* people, not the drives *within* them. Goffman's work on institutionalisation was another influence, along with Erikson's developmental view of human growth and the importance of crises in progressing from one stage of development to the next. A common strand running through these influences is the view that the main problem in 'schizophrenia' is the differentiation and growth of the self from others, especially within the family. Finally, and most significantly, his work is grounded in a phenomenological tradition that had been translated into practice by R.D. Laing, David Cooper and Meddard Boss. Indeed, one reason for setting up Soteria was to create a therapeutic environment capable of testing Laing's theories about madness.

From the outset, Soteria was inspired by the philosophical tradition of Kingsley Hall, where the Philadelphia Association opened a community to help people experiencing psychosis. A belief common to Kingsley Hall and Soteria was the '… innovative conception of the psychotic experience – usually viewed as irrational and mystifying – as one which, if treated in an open, nonjudgmental way, could be valid and comprehensible' (Mosher *et al*, 2004: 4). Unlike Kingsley Hall, which eventually closed in response to pressure from local residents, staff in Soteria worked hard to accommodate the local community.

Being with

'Being with' was the main way of engaging and working with people experiencing psychosis in Soteria, and can be thought of as the practical outcome of Mosher's theory of interpersonal phenomenology. It was the closest thing to an intervention, although it would be quite wrong to describe it as such. It originated in Mosher's readings of existentialism and his interpretation of phenomenology. In practical terms it developed out of the vigil used by Rappaport and Silverman (Rappaport *et al*, 1978), and used in Soteria as a means for interceding in the psychotic process. Rappaport and Silverman's vigil involved pairs of staff (usually one female, one male) spending consecutive shifts of between four to eight hours with the person in crisis, in a comfortable room set aside for the process. The staff had no other demands on their time, so they could spend uninterrupted periods with the person. If the individual wanted to walk about outside they were free to do so accompanied by staff. It was, literally, a case of being with the person continually. Experience indicated that this proved to be a very effective way of engaging with people in acute psychosis.

Being with, '... the basic mode of the Soteria process' (Mosher *et al*, 2004: 169), grew out of the vigil, and took place in three stages. First, staff established and maintained continuous contact with the psychotic person (bonding). The second stage focused on developing ordinary social interactions between the resident and other residents and staff. The third stage encouraged the resident to initiate and engage in activities more generally within and outside the house. This might include involvement in domestic and leisure activities.

Mosher *et al* (2004) provide a detailed description of 'being with' through the vigil of a young man, Chuck. This took place over a period of six weeks, during which time members of staff stayed with him for extended periods of hours and days. During these periods of intense focus, staff set their own needs for sustenance and sleep to one side. This would be impossible to achieve in a conventionally organised acute admissions unit, where staff are constantly changing in the endless cycle of shifts. Reliance on agency and bank staff would confound any opportunity to establish relationships based in being with.

From the descriptions of how staff related to residents in Soteria it is clear that being with involved much more than simply sitting with someone for eight-hour shifts. After all, this happens today on many acute psychiatric inpatient units under the name of 'close observation'. Being with in Soteria demanded a quite specific form of engagement between staff and residents. Some of this was achieved through close physical proximity, and the judicious use of touch and physical contact. It also involved a non-judgemental approach to the experience of another person. This meant that staff had to be open to the world as the resident found it. This openness involved an acceptance of the reality of the other person's experiences, without having to do anything about it, like trying to convince them they were wrong to have the experiences they had. Only from this position, which is a form of concern, is it possible to start the process of entering into the other person's world. There are similarities between being with and Prouty's work on pre-therapy, which is also grounded in existential philosophy (see Prouty *et al*, 2002).

Evaluation of Soteria and Minimal Medication Approaches

At the beginning of this chapter I pointed out that Loren Mosher's work has had little recent influence on mental health services. That is certainly the case in the UK, although the Soteria Network continues to promote his ideas and support local groups who want to set up Soteria-inspired facilities. Elsewhere, Soteria houses survive in Switzerland (Berne), Hungary and Alaska. Loren Mosher faced considerable hostility and antagonism from the psychiatric establishment in the USA, which was falling ever more deeply under the influence of biological psychiatry and the pharmaceutical industry. The idea that it is possible to help people through psychosis without using medication simply didn't sit well with the financial interests of the pharmaceutical industry, and those influential psychiatrists whose careers and professional interests were closely aligned with the industry. His funding was withdrawn and Soteria closed in 1982. Despite this, Mosher managed to publish his initial evaluation of Soteria. In addition, the last twenty years have witnessed the growth of a number of community-based systems of support for people who experience psychosis, particularly in Scandinavia, which share in common with Soteria the idea that it is possible to help people recover from psychosis with minimal or no medication, and by engaging with the stories that they, and their families, have about their experiences.

Mosher *et al* (1995) compared the outcome of Soteria with conventional psychiatric inpatient care for acute psychosis (schizophrenia) at six weeks, but here I will focus on the outcome at two years, since we know from Chapter 3 that a major weakness of treatment studies of schizophrenia is that they rarely extend beyond six weeks. Bola and Mosher (2003) describe the outcome for the subjects described in Mosher *et al* (1995). This study reports the findings of two cohorts. The first consisted of 79 patients in a quasi-experimental design where consecutive admissions were allocated to the two treatment conditions (Soteria versus standard inpatient care) on the basis of available space. The second consisted of a cohort of 100 patients randomly assigned to Soteria or standard inpatient care. In the Soteria group, medications were not used routinely during the first six weeks of treatment. However, there were explicit criteria for their short-term use during this period; 76 per cent (62 of 82) received no antipsychotic medications during the initial 45-day period. After six weeks, decisions about medication were made at a treatment conference that included the client, staff and the consulting psychiatrist.

Outcome measures included readmissions, measures of global psycho-pathology and improvement, living status (independently or with peers), work status, and the social function scale of the Brief Psychiatric Rating Scale (BPRS). The number of subjects completing the two-year trial was 129, and statistical analysis was undertaken for completing subjects (129), endpoint subjects, and for completing subjects adjusted for differential drop-out. The superiority of Soteria noted in the earlier, six-week outcome study (Mosher *et al*, 1995) was maintained at two years. The earlier study found significant and comparable symptomatic improvements in both Soteria and conventional inpatient care, despite the fact that the Soteria group received far less medication.

They discuss the components of Soteria that might contribute to its effectiveness, and single out the quality of the therapeutic relationships as being the key:

> Within staff–resident relationships, an integrative context was created to promote understanding and the discovery of meaning within the subjective experience of psychosis. Residents were encouraged to acknowledge precipitating events and emotions and to discuss and eventually place them into perspective within the continuity of their life and social network. (Bola & Mosher, 2003: 226)

Another important factor was Soteria's social networks, which provided a surrogate family for residents, as well as a client-centred post-discharge support network, which provided peer support for community reintegration. For example, peers helped each other to organise accommodation, educational opportunities, work and social activities.

Calton *et al* (2008) undertook a systematic review to examine the findings of all controlled trials undertaken to assess the efficacy of Soteria for people diagnosed with schizophrenia. They identified twenty published evaluations of 'Soteria' that met their initial inclusion criteria. Of these, three (the two studies described above, and the Soteria Berne study, see, for example, Ciompi *et al*, 1992) met formal criteria for inclusion in terms of experimental design (in essence RCT). These three studies, involving 223 subjects, showed modest benefits for the active treatment group, with five of the US outcomes and two of the Swiss achieving significance at the 0.05 level in favour of the Soteria approach. However, in the US studies, the direction of effects for the remaining comparisons favoured Soteria. This is important because for an ineffective treatment you would expect an equal number of comparisons to favour each treatment. This evidence suggests that Soteria is at least as effective as traditional hospital-based treatment, but without the use of neuroleptic drugs.

Work in Scandinavia, whilst not directly influenced by Soteria, focuses on helping people experiencing acute psychosis in the community, with minimal use of neuroleptic drugs. Alanen *et al* (1991) have developed the needs-adapted approach to helping people suffering from schizophrenia in Turku, Finland. This begins with a joint meeting between the patient, family and team members as soon as possible after admission into the project. The purpose of this is to achieve a shared understanding of the problem, and especially to help the family to see the problem as a shared one that arises from difficulties they have had in living together as a family, rather than seeing it as an 'illness' occurring in a single member. Subsequently a number of psychotherapeutic options may be offered, including family therapy, marital therapy, individual therapy, or a therapeutic community. Medication is used if necessary to help the patient to become accessible, but its use is limited to the minimum amount required to achieve this, and for the shortest period of time possible. The use of long-term medication is avoided. In the first year of the service evaluation, 27 of 31 people received neuroleptic drugs, but this proportion fell to 13 of 25 in the second year. It is difficult to compare their evaluation with other studies because they did not randomly allocate patients.

Cullberg *et al* (2002) have described the evaluation of the Swedish Parachute project, which is influenced by Soteria and the Needs-Adapted model. The aims of the Parachute project are to maximise elements the authors considered to contribute to good outcome, including the avoidance of high doses of neuroleptic medication, continuity of care, focusing on first-episode patients, and the avoidance of hospital care. The project operates according to the following principles:

1. Rapid intervention in the patient's home, after first contact with the clinic.
2. A crisis intervention model that recognises the importance of staff continuity. Depending on needs, psychotherapy (dynamic and cognitive) may subsequently be used.
3. Regular family meetings involving the patient to understand conflicts, and to help the family develop a shared understanding of the psychosis using the vulnerability–stress view.
4. Continuing access to the team over a five-year period.
5. The use of neuroleptic drugs in low optimised doses. As far as possible neuroleptics were avoided for the first 1–2 weeks, and benzodiazepines used for anxiety or insomnia if necessary.
6. Access to small-scale (3 to 6 residents), low-stimulus overnight care if necessary, if the family and or the patient found it difficult to cope. This crisis house was used only for first-episode patients.

The evaluation of the service recruited 253 patients, 69 per cent of whose outcomes were compared with two other groups of people continuously treated as inpatients (n = 71 and 64) one year later. This was not a randomised controlled trial. During the first week, significantly fewer Parachute patients with a diagnosis of schizophrenia spent time in hospital than the control groups. Fewer Parachute patients received neuroleptic drugs (32% vs. 51% and 56%) than controls. At one year, fewer Parachute patients were on neuroleptics (62%) than one of the control groups (62% and 89%). Just over half (54%) of the Parachute patients used inpatient care, for a mean of 12 days, compared with 68 and 62 per cent of the comparison groups (means 30 and 22 days respectively). Although there were no differences in clinical symptoms between the three groups at one year, the Parachute group and one of the comparison groups had significantly better global assessment of function (GAF) scores, which represent a combination of clinical symptoms and social function. Access to the crisis house was associated with higher GAF scores, and patient satisfaction was higher in the Parachute group.

Open dialogue

There are close similarities between Soteria and Open Dialogue (OD), a system of community-based care developed over the last thirty years by Jaakko Seikkula and colleagues in Finland. This is based on a form of psychotherapy influenced by the ideas and work of the Russian pedagogical school of the first half of the twentieth century – particularly the literary critic Mikhail Bakhtin, the Marxist philosopher of language Valentin Voloshinov, and psychologist Lev Vygotsky. Although the theoretical basis is somewhat different from that of Alanen's work and Soteria, there are broad similarities between the approaches. Seikkula *et al* (2006) have described the principal therapeutic elements. The service offers an emergency response in the community to integrate outpatient care with the patient (their expression) and the family's daily activities, the objective being to avoid hospitalisation. The patient is involved right from the outset no matter how psychotic she or he might be. A social network perspective is adopted, which means that the patient, family, and other key members of the patient's social network are immediately involved. Extended social networks might include employers and representatives of statutory organisations like housing, education or health. The staff member who first takes the referral is responsible for coordinating the first meeting in the patient's home, but the team then takes responsibility for the subsequent care, even if it is necessary at some point for this to take place in hospital. This is important for psychological continuity. Meetings take place every day for the first ten to twelve days. This is important in developing the trust necessary to handle the uncertainty that may arise when helping someone who is psychotic in the community.

The final element is dialogism, based in the work of Bakhtin (1981). The purpose of this is to encourage dialogue and promote change in the family. The dialogue creates new understandings between the participants. This is achieved by following the themes raised by the family, and the ways in which they communicate. Another important influence is the work of systemic therapists, although there are important differences: 'The aim in OD is to create a joint space for new language, where things can begin to have different meanings ...'

(Seikkula *et al*, 2006: 216).There are also affinities between OD and the narrative approach to family therapy of White and Epston (1990).

Seikkula *et al* (2003, 2006) have reported very favourable outcomes for acute psychosis at two-year follow-up. The group has recently published the findings of a ten-year outcome for people with first-episode psychosis treated by the service, covering three cohorts recruited at different times (Seikkula *et al*, 2006). A two-year follow-up over two consecutive periods (1992–93 and 1994–97) found that 82 percent of patients had no residual psychotic symptoms. Over 80 per cent had returned to full-time employment. Only one-third of people within these cohorts had used neuroleptics. A third cohort (2003–2005) was studied to replicate these earlier results. What was striking about this study was that the incidence of schizophrenia appeared to have fallen. Fewer people with the diagnosis were identified, and their mean age was significantly lower. Duration of untreated psychosis had shortened to three weeks and the outcomes remained as good as for the first two periods. They concluded that Open Dialogue may also have an influence on the incidence of severe mental health problems in a community.

Barriers to Soteria and minimal medication approaches

Given the evidence that Soteria is at least as effective as conventional psychiatric inpatient care, why has it not been adopted more widely? First, Soteria demedicalised psychosis. It rejected the notion that 'schizophrenia' is a medical condition, but it did so when the influence of psychotherapeutic and social interventions for psychosis was waning. The publication in 1980 of *DSM-III* marked the beginning of a barren period for non-scientific ways of engaging with psychosis. The rise of evidence-based medicine (EBM), and the insistence that interventions must have their efficacy established through controlled trials, have made it even more difficult to argue the case for Soteria. There is a fundamental paradigmatic conflict between the randomisation necessary for EBM, and the emphasis on personal choice that is central to Soteria. Mosher *et al* (2004) give an excellent account of this tension.

Second, there are political factors. Mosher *et al* (2004) describe the political pressures that Soteria encountered in the 1970s and 80s. Some of these persist today, such as the insistence that Soteria conforms to the scientific requirements of evaluation through EBM. There is also the political resistance of a psychiatric profession dominated by the interests of the pharmaceutical industry. But today, in addition, there is the perceived 'dangerousness' of people identified as suffering from schizophrenia, and the perceived role played by medication in 'managing' this risk. Technological psychiatry has created the myth that schizophrenia is a disease amenable to treatment with drugs. Against the context of the risk culture in which we live, this is a powerful factor maintaining the dominance of technological psychiatry (Moncrieff, 1997). The proposition that psychosis does not require treatment with drugs is likely to encounter the question of risk.

The third barrier is the waning influence of psychodynamic and social ways of understanding and responding to madness, although this in turn relates to the rise of positivism in psychiatry. Soteria was explicitly set up to work in a way that did not conform to positivist psychiatry. In addition, since the 1960s and the work of Laing, the influence of existentialism (an important branch of twentieth-century continental philosophy) has waned in British psychiatry. This in part may be because British philosophical thought has been dominated by the analytic tradition.

The fourth barrier is the challenge to professional authority posed by Soteria, which explicitly preferred staff who had no specific mental health knowledge or training. Indeed, former residents who had been through Soteria were frequently employed as staff members. Thus the widespread adoption of Soteria would represent a significant threat to the professional power of psychiatrists, mental health nurses, and other professional groups. In addition to this, staff are expected to work in much more flexible ways than the shift system on conventional in-patient units.

Recommended Reading

Bola, J. & Mosher, L.R. (2003) Treatment of acute psychosis without neuroleptics: Two-year outcomes from the Soteria project. *Journal of Nervous and Mental Disease, 191,* 219–29.

Calton, T., Ferriter, M., Husband, N. & Spandler, H. (2008) A systematic review of the Soteria paradigm for the treatment of people diagnosed with schizophrenia. *Schizophrenia Bulletin, 34,* 181–92.

Corstens, D. & Longden, E. (2013) The origins of voices: Links between life history and voice hearing in a survey of 100 cases. *Psychosis: Psychological, Social and Integrative Approaches, 5,* 270–85. doi: 10.1080/17522439.2013.816337.

Martindale, B. & Summers, A. (2013) The psychodynamics of psychosis. *Advances in Psychiatric Treatment, 19,* 124 –31.

Mosher, L.R., Hendrix, V. & Fort, D. (2004) *Soteria: Through madness to deliverance.* Bloomington, IN: XLibris.

Romme, M. & Escher, S. (1993) The new approach: A Dutch experiment. In M. Romme & S. Escher (Eds.) *Accepting Voices* (pp. 11–27). London: MIND Publications.

Romme, M., Escher, S., Dillon, J., Corstens, D. & Morris, M. (2009) *Living with Voices: 50 stories of recovery.* Ross-on-Wye: PCCS Books.

Seikkula, J., Aaltonen, J., Alakare, B., Haarakangas, H., Keranen, J. & Lehtinen, K. (2006) Five-year experience of first-episode nonaffective psychosis in open-dialogue approach: Treatment principles, follow-up outcomes, and two case studies. *Psychotherapy Research, 16,* 214–28.

Readers should also be aware of the work of the International Society for Psychological and Social Approaches to Psychosis and their journal *Psychosis*: www.isps.org

Community Development and Diversity in Psychiatric Practice   13

In Chapter 5 we examined the troubled relationship between people from black and minority ethnic (BME) communities and mental health services. Brian's story in Chapter 10 added much more detail to this relationship in terms of the interweaving narratives of racism, distress and entanglement with psychiatric services experienced by a young African-Caribbean man. The experiences of people from these communities in mental health services differ markedly from those of people in the majority white communities. These differences depend to some extent upon which particular community the person comes from. Black people are more likely to be diagnosed as suffering from schizophrenia. Black and South Asian people are more likely to be detained under the Mental Health Act than white people, and both BME groups are more likely to receive physical treatment than to be offered psychological help. A recent systematic review of nineteen studies found that black patients were 3.83 times more likely to be detained than whites, and South Asian patients were 2.06 times more likely to be detained (Singh *et al*, 2007). It is, therefore, hardly surprising that high levels of fear, suspicion and mistrust exist between BME communities and mental health services.

There is also evidence that black and South Asian people have different ways of understanding conditions such as schizophrenia (McCabe & Priebe, 2004) and depression (Lavender *et al*, 2006; Bowl, 2007). In broad terms white people appear to favour psychological explanations for depression or biological ones for schizophrenia. In contrast, South Asian and black people see both conditions as having spiritual, supernatural or social origins. It is likely that these differences are related to different cultural understandings of the self. Since Plato, Western thought has been dominated by an individualistic and interiorised view of the self. The origin and development of this notion of selfhood has been explored in great detail by the Canadian philosopher Charles Taylor (1989). South Asian and African cultures appear to understand the self in terms of social and family bonds and connections. Either way, these different understandings of psychosis and distress have implications for the types of responses and support that we might envisage.

The situation is further complicated by the fact that particular groups in society are extremely difficult to engage. Those responsible for commissioning mental health services may be keen to discover what sort of help people want, but the difficulty is that consultation exercises aimed at accessing the views of people who use services and their families tend to access only a limited range of views. Most commissioners will naturally turn to local service user, survivor and advocacy groups if they want to find out what sort of help people in their locality want, but in Chapter 11 we saw that the service user and survivor movement has found it extremely difficult to engage with the views and opinions of people from BME communities. More generally there are certain groups within BME communities, especially women, older people and young people, whose views are particularly difficult to access. Their opinions about what may be helpful for them at times of crisis remain largely invisible to those who need to know about them.

The question that arises is how to overcome this invisibility. Is it possible to access and work with people in these hard-to-access communities? Are there ways of working in and with communities to identify groups and individuals who are concerned about mental health and wellbeing? This is a matter of social justice, for as long as those responsible for commissioning and delivering mental health services continue to assume that the needs of people who are members of BME communities are no different from the needs of the majority, then black and South Asian people will continue to experience inequalities in mental health. In this chapter I will examine the role of community development (CD) and community development workers (CDWs) in tackling the questions above. First, I will describe community development, and then provide an example through the work of a project specifically set up to work with BME communities, Sharing Voices Bradford.

Community Development

Most mental health interventions these days focus on the individual. In Chapter 2 we saw that the technological paradigm assumes that psychosis and distress arise through biological or psychological dysfunction in the person. A consequence of this is that it downplays the importance of social, cultural and other contexts. In Chapter 3 we saw that interventions based on this paradigm are intended to rectify these dysfunctions, either through drugs or individual psychotherapies of one sort or another. But Chapters 4 and 5 examined the role of contexts of adversity, socio-economic status, oppression, discrimination and racism, in understanding the experiences of psychosis and distress. These contexts shape the stories and experiences of individuals, but they are also shared by large numbers of people. We may think of these larger numbers or groups as communities that have particular experiences in common. This opens up the possibility of a role for community development.

Community development represents a different way of thinking about and responding to distress. This is because the focus is not primarily on the individual (although it may include elements of individual support) but on the groups and networks in which individuals exist. Alison Gilchrist, an experienced CDW and trainer, writes:

> Community development is distinguished from social work and allied welfare professions through its commitment to *collective ways of addressing problems*. Community development helps community members to identify unmet needs, to undertake research on the problems and present possible solutions. (Gilchrist, 2004: 34, emphasis added)

There are, to put it very simply, two main ways in which we can think about communities – geographically, or as communities of interest. Geographical communities are identifiable by virtue of sharing a location in a particular part of a town or a city, such as a neighbourhood, a group of streets, a suburb or an estate. Communities of interest exist in diffusely distributed groups who may be found throughout a country, or internationally. They share a particular set of experiences, concerns and interests. This is what most people refer to when they speak, for example, about the black community or the Muslim community. Communities of interest cover a wide range of groups, many of whom share, in common, experiences of exclusion and oppression by the majority, for example, lesbian, gay, bisexual and transgender (LGBT) communities, asylum seekers and refugees. There may be considerable difference and diversity within these more diffuse groupings, but in broad terms they involve particular features that tie group membership to personal identity in powerful ways, often involving religious belief, culture, language, lifestyle, the ways in which sexuality is expressed, and values. Another important feature of communities of interest is that they are often numerically small, and within the population as a whole they may be seen as minorities. Historically such groups have found it extremely difficult to have their interests and preferences taken seriously by the majority. And even within these minority groups there are yet more minorities who share particular perspectives and experiences that contrast with those of the dominant minority, for example, the position and experiences of South Asian women within their communities, or LGBT people in African and African-Caribbean communities. This is particularly important in health care. Their position as minorities also tends to be associated with particular experiences, some of which may be positive and affirmative, and some of which may be negative and oppressive. Examples of the latter include racism, homophobia and Islamophobia.

Community development is a way of working with groups and individuals who are members of geographical communities and communities of interest. The values that underpin community development in Britain are deeply rooted in our history and culture. They include the work of religious groups like the Quakers, the work of the Welsh social reformer Robert Owen (one of the founders of socialism and the Co-operative movement in England), and the philanthropy that gave rise to the Mechanics' Institutes, and subsequently the Workers' Educational Association, both of which sought the advancement of working-class men and women. Another important strand linking community development to health is to be found in the work of the Peckham Experiment, which ran from 1926 to 1950. This was set up by two doctors, George Scott Williamson and Innes Pearse, who recognised that health promotion depended on families and communities, not individuals. Local families paid a small annual subscription to attend the centre, which Williamson and Pearse set up in an old industrial building in Peckham, London. There they had health check-ups, access to locally grown food, and a wide range of social activities. The project demonstrated that people thrive when they are given the freedom to make choices about their activities. Furthermore, when they are given opportunities and resources through their communities to enable them to grow, they can then become active in their communities for the benefit of others. This idea is at the heart of community development.[1]

After World War Two community development became an important feature of social work, where it had a preventative role. But the political transformations that came about in the 1960s, especially the rise to prominence of civil and human rights, resulted in community development becoming politicised. In England and Scotland, community development supported the welfare rights movement, and also worked to engage ordinary people in planning public services. At the same time community development (CD) was influenced by the experiences of the disability movement and the work of black activists and communities in challenging the assumptions and power structures that excluded them from society. Thus CD fell under the influence of a variety of equality perspectives, making it more committed to the engagement, participation and empowerment of marginalised groups (Gilchrist, 2004).

Until recently, the work of CDWs was overseen and supported by two organisations, the Community Development Exchange (CDX) and the Federation for Community Development Learning (FDCL). The former was originally established as a charity in 1987, and functioned as a strategic partner with the government. However, it lost its funding in 2011 and closed in 2012 (a fascinating account of the CDX's history and work is available at http://www.iacdglobal.org/files/cdx_retro_paper.pdf).[2] The FCDL, based in Sheffield, sets professional standards and qualifications for CDWs (FCDL, 2009), and gives the following definition of CD:

---

1. For further details, see http://thephf.org/index.php/history/what-was-the-peckham-experiment. Accessed on 11th September 2013.

2. There is a deep irony and cause for anger and scepticism that an organisation that worked hard for a quarter of a century to support and advocate for community development should lose its funding a year after a prime minister, who once spoke endlessly about 'the Big Society' came to power.

Community Development is a long-term value based process which aims to address imbalances in power and bring about change founded on social justice, equality and inclusion.

The process enables people to organise and work together to:
- identify their own needs and aspirations
- take action to exert influence on the decisions which affect their lives
- improve the quality of their own lives, the communities in which they live, and societies of which they are a part. (FCDL, 2009)

Armstrong and Henderson (1992) describe the key characteristics of community development as follows:

- Knowing about community strengths: mapping of needs and resources is an essential first step to working in partnership with local groups and organisations.
- Empowerment: peer groups, increased participation in decision making forums, facilitating community enterprise all enhance scope for self-determination.
- Enhancing community support and networks: community development techniques can facilitate positive networks and help to address oppressive behaviour.
- Contracting: through capacity building on both sides, community development workers can increase opportunities for devolving services to small organisations.
- Training for [statutory sector] staff: this can promote understanding of local communities. (Adapted from Armstrong & Henderson, 1992, cited by Seebohm et al, 2005: 26)

It is worth noting that there are different models of CD, and these models, as Alison Gilchrist (2004) points out, have implications for the relationships between communities and statutory services. The consensus model focuses on self-help and supporting communities to become involved in consultation exercises with providers of statutory services. This model leaves unchallenged imbalances in resources and power. The liberal or pluralist model attaches greater importance to challenging disadvantage and social exclusion by drawing attention to the interests of the participants (communities, statutory services) with particular emphasis on the self-defined needs of communities. The third, or 'radical', model emphasises civil rights and focuses on raising the political consciousness of communities so they can challenge those in authority and work towards the redistribution of power and resources. This model resonates strongly with the critical pedagogy of Paulo Freire (1996). In practice CDWs rely on all three models depending upon the circumstances. It follows that organisations like mental health service providers and commissioners will feel more at home with the consensus model, whereas community groups may want a radical approach. This tension was apparent in the evaluation of the work of Sharing Voices Bradford (Seebohm *et al*, 2005).

The position that Pat Bracken and I adopted when we started working with Bradford's communities was that community development is valuable because it represents a principled and ethical way of working with communities. And the principle at the heart of community development is that of social justice. Prilleltensky (2012) argues convincingly that health and wellbeing are primarily matters of social justice. The fundamental problem with the concept of wellness or wellbeing in medicine and psychology is that it individualises it. It overlooks the extent to which social relationships, of power, domination and inequality, lie at the heart of the way we feel about ourselves. This applies to the way we think about ourselves internally (intrapersonal), our relationships with others (interpersonal), our communities, and different groups within our societies. For this reason, Prilleltensky argues that we should think of wellness primarily in terms of fairness and thus justice, or social justice.

> By placing justice squarely in the center of wellness, I am saying that psychosocial determinants of health are not naturally distributed among people, but rather given to power dynamics, political disputes, and ethical considerations. (Prilleltensky, 2012: 18)

My argument here is that CD offers communities a way of engaging and intervening directly with power dynamics that affect their wellbeing. This ethical, or values-based, argument in support of community development is important because there is little if any empirical evidence for 'effectiveness'. If we set to one side the conceptual problems that surround the empirical evaluation of complex socio-political projects, the position that we advocated in 'postpsychiatry' is that of ethics before effectiveness (Bracken & Thomas, 2001). However, there is work that links social adversity and mental health in ways that enable us to advance the case for community development from a slightly different theoretical perspective, and I want to consider this briefly before I move on to describe in some detail the work of Sharing Voices Bradford. That perspective is the concept of social capital.

Kwame McKenzie and colleagues (2002) point out that the idea that the structure of society has a powerful influence on psychological health is not a new one. They draw attention to the work of the sociologist Emil Durkheim at the end of the nineteenth century, and in the twentieth century the work of Faris and Dunham (1965) who showed that the incidence of schizophrenia was much higher in the poor inner-city districts of Chicago compared with the more prosperous suburbs. In recent years, sociologists and epidemiologists have turned to the concept of social capital to understand the links between poverty and health, especially mental health.

Social capital may be thought of as the glue that binds societies together.

Robert Putnam, the political scientist who has written extensively about social capital, describes it thus:

> By 'social capital', I mean features of social life – networks, norms, and trust
> – that enable participants to act together more effectively to pursue shared
> objectives. (Putnam, 1996, cited by McKenzie *et al*, 2002: 280)

Again, it is important to recognise that social capital is not a property of individuals. It is a property of social groups, such as communities. In reviewing the literature, McKenzie *et al* (2002) describe four main features of social capital: collective efficacy, social trust and reciprocity, participation in voluntary organisations and activities, and social integration for mutual benefit. They write:

> These may bond individuals in groups to each other, bridge divides between
> societal groups or vertically integrate groups with different levels of power and
> influence in a society, leading to social inclusion. (McKenzie *et al*, 2002: 280)

Like community development, it is extremely difficult to evaluate the part played by social capital in health and mental health. It is almost impossible to investigate it scientifically in ways that give rise to 'evidence' in support of its usefulness in health and wellbeing. For example, trust can be both an important constituent of social capital and an outcome of it. This is because social capital, like community development, is a complex phenomenon that is not readily reducible to finite individual components whose relationships and interactions can be isolated and investigated causally through scientific inquiry. Despite this, measures of trust in communities have been developed, and these have figured prominently in health research (see, for example, the work of Wilkinson and Pickett in Chapter 4, this volume). Another difficulty referred to by Kwame McKenzie *et al* (2002) is that most studies of social capital are based on aggregated characteristics of people living in particular areas, and thus concern geographical communities. There have been few if any contextual studies of social capital, for example, in communities of interest such as black people. Contexts are vitally important in this. They point out that homogeneous communities in a particular location may appear to have high levels of social capital, but they may be extremely intolerant of minority groups in their midst. Such minorities are likely to experience marginalisation and persecution unless they are seen to 'conform'.

There has been little research on the relationship between social capital and mental health, but the work of Wilkinson and Pickett (2009) suggests that there are important links. The problem is that these relationships are complex and thus difficult to study empirically, but there is evidence that there are relationships between mental health and social capital. McCulloch (2001) found that men living in areas characterised by low social capital were almost twice as likely to be identified as 'cases' on the General Health Questionnaire (a screening instrument for depression and anxiety widely used in epidemiological research). Other studies have found that higher levels of social capital on college campuses are linked to lower levels of problem behaviours such as binge drinking (Weitzman & Kawachi, 2000), and that ethnic communities that have lower levels of social capital have a higher incidence of schizophrenia (Boydell *et al*, 2001).

There may be a paucity of empirical evidence that community development is an 'effective' intervention, but my argument is that it is a principled and value-based way of helping and supporting people and communities facing adversity. This will become clear from the following account of the work of Sharing Voices Bradford (SVB).

Community Development in Practice – Sharing Voices Bradford[3]

The Sharing Voices Initiative opened in 2002, funded to the extent of £100,000 by Bradford City Teaching Primary Care Trust, but managed under the aegis of the Asian Disability Network (ADN), a leading voluntary sector organisation in the city. In 2004 the project changed its name to Sharing Voices Bradford (SVB) and became a Company Limited by Guarantee, with its own management committee.[4] The membership of the committee included members from the local community (through ADN), and expertise on community development (Paul Henderson), and equality and diversity (Professor Udy Archibong, from Bradford University). In 2006 it successfully applied for charitable status. It has thus functioned independently of the statutory sector since its inception, and continues to do so as a charity. It also adopted an explicitly critical perspective on mainstream psychiatric practice informed by *Postpsychiatry* (Bracken & Thomas, 2001, 2005). In particular it questions the appropriateness of mental health theory and practice based in Western understandings of the self for people from non-Western traditions.

The project was set up to address the mental health inequalities experienced by members of Bradford's BME communities. The population of the city in the 2001 census was just under 468,000, of whom 14.5 per cent described themselves as Pakistani, 2.7 per cent Indian and 1.1 per cent Bangladeshi. The city has a significant Muslim community; at the time it was the fourth highest figure in the country (16.1%). The demography of the city's BME community is evolving, with growing numbers of British-born Muslims, Hindus and Sikhs. However,

---

3. It is impossible in the space available to provide a detailed account of all the project's activities, but further information is available on the website: http://sharingvoices.org.uk/about-us.html

4. Pat Bracken and I were closely involved with the project from its earliest days. We both contributed to the original project proposal. Pat was the first Chair of the organisation, from 2002 to 2004, when he left to work in Ireland and I took over in that capacity.

these figures fail to reveal the way in which the city's BME communities are concentrated in the inner city areas. Two wards, City (the area around the city centre and university, population 18,579) and Manningham (to the north of the city centre, population 16,863) have the highest proportion of people of Pakistani origin at 60 per cent.

The project started work with a manager and two community development workers. The manager, Salma Yasmeen, was a second-generation West Yorkshire Muslim, trained as a community psychiatric nurse, and who had worked previously with Bradford Home Treatment Service. The community development workers were Fozia Sarwar from Manningham, who trained as a CDW, and Jennifer Powell of mixed heritage from Huddersfield, who had trained as a social worker. Jennifer had experience of third-sector community work in mental health, having worked as an outreach worker with the Manchester African and Caribbean Mental Health Services.[5] The project rapidly grew and expanded largely owing to the passion, enthusiasm and commitment of its three workers. In 2005 the manager left to work with the PCT to manage the 'Delivering Race Equality' Focused Implementation Site in Bradford. In her place, Mohammad Shabbir, a second-generation Bradford Muslim with extensive experience in community development (he previously worked with the Asian Disability Network), was appointed.

When the Department of Health launched its policy, Delivering Race Equality, Bradford became one of fifteen focused implementation sites. The policy funded over five hundred CDW posts to implement community engagement aimed at tackling the health inequalities experienced by BME communities. The local health commissioners in Bradford decided to invest most of their share of this money in SVB and Roshni Ghar (a sister organisation working with South Asian women in the town of Keighley)[6] because the project had been running for nearly four years and was being evaluated by the Sainsbury Centre. As a result SVB was able to employ an additional four CDWs to work with asylum seekers and refugees, BME elders, children and young people, and Eastern European diasporas, and to establish a closer working relationship with Roshni Ghar.

Although community development has always been at the heart of its work, the project recognised the importance of working alongside and within statutory mental health services from the outset. This resulted in some tensions within the project. Simply put, CD traditionally does not work with individuals; it works with communities, while on the other hand, mental health practice primarily involves working with individuals. The project recognised that there would be an expectation held by mental health services that it would engage in one-to-one work, and so this was offered. However, the priority from a community development perspective continues to be to help individuals who, for a variety of

5. See http://www.voluntarysectorhealth.org.uk/?q=node/157

6. See http://www.roshnighar.org.uk

complex reasons, have become isolated and disengaged from their communities to become re-engaged.

The project's original aims were:

1. To liaise with statutory service providers and to work together to improve the range and quality of services

2. To stimulate voluntary sector activity in the area of mental health and well-being, by developing capacity within communities and supporting the development of self-help/support groups and networks

3. To stimulate a wider debate locally about the nature of mental health. To contribute to debates nationally/internationally about the nature of mental health, diverse perspectives and ethnicity. (From Seebohm *et al*, 2005: 40)

In October 2004 the Sainsbury Centre for Mental Health (SCMH) began a nine-month evaluation of SVB, using participatory action research (Winter & Munn-Giddings, 2001). Community researchers, many of whom were volunteers with the project, were trained in qualitative research methods. The first stage of the evaluation audited all those in contact with the project in November 2004 (Seebohm *et al*, 2005). Of the 125 people who completed audit forms, 41 per cent were involved in one of the six peer-support groups, 14 per cent received support on a one-to-one basis, and 14 per cent were volunteers. The rest had participated in workshops or other activities. The majority of people (about three-fifths of the total) identified themselves as Pakistani. It is worth noting that about a third of those in contact with the project were aged less than 25 years, and about 60 per cent were women with childcare responsibilities. This suggests that with the exception of older people, the project was successful in working with difficult-to-access groups. Only two-fifths of participants had used specialist mental health services, whereas two-thirds had consulted a GP in connection with a mental health problem.

At the time of the evaluation the project was involved in five main areas of activity (Thomas *et al*, 2006):

1. *Peer-group activities*
   There were seven peer-support groups attended by sixty-seven people. These included five women-only groups (one for Muslim women, two for South Asian women of any faith, two for women of any faith or ethnicity), one group for men and women of any faith or ethnicity, and one group for men of any faith or ethnicity.

2. *Individual support*
   Eighteen volunteers received support from CDWs, eight of these on a regular basis. In addition, eighteen people who were neither volunteers nor peer-group members received one-to-one support. Most of these (fifteen) had either used mental health services, or had contact with their GPs for reasons related to their mental health. Individual support included outreach sessions, and supported access to external

resources, such as fitness groups, music groups and creative expression groups. Other forms of individual support included attendance at an employment project which assisted fifteen participants back into employment, a further nine into education or training, and six into other daytime activities.

3. *Partnerships and networks*

This work included a two-year agreement to deliver community engagement for the local Primary Care Trust in the early stages of Delivering Race Equality (DRE)[7] and a one-year pilot with the National Institute for Mental Health in England (North East) to deliver community engagement, and research on community participation with Bradford University, and participation in a range of local health networks (African Network, Black Health Forum). Subsequently (in 2007–2009), SVB collaborated in a major project undertaken with the Bradford Primary Care Group and the University of Central Lancashire funded by the DRE Focused Implementation Site in Bradford, under the management of Salma Yasmeen. I will describe this work in some detail shortly.

4. *Increasing participation*

Individual participants in contact with local mental health services were encouraged and supported to become engaged in their own care plans. The project also ran focus groups with local communities on behalf of the main mental health service provider, Bradford District Care Trust, as part of its citizenship and mental health work.

5. *Dialogue and debate*

The project participated in local seminars on spirituality, and contributed to debates in local radio and press. One of the CDWs had a regular programme on the local community radio dealing with BME mental health. More widely, members of the project presented the projects' work at national events, including the Black Mental Health Forum, BME Mental Health Forum, the annual general meeting of the Royal College of Psychiatrists, and international events (e.g., Mental Health Europe).

Two Examples: Commissioning and Outcomes

We have already considered one example of SVB's work in Chapter 8, where we encountered the work of Hamdard. This chapter will conclude with a quite different example of the project's work, which lies at the heart of community development. This concerns the work of the project in collaboration with NHS Bradford and Airedale and the University of Central Lancashire (UCLan) in developing a model of engagement and consultation in commissioning and evaluating the outcome of mental health services for Bradford's BME communities.

---

7. DRE was a policy run by the Department of Health from 2005 to 2010, aimed at improving outcomes for BME people using mental health services. It included the appointment of over 500 community development workers, and established 17 'demonstration' sites, one of which was in Bradford (see below).

Commissioning and outcomes

Barriers exist that make it difficult for people from BME communities to participate in decision-making processes that influence health and social care. Bradford is no different from any other large British city in this respect, and earlier research, undertaken by the University of Bradford with the help of SVB, found that the main barrier to community involvement with local statutory services was a lack of trust, and the belief that statutory services would not listen, or that change would not follow (Blakey, 2005; Blakey et al, 2006). The purpose of the commissioning and outcomes project (Seebohm et al, 2009) was to create sustainable change in the provision of help and support for people from BME communities who experience mental health problems, by embedding their views in the commissioning process. Its aims were:

1. To involve members of BME communities, particularly service users and carers, in developing a commissioning framework to shape the outcomes delivered by local mental health services.
2. To develop and pilot a model for participation which enabled BME communities and mental health service commissioners to work together to commission relevant and culturally appropriate mental health services. (Seebohm et al, 2009: 8)

Sharing Voices Bradford played a central role in the project. It recruited and supported the community researchers, who in turn, through their personal networks in their communities, recruited subjects whose experiences, views and opinions were sought. Some members of the community research team also attended workshops to develop the strategy of involvement, and some contributed to the UCLan training for commissioners. Other volunteers attended meetings with the local commissioners, the project steering group, and visitors from the national Delivering Race Equality programme.

The project proposal received ethical approval from the Bradford Local Research Ethics Committee in August 2007, and shortly after that, the project began to recruit participants. Of the twenty-four people who joined, sixteen were women and eight were men. Their ages ranged from 22 to 57 years old. A third of participants were current or past users of mental health services; nearly a third were carers of people with mental health problems. Others recruited included asylum seekers, refugees, women with experience of domestic abuse, and people working or wishing to work with people with mental health problems. Participants came from a wide range of ethnic backgrounds: thirteen South Asian (Pakistani, Bangladeshi, Kashmiri), four African-Caribbean/black British, two Irish (one born in Bradford, one in Ireland), two Polish (one born in Bradford, one in Poland), one African, one Iranian and one Iraqi.

The primary purpose of the research was to inform the commissioning framework by gathering the views of local people from BME communities. The mental health commissioners wanted to find out from local BME groups what factors contribute to their emotional wellbeing, and, if they felt sad or distressed or experienced an emotional crisis and were unable cope with their life, what helped them to regain a sense of wellbeing. Nine of the twenty-four project participants chose to become community researchers and they attended weekly meetings over six months. Community researchers were trained to run focus groups, and with the support of SVB, identified sites within their communities where these could take place. CDWs and other community workers facilitated access to local people and in some cases took a lead role in organising the groups. Individual interviews were offered to Gypsies and Travellers and Muslim women with experience of domestic violence, because this was their preference. In total, the community researchers held sixteen focus groups and sixteen one-to-one interviews, involving a total of 135 people, 59 men (44%) and 76 women (56%). Ages ranged from under 22 to over 60. The ethnicity of participants is given in Table 13.1.

Table 13.1: Ethnicity of participants in focus groups and interviews

South Asian (63)	Pakistani (34) Bangladeshi (15) Indian (7) Other South Asian (Iranian, Iraqi) (7)
Black/African (29)	Black African (12) Black Caribbean (16) Black Other (1)
Mixed heritage (9)	Caribbean/White (7) African/White (1) Black/Other (1)
White Other (16)	Polish (11) Gypsy or Romany (4) Irish (1)
Other (18)	Data not given

The project attached considerable importance to sustainability. This was achieved by investing in the social capital of the communities in a number of ways. One offered participants an opportunity to study for a Certificate in Policy and Participation, which was developed and delivered by staff in the Centre for Ethnicity and Health, who had considerable experience in developing higher education opportunities for people from BME communities. This developed students' awareness of social policy and the organisational structures found in the public sector, and helped to develop the skills and knowledge necessary for effective engagement with statutory sector agencies. Twenty of the twenty-four participants were awarded university certificates, with four distinctions and five merits.

Participant feedback was positive. People valued opportunities to meet commissioners, conduct research and learn more about mental health services. Several said that they gained a good background to statutory services and greater confidence in helping to improve them. They valued the skills and knowledge that they gained. The most frequently mentioned benefit of the project was the opportunity to meet and work with such a wide variety of people. Participants were surprised to find how much they had in common with people from very different backgrounds. This was a strongly cohesive experience for the participants. Six progressed in their careers during the project, with five taking up full, part-time or sessional employment. Involvement in the project may have been a contributory factor in this. Opportunities for involvement and engagement with statutory services, if well supported by community workers and NHS staff, will help people from minority communities to achieve what they want in their life.

Recommended Reading

Armstrong, J. & Henderson, P. (1992) Putting the community into community care. *Community Development Journal, 27*(2), 189–92.

Gilchrist, A. (2004) *The Well-Connected Community: A networking approach to community development.* Bristol: Policy Press.

Prilleltensky, I. (2012) Wellness as fairness. *American Journal of Community Psychology, 49*, 1–21.

Seebohm, P., Henderson, P., Munn-Giddings, C., Thomas, P. & Yasmeen, S. (2005) *Together We Will Change: Community development, mental health and diversity.* London: Sainsbury Centre for Mental Health.

Thomas, P., Seebohm, P., Henderson, P., Munn-Giddings, C. & Yasmeen, S. (2006) Tackling race inequalities: Community development, mental health and diversity. *Journal of Public Mental Health, 5*, 13–19.

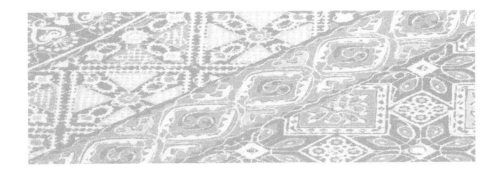

Section 6

Conclusions

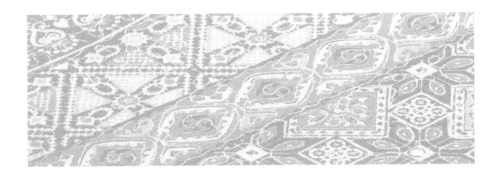

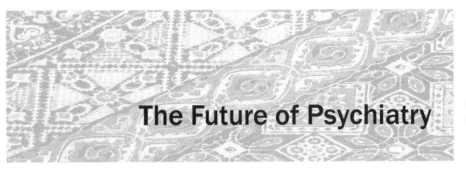

The Future of Psychiatry 14

There is a view that psychiatrists have no future role in mental health services. The growing influence of neuroscience and molecular genetics is a barrier between psychiatrists and those who use mental health services. Neuroscientific insights into psychosis and distress seem irrelevant when people are struggling with tragic histories of trauma and suffering, and living in contexts of adversity. If after 150 years science has failed to find a biological basis for psychosis it is difficult to estimate the probability that the future of psychiatry really lies in the direction of a 'medicine of the brain' as some claim. That said, there are some positive developments in neuroscience that recognise the sterility and futility of the reductionism and determinism we encountered in Chapter 6. Some, however, take the failure of scientific psychiatry a stage further, arguing that there is no role for medically qualified doctors in the field of mental health. This is an understandable position, and one that most critical psychiatrists will admit that they have thought long and hard about. Does medicine have anything to offer those who experience pain and suffering that involve their thoughts, emotions and relationships?

Fifty years ago Thomas Szasz famously answered this question with a resounding 'no'. My position is slightly different. It seems to me that psychiatry has no future as a 'medicine of the mind' based in neuroscience or molecular genetics, but I depart from Szasz's argument that there is no role for medically trained doctors in the field of mental health. The position I put forward in this book is that doctors do have a valuable contribution to make to the care of people who use mental health services, not necessarily as consultant psychiatrists, and certainly not from the position of dominance or team 'leadership' that some prominent psychiatrists feel is under threat today. In this final chapter I want to set out the basis for a prospectus on the role of doctors in mental health care by referring to recent critiques of Szasz's work. I will end by outlining four key areas of work in which doctors have an important future role.

Pat Bracken and I (Bracken & Thomas, 2010; Thomas & Bracken, 2011) have compared and contrasted the ideas of Thomas Szasz with those of Michel

Foucault. Most mainstream psychiatrists would see both as antipsychiatrists, although both would reject the label. To dismiss their work in this way is to obscure important differences between the two. This text has already considered the value of Foucault's work on power and subjectivity in Chapter 11. Here I will focus on Szasz. His critiques of psychiatry are powerful and lucid. He challenges psychiatric practice in several areas, including its role in coercion and its use in the insanity defence, and I broadly agree with his arguments. However, at the heart of his work is his perception of a clear boundary between medicine and psychiatry. Throughout his career he consistently argued (Szasz 1960, 2007) that there are limits to what might legitimately be considered as illness. Doctors rightly consider disturbances in bodily function in terms of pathology, but it is incorrect, even illogical, to consider disturbances in our mental worlds as pathological and evidence of mental illness. Such problems, he argues, are best thought of as moral problems or problems in living. In his best-known paper, The Myth of Mental Illness (Szasz, 1960), he draws attention to the confusion that has existed in psychiatry over the relationship between the physical and mental worlds. In his later work he uses an analogy between a television set and the programme we watch on it, to make this point:

> I maintain that mental illness is a metaphorical disease: that bodily illness stands in the same relation to mental illness as a defective television set stands to a bad program. (Szasz, 2007: 6)

This means that we require two different ways of speaking and understanding; one to describe the malfunction of the television set, and another to describe the quality of the programme. He then extends the analogy back to the concept of mental illness, arguing that we cannot 'cure' problems in our mental worlds by interfering with the physical function of the body of the person who is in distress, just as interfering with the internal components of the television will not result in a better programme. Therefore it is inappropriate to conceptualise psychological and emotional distress as though it were a brain (physical) problem.

This is fine, and the arguments developed in this book are consistent with Szasz's argument to this point – broadly in agreement with his analysis of the problems of the brain in psychiatry. However, his solution to the problem of the relationship between body and mind in psychiatry and medicine is strictly dualistic and has unforeseen consequences. His insistence that body and mind are separate domains to be spoken about only in their own terms is to deny the symbolic meaning of the body and biology in our lives. He correctly points out that the concept of mental illness is a metaphor, but he fails to acknowledge that we use metaphor continually to talk about ourselves and our physical illnesses. Many years ago I worked for a week as a locum GP in rural Hampshire. An elderly lady came into the surgery accompanied by her daughter. 'My head's a charnel house full of mortifying bones,' she replied when I asked her what the matter was.

I was flummoxed. It was only when I asked her daughter and looked back through her medical record that I discovered she was suffering from chronic sinusitis, which explained the unpleasant smell she experienced. I didn't understand the significance of what she was saying in medical terms, but I understood vividly how her physical condition made her feel.

Of course, mental illness is a metaphor, but then the language we use to convey the way we feel, our fears and anxieties, our experiences of psychosis, abounds with metaphor, and the same holds for our experiences of physical disease. If someone says they feel full of sadness, we do not interpret such a statement as a literal truth any more than we do when someone describes their experience of arthritic pain as being stabbed with a red hot knife. In Chapter 7 we saw that we can think of a great deal of psychiatric theory as having metaphorical significance. The idea that our distress arises from a chemical imbalance may be helpful for some people, but this does not mean to say that we have to accept it as a literal truth. Metaphor, as a key component of narrative, has an important role to play in helping us to understand the stories we tell about ourselves.

Szasz argues that doctors should restrict their practice to physical illnesses affecting the body, and nothing else; that they have no role to play in helping people who experience psychosis and distress, and that people who experience these problems should turn to psychotherapy and enter into a contract with a therapist. However, Szasz appears incapable of peering beyond the walls of his consulting room. Indeed, he would rather not do so. He sees the world outside, especially the state, as a threat to the autonomy of his clients and their freedom to negotiate contracts with their therapists. This raises another aspect of Szasz's dualism. In Chapter 3 of *The Myth of Mental Illness*, he asserts that culture has no role to play in relation to physical illness and medicine (Szasz, 1974), and that the manifestations of physical diseases are largely independent of culture or socio-political conditions in general: 'A diphtheritic membrane was the same and looked the same whether it occurred in a patient in Czarist Russia or Victorian England' (*ibid*: 48). He maximises this polarisation between mental and physical illness by asserting that although the 'phenomenology' of bodily illness such as tuberculosis is not influenced by socio-cultural factors, this is most certainly the case as far as mental illness is concerned:

> ... the phenomenology of so-called mental illness ... depend[s] upon and var[ies] with the educational, economic, religious, social and political character of the individual and the society in which it occurs. (*ibid*: 48–9)

Again, this chapter concurs with Szasz as far as the influence of culture on phenomenology in psychiatry is concerned, but strongly disputes his insistence that the body is beyond culture. It may be true that when people from different cultural backgrounds become ill, their bodies display the same physical derangements, but the weakness with Szasz's position is that to deny the role of culture in illness is to deny the importance of the personal meaning and significance of bodily disease. Szasz engineers a radical disconnection between the world of culture and medicine, which in his analysis can only be spoken about in terms given to us by natural science. In effect he dismisses the work of medical anthropologists and writers[1] in the field of medical humanities, who have shown that diseases have meanings for us, and that the interaction between meaning and pathology is a complex and vital factor in understanding the outcome of disease and treatment.

In any case, to those accustomed to working in the British NHS, Szasz's position seems absurd. Many patients who are seen in general practice have a complex mixture of problems, combinations of incurable medical conditions such as arthritis, chronic pain, and chronic diseases affecting lungs and heart, which are held in a matrix of unsatisfactory or abusive personal relationships that more often than not originate in childhood adversity, and all overlain by financial adversity and poverty, and lives lived in desolate, cheerless concrete environments that threaten and instil fear. There is a considerable overlap between a GP's work and that of a psychiatrist. For many years in the UK it has been recognised that GPs and psychiatrists have a role in helping and supporting people with such complex problems. Although this role may not always have been carried out in ways that are helpful or effective (for example, the problem of overprescription of benzodiazepines and more recently antidepressants), nevertheless doctors do support people struggling with adversity. Listening to stories, bearing witness to suffering, and the occasional judicious short-term use of medication to help sleep and reduce anxiety at the height of a crisis have always been an important aspect of medical care in the GP's surgery or psychiatrist's office. The central issue here is that our experience of suffering is embodied. It may be possible to separate out mental pain from physical pain on ideological grounds as Szasz does, but human beings do not suffer in separate mental or physical domains. Emotional pain and suffering may have a serious impact on physical health through stress and immunological mechanisms. Physical illnesses have profound existential significance for us.

It is worth noting that Szasz's view of the doctor's role in helping people who experience emotional distress was shaped by the very factors that he considered irrelevant in understanding illness. After escaping from Hungary at the age of 18, he lived in the USA, a culture that has always been deeply suspicious about state intrusion into the lives of individuals, and which valued personal freedom and autonomy (as long as you have the means to pay for it). It is, of course, just

---

1. An excellent example is to be found in the work of Thomas Csordas whose account of Dan, a Navajo Indian who experienced a psychosis following neurosurgery for intractable epilepsy, demonstrates the inseparability of culture, neurological impairment and experience (voices) (Csordas, 1994). Frank's (1995) work on illness and narrative (see Chapter 7, this volume) confirms that there are deep links between pathology, our experiences of illness, and culture.

as true that *my* view of the doctor's role in psychosis and distress is shaped by *my* culture, but here the values are quite different. Until recently in this country there was a strong view that we have a collective and mutual responsibility to help and support those less fortunate than ourselves. This responsibility is realised through the welfare state and the provision of health care free at the point of delivery through the NHS, a view that is anathema to American sensibilities. At least these have been the values that held sway in the post-war years, with the introduction of the welfare system and NHS in 1948. Many argue that the last ten to fifteen years have seen many of the principles of welfare provision and a public national health service whittled away. Nevertheless the central point stands; we live in different cultures that bring different values about disease, distress, illness and what we should do about it. We cannot shrug off culture and dismiss its influence on how we understand the meaning of health care.

This book argues against reductionist scientific models of psychosis because they are, it is suggested, not capable of generating insights that might be helpful in mental health work. Nevertheless, the embodied complexity of suffering – the interweaving of our physical and mental worlds, means that it is clear that medically qualified practitioners will continue to play a valuable role alongside professionals from other backgrounds in the future. In short, my argument is that medical practitioners do not need to justify their involvement in helping people who experience psychosis and distress on the basis of a putative future 'medicine of the brain'.

If not as a neuroscientific psychiatry then what is the future role of the doctor in mental health care? Narrative psychiatry and engaging with communities are two aspects of this role that we have already considered. I will end by outlining briefly some key areas of work that I haven't had the opportunity to cover. Some of this work is in progress. It includes non-technological modes of care, placing ethics before technology, physical health care in mental health, and science and psychiatry. These areas overlap and are not mutually exclusive.

Non-technological Models of Care

This refers to engaging and working with people in ways that prioritise the value of ordinary human relationships. Narrative psychiatry is one aspect of this, but there is more to narrative psychiatry than just sitting down listening sympathetically to someone's story. It goes without saying that trust is necessary if someone is to tell their story, and in developing trust it is important that the person feels cared for. Caring has had a difficult time in the NHS in recent years. We think we know what it means, but pressures of time, the value base of NHS work with its emphasis on achieving and measuring outcomes, the increasingly technological nature of health care, and the emphasis on scientific knowledge in professional training all mean that we are in danger of overlooking the value of caring. I don't want to dwell on this in any detail, other than to say that there are ways of understanding caring through philosophy that help us to understand its relationship both to technological modes of care and narrative (Thomas & Longden, 2013).

The importance of caring in positive therapeutic relationships has emerged in recent work on the placebo effect. A team at Harvard University led by the Professor of Medicine, Ted Kaptchuk, is investigating the different components of the placebo effect. One study (Kaptchuk *et al*, 2008) investigated whether the placebo response could be broken down into three components – assessment and observation, a therapeutic ritual (administration of placebo), and a caring therapeutic relationship. These three elements were assessed individually and in combination in 262 adults with irritable bowel syndrome is a six-week, blind, three-arm randomised controlled trial. One arm involved waiting list only (observation); the second arm, 'placebo' acupuncture (limited); and the third, placebo acupuncture with enhanced warmth, attention and conference (augmented – caring). The augmented group had consistently better outcomes at six weeks in terms of symptom severity scores, relief of symptoms, and global improvement. They concluded that the therapeutic relationship is the most robust component of the placebo effect.

This view of the value of caring has implications for the way we understand recovery in mental health work. Elsewhere, Pat Bracken and I have written about the role of narrative in the process of recovery (Bracken & Thomas, 2005). Since those chapters were written nearly ten years ago, many of us have become increasingly concerned about the 'professionalisation' of recovery. This takes different forms, including the appropriation of the word 'recovery' by mental health services that adopt it as a form of corporate branding, without really engaging with the full complexity of meanings that the word has for people who use mental health services. Recovery is an idea that emerged from the struggle of the service user and survivor movement to have individual and collective voices about their experiences, to tell their stories of recovery *despite* interventions by psychiatrists and mental health services. There is a deep paradox in the idea that mental health services can be recovery-based if all they do is diagnose and prescribe drugs. For this reason I prefer to speak of *healing* rather than recovery. Caring is an important component of healing relationships because it draws attention to the dialogical and thus primarily interpersonal and ethical basis of clinical practice (Thomas & Longden, 2013). Recovery isn't something that professionals (or for that matter other survivors) *do* to suffering people, but increasingly there is a tendency to present it that way. In contrast, healing occurs through caring relationships and environments, and this leads to another important non-technological aspect of care.

The mad were once cared for in large Victorian asylums dotted around the perimeters of our large cities and towns, with fields, farms and orchards that provided residents with contact with nature. These institutions have long since disappeared, and mental health care now takes place on windswept post-war council estates, in concrete modernist monstrosities that warehouse those who live in inner cities, and the confusing maze of postmodern passageways that seem to lead nowhere on estates built in the 1970s and 80s. Rex Haigh, a psychiatrist experienced in working in therapeutic communities with people identified as having 'personality disorders', has written recently about the value of thinking about therapeutic work and healing in terms of 'greencare'. He sees this as a way of offering a moral treatment for the twenty-first century (Haigh, 2012). He points out that recent social policy in Europe draws attention to the importance of sustainability and contact with nature in health care, and the value of 'green' elements in therapeutic programmes. Contact with nature has beneficial effects on wellbeing in the physical, emotional and spiritual aspects of our lives. In addition, mutual and peer support described in Chapter 11 (this volume) is sustainable and thus fits well with the values of greencare. He also draws attention to the parallels between therapeutic communities and greencare, through metaphors of change, growth and transformation. He continues:

> *Pruning.* Needs to be undertaken in order to cut back unhealthy or outdated coping mechanisms and keep the work within safe boundaries.
>
> *Watering.* Sometimes work in a therapeutic community becomes arid and dry and needs irrigation. The psychological equivalent of this is having a range of different activities within the treatment programme.
>
> *Feeding.* Little growth is possible without suitable nourishment, and this 'fertiliser' can be found either in developing relationships between members of the community itself or with staff. Often this is accomplished by people who have moved on through the programme coming back and helping to nurture those earlier on in the process.
>
> *Rotation.* Crops thrive best when subject to rotation or mixed planting in small domestic settings: therapeutic community programmes often benefit from 'refreshing' by changing the therapy ingredients (the mixture of types of groups); different talents can be used from individual members to contribute to the health and wellbeing of the whole community. (Haigh, 2012: 129–30)

Greencare provides a powerful set of metaphors for a non-technological form of care that is genuinely holistic. In addition, the value it attaches to democratic structures and peer support has much in common with Soteria.

Ethics Before Technology

Pat Bracken and I first used this expression in relation to postpsychiatry (Bracken & Thomas, 2001), and this ethical imperative permeates not only this book, but most of what has been written by critical psychiatrists over the last twenty years or so. Chapter 7 (this volume) set out in some depth an ethical basis for psychiatric practice through narrative, but there is much more to it than that. There are two important areas that I want to refer to briefly here. These involve the ethical use of medication, and attempts to uncouple care from coercion.

The ethical use of psychotropic medication is perhaps the single most important aspect of psychiatric care that requires urgent attention. Fortunately much of the ground has been prepared for this by Joanna Moncrieff's work on the disease-centred and drug-centred models of drug action (Moncrieff, 2008). The two models cast the relationship between doctor and patient in a very different light. In the former the doctor is the expert by virtue of his or her possession of specialist knowledge about the supposed mode of action and properties of psychotropic drugs. This puts the doctor in a position of considerable authority and power, and a consequence of this is that the lack of evidence in support of this model is rarely acknowledged. My experience is that many people who see psychiatrists bitterly resent the fact that their doctors rarely listen to their experiences of taking medication. This is particularly likely to happen when the drugs appear not to work, or when the side effects of the drugs do not conform to those that the doctor expects from his or her reading of the scientific literature.

In contrast, the drug-centred model constructs the doctor–patient relationship very differently. Apart from some very early studies made when these drugs were first introduced, there has been little in the way of systematic scientific study of the subjective effects of these drugs in healthy people. This means that the most appropriate source of evidence for drug-centred practice in psychiatry is the patient's testimony. We have to attach much greater significance to what patients tell us about the effects that psychotropic drugs have on them. We must set aside our own assumptions and biases about the properties of these drugs and how we think they work. As Moncrieff points out in Chapter 13 of *The Myth of the Chemical Cure* (2008), this represents a move to a democratic form of drug treatment. It also has important implications for drug-related research which I will consider shortly.

The drug-centred model helps us to understand how some people may gain benefit from psychiatric drugs at least in the short term, through the idea that they induce an abnormal state in the central nervous system. It is, in effect, a form of intoxication similar to the effects of self-medicating anxiety with alcohol. For this reason, it seems reasonable and appropriate to offer those who experience psychosis and other forms of distress neuroleptics or antidepressants from within a drug-centred framework, but this should only be for short periods of time, on a 'suck it and see' basis for up to a maximum of a month. There is no justification for telling people they must remain on these drugs for any longer than this. We have a responsibility to help people find more appropriate long-term ways of coping with their problems, particularly when we consider the harm associated with the long-term use of neuroleptic drugs.

Deep concern about the problems of drug treatment in psychiatry and the historical inertia of professional organisations like the Royal College of

Psychiatrists and NICE are reasons why survivors, observers of psychiatry, and concerned mental health professionals are taking action. James Davies, author of *Cracked* (2013), and a group of others concerned about drug treatment in psychiatry have established the Council for Evidence-based Psychiatry (CEP) to disseminate more widely the evidence for the harmfulness of these drugs, and to stimulate a much wider debate about this. The evidence needs to be brought out from the darker recesses of specialist journals into the light of the public gaze (http://cepuk.org/). Another initiative, the Coming Off project, is in the process of collecting survivor and service user narratives about their experiences of coming off or reducing neuroleptic medication, some of which will be published by Palgrave Macmillan or on the Coming Off website (http://www.comingoff. com/index.php?).

There are important implications here for the use of coercion in psychiatric practice. In a nutshell it is not possible to justify compulsion either through categories of mental disorder that have no scientific validity, or by the use of forced 'treatment' that is limited in effectiveness and may cause serious harm to health in the long term. There is an urgent need to uncouple psychiatric care from coercion, all the more so since the introduction of community treatment orders in 2008 shifted the locus of the forced administration into the community. This isn't something that psychiatrists alone can achieve. Only a concerted series of campaigns involving a broad alliance of various interest groups dealing with different aspects of the problems raised by coercion (a human rights perspective, the scientific evidence on the problems of neuroleptics, and so on) is likely to bring about ultimate changes in the law.

There are practical steps that psychiatrists and other mental health professionals can do to reduce the impact of coercion. There is an extensive literature on the use of advance statements (ASs) in mental health care, and at the turn of the millennium there was considerable interest in their use. It was hoped that they might offset some of the consequences of what were increasingly coercive proposals to change the Mental Health Act, for example, by reducing rates of compulsory admission to hospital. One randomised controlled trial of ASs found no evidence that they did so (Papageorgiou *et al*, 2002), but in contrast a randomised trial carried out by Henderson and colleagues (2004) found a significant reduction in the use of the Mental Health Act in an experimental group of patients who had joint crisis plans (a form of AS) compared with the control group. Of the former group, 13 per cent experienced compulsory admission or treatment in the follow-up period, compared with 27 per cent of the control group.

The difficulty in implementing and evaluating a complex intervention like advance statements is that the process is deeply embedded in a wide range of competing political interests and perspectives that may adversely influence the outcome of the process. Anne Cahill and I wrote an editorial in the *British Medical Journal* accompanying the Henderson *et al* paper, in which we described the difficulties we had experienced in implementing and evaluating advance statements in Bradford (Thomas & Cahill, 2004). Although a few people had negotiated advance statements individually with their consultants, two years of extensive development work with service users and mental health professionals generated a disappointingly low uptake of advance statements. Of seventy service users who attended presentations on advance statements only one took up the opportunity. This is puzzling. Why were service users reluctant to get involved? Perhaps they see little point in planning ahead because they feel demoralised, disempowered and oppressed by years of compulsion in the mental health system.

Physical Health and Mental Health

In Chapter 3 we saw that neuroleptic drugs have serious adverse effects on the physical health of those who take them. Their use is associated with obesity, diabetes and cardiovascular disease. There is also evidence that the life expectancy of people with the diagnosis of schizophrenia and other psychoses is much lower than that of people who do not have these diagnoses. It is of course extremely difficult to disentangle these relationships. The lives of many people who have a diagnosis of schizophrenia are blighted by poverty and this too is associated with a wide range of factors that reduce life expectancy, including poor diet, smoking, and lack of opportunity for physical exercise. They are less likely to present to primary care, and when they do so their complaints may not be taken seriously or investigated. All these factors may contribute to reduced life expectancy.

A recent report by Rethink (2013) found that although over 40 per cent of all tobacco is smoked by people with mental health problems, they are less likely to be given help to stop smoking. Fewer than 30 per cent of people with a diagnosis of schizophrenia receive a basic annual physical health check. Despite the serious problems associated with weight gain on neuroleptics, up to 70 per cent of people on these drugs do not have their weight monitored. In addition, the report found that many health professionals fail to take people with mental health problems seriously when they raise concerns about their physical health.

This disparity in life expectancy demands attention and action. It is, as Thornicroft (2011) has observed, a human rights issue, and the Rethink report makes a number of recommendations to tackle the problem. However, psychiatrists as medical practitioners involved in mental health care, are ideally placed to improve the physical health care of people with psychiatric diagnoses. I often found myself struggling to deal with my patients' physical health problems when I worked as a consultant, and I frequently had to act as an advocate on my patients' behalf with GPs or hospital specialists, as medical staff were not taking my patients' physical illnesses seriously because he or she was a psychiatric patient. I also felt there was something lacking in my training as a psychiatrist, especially general practice, neurology and public health medicine. The point here is that an important aspect of the work of medically qualified practitioners in mental health is to deal with the complex interactions between mental health, environment and physical health, and this should be reflected in the training of psychiatrists and their work. There should be much greater flexibility in training and job descriptions so that psychiatrists are exposed to these three areas of work in their training. In this respect I would broadly agree with Oyebode and Humphreys (2011) on the importance for psychiatrists of a sound basis in neurology and general medicine.

Science and Psychiatry

Chapter 6 set out a critique of the naive reductionism and determinism that characterise much research into the scientific basis of psychosis. Scientific inquiry does have a role in exploring consciousness and subjectivity in 'normal' states as well as those of psychosis and distress. We saw that one of the main problems of neuroscientific research into psychosis is that it does not engage with subjective experience. It turns away from what in personal terms are the most important and significant aspects of consciousness in psychosis – the uniquely subjective nature of the experience. This is partly because it is not informed by philosophical insights into the nature of consciousness, especially the problems of brain–mind and mind–world dualisms. In recent years, philosophers of neuroscience have started to engage with these problems and are developing more sophisticated ways of conceptualising the relationships between brain and mind, and mind and world, through what is broadly called 'enactivism' (Varela *et al*, 1991; Noë, 2012). There are also signs that those engaged in neuroscientific research in psychiatry are beginning to grapple with these problems.

Harland *et al* (2004) draw attention to the gap that exists between our understanding of social factors that we know are important in psychosis, the phenomenology of psychosis, and its neurobiology. They propose that insights from phenomenology and anthropology can help to create a framework to study the relationship between subjective experience, social factors such as migration, and the biological basis of psychosis. Referring briefly to the hermeneutic phenomenology of Heidegger, Ricoeur's work on time and narrative, and the interpretive anthropology of Geertz, they argue that the adjustments demanded by migration can be seen in terms of cultural shifts in meaning and moral frameworks, which are also consistent with biological theories of psychosis in terms of neural plasticity. They propose that a coming together of neuroscience and phenomenology, starting with '… a description of the phenomena of lived experience …' (*ibid*: 362) may make it possible to establish testable hypotheses that help to establish the correlates of experience in the brain. Although I have reservations about this, it is encouraging to see scientific psychiatry acknowledge that there is a gap between the values and methods of science, and that of lived experience. This has the potential to take us beyond the simplistic and reductionist neuroscience we considered in Chapter 6. Ultimately, however, the world of meaningful human experience is beyond the explanatory power of neuroscience, which as Pat Bracken has recently argued (Bracken, 2014), is why psychiatry requires a shift to hermeneutics

A more sophisticated form of scientific inquiry more closely engaged with subjective experience is also necessary for future investigations of the drug model of psychotropic drug action and the placebo effect. There have been very few studies of the subjective effects of psychotropic drugs in non-psychotic subjects. An exception is work by David Healy on the effects of the neuroleptic droperidol on healthy volunteers (I was one of the volunteers who took the drug in this study, see Healy & Farquhar, 1998). One of the conclusions of Moncrieff's work is that there is an urgent need for more research of this nature, to clarify and deepen our understanding of the relationship between the subjective side effects of these drugs and their pharmacological properties.

Chapter 3 indicated that the non-specific placebo effect has at least as large an effect on outcome as specific drug treatments. The placebo effect brings together culture and biology in a way that Szasz's work fails to grapple with. For many years the use of placebos in clinical practice has been frowned upon because of its association with quackery, but this is starting to change. A themed issue of the *Philosophical Transactions of the Royal Society* (Meissner *et al*, 2011) was recently devoted to the subject. Understanding the neurobiology of the placebo effect has the potential to offer another way of drawing together culture and biology (McQueen & Smith, 2012), only here the emphasis is on the factors, phenomenological, cultural and biological, that are important in the processes of healing. We have already seen how the work of the Harvard team under Kaptchuk (2008) is drawing attention to the importance of caring therapeutic relationships as part of the placebo response in the management of conditions like irritable bowel syndrome. It is inconceivable that this does not also hold for people who experience psychosis and distress. Work in this area has the potential to yield valuable insights into how we can best help people who experience psychosis in ways that are both effective and much less harmful than current psychiatric treatment.

Coda

Our culture swings crazily from one extreme to another. Less than fifty years ago we teetered on the edge of revolution. Students and workers joined forces against exploitation and injustice. Black people renewed the call for civil rights in the USA, a call reinvigorated by the radical politics of Stokely Carmichael and Malcolm X. The women's movement and radical feminists challenged patriarchal orthodoxies and in doing so gave rise to new ways of thinking about human relationships (Gilligan, 1982). A new world emerged as people who were formerly seen as 'colonial' subjects across the globe fought for and were granted liberation. After the horrors of genocide in the Second World War, as well as Hiroshima and Nagasaki, people realised that the idea of the advancement of society through scientific knowledge was a bitter-sweet promise, a tragedy saturated with the most terrible irony. This realisation together with the liberatory movements placed the question of values, ethics and epistemology at the forefront of human affairs. What do we really consider to be important about how we relate to one another? How can we find a moral basis for guiding our relationships when we are blinded by the spell of science? What systems of knowledge are most appropriate for engaging with the suffering that is an inevitable consequence of existence?

The world has revolved and changed. Today, such questions are dismissed in a neo-liberal, rational society hellbent on progress and profit, in which science is sovereign because we still believe that science is capable of solving all our problems. In medicine it is common to speak today of evidence-based medicine as the gold standard. We believe that we have created an empirical empire glittering with facts. But by themselves facts are little more than fool's gold, and we are seduced by them. Trisha Greenhalgh and Brian Hurwitz, in a paper on the value of narrative in medicine, write:

> At its most arid, modern medicine lacks a metric for existential qualities such as the inner hurt, despair, hope, grief, and moral pain that frequently accompany, and often indeed constitute, the illnesses from which people suffer. (Greenhalgh & Hurwitz, 1999: 50)

This is true for psychiatric practice dominated by science. A scientific psychiatry that fails to engage with the pain and suffering of those who experience psychosis and distress impoverishes not only our patients, but ourselves as doctors. Caring, and the imagination it takes to care for others, is as Kleinman (2008) points out, an existential quality of human *being*; it is a foundational component of our lives as *moral* beings. Imagination and our capacity for moral imagination must be at the centre of our attempts to help those who suffer (Thomas & Longden, 2013). In the preface to this book we encountered Philomela's struggle to tell the story of her violation and trauma, something she managed to achieve by weaving her narrative. The story will out one way or another, and we must wait, watch, listen and wait again. The time that binds our lives is infinitely precious.

References

Aderhold, V., Stastny, P. & Lehmann, P. (2007) Soteria: An alternative mental health reform movement. In P. Stastny & P. Lehmann (Eds.) *Alternatives Beyond Psychiatry* (pp. 14–60). Berlin/Eugene, OR/Shrewsbury: Peter Lehmann Publishing.

Alanen, Y.O., Lehtinen, K., Rakkolainen, V. & Aaltonen, J. (1991) Need-adapted treatment of new schizophrenic patients: Experiences and results of the Turku Project. *Acta Psychiatrica Scandinavica, 83*, 363–72.

Allen, P., Modinos, G., Hubl, D., Shields, G., Cachia, A., Jardri, R. *et al* (2012) Neuroimaging auditory hallucinations in schizophrenia: From neuroanatomy to neurochemistry and beyond. *Schizophrenia Bulletin, 38*, 695–703. doi: 10.1093/schbul/sbs066.

Allers, R. (1961) *Existentialism and Psychiatry*. Springfield, IL: Charles C. Thomas.

Anckarsäter, H. (2010) Beyond categorical diagnostics in psychiatry: Scientific and medicolegal implications. *International Journal of Law and Psychiatry, 33*, 59–65.

Andreasen, N. (1979) Thought, language and communication disorders: II. Diagnostic significance. *Archives of General Psychiatry, 36*, 1325–30.

Andreasen, N. (1995) The validation of psychiatric diagnosis: New models and approaches. *American Journal of Psychiatry, 152*, 161–2.

Andrews, G. (2001) Placebo response in depression: Bane of research, boon to therapy. *British Journal of Psychiatry, 178*, 192–4.

Armstrong, J. & Henderson, P. (1992) Putting the community into community care. *Community Development Journal, 27*(2) 189–92.

Bachelor, A. & Horvath, A. (1999) The therapeutic relationship. In M.A. Hubble, B.L. Duncan & S.D. Miller (Eds.) *The Heart and Soul of Change: What works in therapy* (pp. 133–78). Washington, DC: American Psychological Association.

Bagley, D. (1971) The social aetiology of schizophrenia in inpatient groups. *International Journal of Social Psychiatry, 17*, 292–304.

Baker, L. (2008) History of anthropology. In J. Moorem (Ed.) *Encyclopedia of Race and Racism, Vol 1* (pp. 93–7). Detroit: Thomson Gale.

Baker, P. (1993) The British experience. In M. Romme & S. Escher (Eds.) *Accepting Voices* (pp. 28–37). London: MIND Publications.

Baker, P. & Eversley, J. (Eds.) (2000) *Multilingual Capital*. London: Battlebridge.

Bakhtin, M.M. (1981) *The Dialogic Imagination: Four essays* (Trans. C. Emerson & M. Holquist; Ed. M. Holquist). Austin, TX: University of Texas Press.

Baldessarini, R.J. & Viguera, A.C. (1995) Neuroleptic withdrawal in schizophrenic patients. Commentary in *Archives of General Psychiatry, 52*, 189–92.

Bartels, A. & Zeki, S. (2000) The neural basis of romantic love. *NeuroReport, 11*, 3829–34.

Bebbington, P., Feeney, S., Flannigan, C. *et al* (1991) Inner London collaborative audit of admissions in two health districts. II: Ethnicity and the use of the Mental Health Act. *British Journal of Psychiatry, 165*, 743–9.

Bebbington, P., Bhugra, D., Brugha, T., Singleton, N., Farrell, M., Jenkins, R. *et al* (2004) Psychosis, victimization and childhood disadvantage: Evidence from the second British National Survey of Psychiatric Morbidity. *British Journal of Psychiatry, 185*, 220–6.

Beck, A.T., Ward, C., Mendelson, M., Mock, J. & Erbaugh, J. (1962) Reliability of psychiatric diagnoses: 2. A study of consistency of clinical judgements and ratings. *American Journal of Psychiatry, 119*, 210–16.

Beck, A.T. (1993) Cognitive therapy: Past, present, and future. *Journal of Consulting and Clinical Psychology, 61*, 194–8.

Beeforth, M., Conlan, E. & Graley, R. (1994) *Have We Got Views for You: User evaluation of case management*. London: Sainsbury Centre for Mental Health.

Bentall, R.P. (Ed.) (1990) *Reconstructing Schizophrenia*. London: Routledge.

Bentall, R.P. (2003) *Madness Explained: Psychosis and human nature*. London: Allen Lane.

Bentall, R.P. & Jackson, H. (1988) Abandoning the concept of 'schizophrenia': Some implications of validity arguments for psychological research into psychotic phenomena. *British Journal for Clinical Psychology, 27*, 303–24.

Berne, E. (1964) *Games People Play: The psychology of human relationships*. New York: Penguin.

Beveridge, A. (2011) *Portrait of the Psychiatrist as a Young Man: The early writing and work of R.D. Laing, 1927–1960*. Oxford: Oxford University Press.

Bhugra, D., Hilwig, M., Hossein, B., Marceau, H., Neehall, J., Leff, J. *et al* (1996) First-contact incidence rates of schizophrenia in Trinidad and one-year follow-up. *British Journal of Psychiatry, 169*, 587–92. doi: 10.1192/bjp.169.5.587.

Bhui, K. & Bhugra, D. (2002) Mental illness in Black and Asian ethnic minorities: Pathways to care and outcome. *Advances in Psychiatric Treatment, 8*, 26–33.

Bhui, K., Brown, R., Hardie. T. *et al* (1998) African-Caribbean men remanded to Brixton prison. *British Journal of Psychiatry, 172*, 337–44.

Bhui, K., Bhugra, D., Goldberg, D. *et al* (2001) Common mental disorders among Punjabi and English subjects in primary care: Prevalence, detection of morbidity and pathways into care. *Psychological Medicine, 29*, 475–83.

Bifulco, A., Bernazzani, O., Moran, P.M. & Jacobs, C. (2005) The childhood experiences of care and abuse questionnaire (CECA.Q): Validation in a community series. *British Journal of Clinical Psychology, 44*, 563–81. doi: 10.1348/014466505X35344.

Black, D., Morris, J.N., Smith, C. & Townsend, P. (1982) *Inequalities in Health: The Black Report*. Harmondsworth: Penguin.

Blackman, L. (2001) *Hearing Voices: Embodiment and experience*. London: Free Association Books.

Blakey, H. (2005) Participation, Why Bother? The views of black and minority ethnic mental health service users on participation in the NHS in Bradford: ICPS Working Paper 2. Bradford: Bradford University.

Blakey, H., Pearce, J. & Chesters, G. (2006) *Minorities within Minorities: Beneath the surface of South Asian participation*. York: Joseph Rowntree Foundation.

Blashfield, R. (1973) An evaluation of the *DSM-II* classification of schizophrenia as a nomenclature. *Journal of Abnormal Psychology, 82*, 382–9.

Bleuler, M. (1978) *The Schizophrenic Disorders: Long-term patient and family studies*. New Haven, CT: Yale University Press.

BNP (2009) Shock as government report claims schizophrenia is 'epidemic' amongst Africans in Britain. Accessed on 18th December 2009 at http://bnp.org.uk/2009/12/shock-as-government-report-claims-schizophrenia-is-epidemic-amongst-africans-in-britain/

Bola, J. & Mosher, L.R. (2003) Treatment of acute psychosis without neuroleptics: Two-year outcomes from the Soteria project. *Journal of Nervous and Mental Disease, 191*, 219–29.

Bola, J., Lehtinen, K., Cullberg, J. & Ciompi, L. (2009) Psychosocial treatment, antipsychotic postponement, and low-dose medication strategies in first-episode psychosis: A review of the literature. *Psychosis, 1*, 4–18.

Bola, J., Kao, D., & Haluk, S. (2012) Antipsychotic medication for early-episode schizophrenia. *Schizophrenia Bulletin, 38*(1), 23–5.

Bolton, D. & Hill J. (1996) *Mind, Meaning and Mental Disorder*. Oxford: Oxford University Press.

Boney-McCoy, S. & Finkelhor, D. (1995) Psychosocial sequelae of violent victimization in a national youth sample. *Journal of Consulting and Clinical Psychology, 63*, 726–36.

Boss, M. (1963) *Psychoanalysis and Daseinanalysis*. New York: Basic Books.

Bowl, R. (2007) Responding to ethnic diversity: Black service users' views of mental health services in the UK. *Diversity in Health and Social Care, 4*, 201–10.

Bowles, N., Dodds, P., Hackney, D., Sutherland, C. & Thomas, P. (2002) Formal observation and engagement: A discussion paper. *Journal of Psychiatric and Mental Health Nursing, 9*, 255–60.

Boydell, J., van Os, J., McKenzie, K. *et al* (2001) Incidence of schizophrenia in ethnic minorities in London: Ecological study into interactions with environment. *British Medical Journal, 323*, 1336–8.

Boyle, M. (2002) *Schizophrenia: A scientific delusion?* (2nd ed.). London: Routledge.

Bracken, P. (2014) Towards a Hermeneutic Shift in Psychiatry. In Press, World Psychiatry, June.

Bracken, P. & Thomas, P. (2000) Cognitive therapy, Cartesianism and the moral order. *European Journal of Psychotherapy, Counselling and Health, 2*, 325–44.

Bracken, P. & Thomas, P. (2001) Postpsychiatry: A new direction for mental health. *British Medical Journal, 322*, 724–7.

Bracken, P. & Thomas, P. (2002) Time to move beyond the mind–body split. *British Medical Journal, 325*, 1433–4.

Bracken, P. & Thomas, P. (2005) *Postpsychiatry: Mental health in a postmodern world*. Oxford: Oxford University Press.

Bracken, P. & Thomas, P. (2010) From Szasz to Foucault: On the role of critical psychiatry. *Philosophy, Psychiatry and Psychology, 17*(3), 219–28.

Bracken, P., Thomas, P., Timimi, S., Asen, E., Behr, G. *et al* (2012) Psychiatry beyond the current paradigm. *British Journal of Psychiatry, 201*: 430–4. doi: 10.1192/bjp.bp.112.109447.

Brentano, F. (1874/1995) *Psychology from an Empirical Standpoint* (Trans. A. Rancurello, D. Terrell & L. McAlister). London: Routledge.

Brockington, I., Kendell, R. & Leff, J. (1978) Definitions of schizophrenia: Concordance and prediction of outcome. *Psychological Medicine, 8*, 399–412.

Brown, G. & Harris, T. (1978) *The Social Origins of Depression: A study of psychiatric disorder in women*. New York: The Free Press.

Brown, G., Harris, T. & Copeland, J. (1977) Depression and loss. *British Journal of Psychiatry, 130*, 1–28.

Bruce, M.L., Takeuchi, D.T. & Leaf, P.J. (1991) Poverty and psychiatric status. *Archives of General Psychiatry, 48*, 470–4.

Brunner, E. (1997) Socioeconomic determinants of health: Stress and the biology of inequality. *British Medical Journal, 314*, 1472–6.

Bullmore, E., Fletcher, P. & Jones, P. (2009) Why psychiatry can't afford to be neurophobic. *British Journal of Psychiatry, 194*, 293–5. doi: 10.1192/bjp.bp.108.058479.

Burnett, R., Mallett, R. & Bhugra, D. (1999) The first contact of patients with schizophrenia with psychiatric services: Social factors and pathways to care in a multi-ethnic population. *Psychological Medicine, 29*, 475–83.

Bush, G. (1990) *Project on the Decade of the Brain: Presidential Proclamation 6158*. Accessed on 8th May 2012 at http://www.loc.gov/loc/brain/proclaim.html

Button, K., Ionnadis, J., Mokrysz, C., Nosek, B., Flint, J., Robinson, E. & Munafò, M. (2013) Power failure: Why small sample size undermines the reliability of neuroscience. *Nature Reviews Neuroscience, 14*, 365–76. doi: 10.1038/nrn3475.

Callan, A. & Littlewood, R. (1998) Patient satisfaction: Ethnic origin or explanatory model? *International Journal of Social Psychiatry, 44*, 1–11.

Callard, F., Smallwood, J. & Margulies, D. (2012) Default positions: How neuroscience's historical legacy has hampered investigation of the resting mind. *Frontiers in Psychology, 3*, 1–6. doi: 10.3389/fpsyg.2012.00321.

Calton, T., Ferriter, M., Husband, N. & Spandler, H. (2008) A systematic review of the Soteria paradigm for the treatment of people diagnosed with schizophrenia. *Schizophrenia Bulletin, 34*, 181–92.

Campbell, M. & Morrison, A. (2007) The relationship between bullying, psychotic-like experiences and appraisals in 14–16-year-olds. *Behaviour Research and Therapy, 45*, 1579–91.

Campbell, P. (1989) The self-advocacy movement in the UK. In A. Brackx & C. Grimshaw (Eds.) *Mental Health Care in Crisis* (pp. 206–13). London: Pluto Press.

Campbell, P. (1996) Challenging loss of power. In J. Read & J. Reynolds (Eds.) *Speaking Our Minds: An anthology* (pp. 56–62). London: Macmillan/Open University.

Campbell, P. (2009) The service user/survivor movement. In J. Reynolds, R. Muston, T. Heller, J. Leach, M. McCormick, J. Wallcraft & M. Walsh (Eds.) *Mental Health Still Matters* (pp. 46–52). Basingstoke/Milton Keynes: Palgrave Macmillan/Open University.

Carmichael, S. (1968) Black Power. In D. Cooper (Ed.) *The Dialectics of Liberation* (pp. 150–74). Harmondsworth: Penguin.

Carr, D. (1986) *Time, Narrative, and History*. Bloomington, IN: University of Indiana Press.

Cartwright, S. (1843) Essays (Natchez, MS), p. 12 cited in William S. Jenkins' *Pro-Slavery Thought in the Old South* (Chapel Hill: University of North Carolina Press, 1935) p. 251, cited by Deutsch 1944, p. 471.

Cartwright, S. (1851) Report on the diseases and physical peculiarities of the Negro race. *The New Orleans Medical and Surgical Journal*, 691–715. Republished in A. Caplan., H. Engelhardt, & J. McCartney (Eds.) (1981) *Concepts of Health and Disease: Interdisciplinary perspectives* (pp. 305–25). Reading, MA: Addison-Wesley.

Casey, D., Rodriguez, M., Northcott, C., Vickar, G. & Shihabuddin, L. (2011) Schizophrenia: Medical illness, mortality, and aging. *International Journal of Psychiatry in Medicine, 41*, 245–51.

Castle, D., Wessely, S., Der, G. & Murray, R. (1991) The incidence of operationally defined schizophrenia in Camberwell, 1965–84. *British Journal of Psychiatry, 159*, 790–4. doi: 10.1192/bjp.159.6.790.

Chahal, K. & Julienne, L. (1999) *'We Can't All Be White!' Racist victimisation in the UK*. London: York Publishing Services.

Chang, C.-K., Hayes, R., Perera, G., Broadbent, M., Fernandes, A., Lee, W. *et al* (2011) Life expectancy at birth for people with serious mental illness and other major disorders from a secondary mental health care case register in London. *PLoS ONE, 6*(5), e19590. Accessed on 14th February 2012 at http://www.plosone.org/article/info:doi/10.1371/journal.pone.0019590

Ciompi, L. (1980) The natural history of schizophrenia in the long term. *British Journal of Psychiatry, 136*, 413–20.

Ciompi, L., Dauwalder H.P., Maier C. *et al* (1992) The pilot project 'Soteria Bern': Clinical experiences and results. *British Journal of Psychiatry, 161*, 145–53.

Coid, J., Kahtan, N., Gault, S. *et al* (2000) Ethnic differences in admissions to secure forensic psychiatry services. *British Journal of Psychiatry, 177*, 241–7.

Colombo, A., Bendelow, G., Fulford, B. & Williams, S. (2003) Evaluating the influence of implicit models of mental disorder on processes of shared decision making within community-based multi-disciplinary teams, *Social Science and Medicine, 56*, 1557–70.

Corstens, D. & Longden, E. (2013) The origins of voices: Links between life history and voice hearing in a survey of 100 cases. *Psychosis: Psychological, Social and Integrative Approaches, 5*, 270–85. doi: 10.1080/17522439.2013.816337.

Corstens, D., Longden, E. & May, R. (2012) Talking with voices: Exploring what is expressed by the voices people hear. *Psychosis, 4*, 95–104. doi: 10.1080/17522439.2011.571705.

Craddock, N., Antebi, D., Attenburrow, M.-J., Bailey, A., Carson, A. *et al* (2008) Wake-up call for British psychiatry. *British Journal of Psychiatry, 193*, 6–9. doi: 10.1192/bjp.bp.108.053561.

Crawford, M., Rutter, D., Manley, C., Weaver, T., Bhui, K., Fulop, N. & Tyrer , P. (2002) Systematic review of involving patients in the planning and development of health care. *British Medical Journal, 325*, 1263–5. doi: 10.1136/bmj.325.7375.1263.

Crow, T.J., Done, D.J. & Sacker, A. (1994) Childhood precursors of psychosis as clues to its evolutionary origins. *European Archives of Psychiatry and Neurological Sciences, 245*, 61–9.

CSIP/NIMHE (2008) *Three Keys to a Shared Approach in Mental Health Assessment*. Warwick: University of Warwick. Accessed on 13th September 2013 at http://www2.warwick.ac.uk/fac/med/study/research/vbp/resources/three_keys_to_a_shared_approach.pdf

Csordas, T. (1994) Words from the holy people: A case study in cultural phenomenology. In T. Csordas (Ed.) *Embodiment and Experience: The existential ground of culture and self* (pp. 269–90). Cambridge: Cambridge University Press.

Cullberg, J., Levander S., Holmqvist, R., Mattsson, M. & Wieselgren, I.-M. (2002) One-year outcome in first episode psychosis patients in the Swedish Parachute project. *Acta Psychiatrica Scandinavica, 106*, 276–85.

Curtis, C., Shah, S., Chin, S-F., Turashvili, G., Rueda, O., Dunning, M., Speed, D. *et al* (2012) The genomic and transcriptomic architecture of 2,000 breast tumours reveals novel subgroups. *Nature, 486*(7403), 346–52. doi: 10.1038/nature10983.

David, S., Ware, J., Chu, I., Loftus, P., Fusar-Poli, P., Radua, J., Munafo, M. & Ioannidis, J. (2013) Potential reporting bias in fMRI studies of the brain. *PLoS ONE, 8*(7), e70104. Accessed on 3rd December 2013 at http://www.plosone.org/article/fetchObject.action?uri=info%3Adoi%2F10.1371%2Fjournal.pone.0070104&representation=PDF

Davies, J. (2013) *Cracked: Why psychiatry is doing more harm than good.* London: Icon Books.

Davies, P., Thomas, P. & Leudar, I. (1999) Dialogical engagement and verbal hallucinations: A single case study. *British Journal of Medical Psychology, 72*, 179–87.

Davies, S., Thornicroft, G., Lease, M. *et al* (1996) Ethnic differences in the risk of compulsory psychiatric admission among representative cases of psychosis in London. *British Medical Journal, 312*, 533–7.

Department of Health (2005a) *New Ways of Working for Psychiatrists: Enhancing effective, person-centred services through new ways of working in multidisciplinary and multi-agency contexts.* London: Department of Health. Accessed on 20th November 2013 at http://eprints.nottingham.ac.uk/788/1/NWW_Psychs.pdf

Department of Health (2005b) *Delivering Race Equality in Mental Health Care: An action plan for reform inside and outside services and the government's response to the independent inquiry into the death of David Bennett.* London: Department of Health.

Deutsch, A. (1944) The first US Census of the Insane (1840) and its use as pro-slavery propaganda. *Bulletin of the History of Medicine, 15*, 469–82.

Dill, D.L., Chu, J.A., Grob, M.C. & Eisen, S.V. (1991) The reliability of abuse history reports: A comparison of two inquiry formats. *Comprehensive Psychiatry, 32*(2), 166–9. doi: 10.1016/0010-440X(91)90009-2.

Dillon, J. (2011) The personal is the political. Chapter 11 in M. Rapley, J. Moncrieff & J. Dillon (Eds.), *De-Medicalising Misery: Psychiatry, psychology and the human condition* (pp. 141–57). Basingstoke: Palgrave Macmillan.

Dillon, J. & Longden, E. (2012) Hearing voices groups: Creating safe spaces to share taboo experiences. In M. Romme & S. Escher (Eds.) *Psychosis as a Personal Crisis: An experience-based approach* (pp. 129–39). London: Routledge.

Double, D. (2002) The overemphasis on biomedical diagnosis in psychiatry. *Journal of Critical Psychology, Counselling and Psychotherapy, 2*, 40–7.

Double, D. (2007) Adolf Meyer's psychobiology and the challenge for biomedicine. *Philosophy, Psychiatry and Psychology, 14*, 331–9.

Duncan, B., Miller, S. & Sparks, J. (2004) *The Heroic Client.* San Francisco: Jossey-Bass.

Eagles, J. (1991) The relationship between schizophrenia and immigration. Are there alternatives to psychosocial hypotheses? *British Journal of Psychiatry, 159*, 783–9. doi: 10.1192/bjp.159.6.783.

EBMWG (Evidence-Based Medicine Working Group) (1992) Evidence-based medicine: A new approach to teaching the practice of medicine. *Journal of the American Medical Association, 268*, 2420–5.

Elkin, I., Shea, M., Watkins, J., Imber, S., Sotsky, S., Collins, J. *et al* (1989) National Institute of Mental Health Treatment of Depression Collaborative Research Program: General effectiveness of treatments. *Archives of General Psychiatry, 46*, 971–82.

Ellenberger, H. (1970) *The Discovery of the Unconscious: The history and evolution of dynamic psychiatry.* London: HarperCollins.

Engel, G. (1977) The need for a new medical model: A challenge for biomedicine. *Science, 196*(4286), 129–36.

Escher, S. (1993) Talking about voices. In M. Romme & S. Escher (Eds.) *Accepting Voices* (pp. 50–8). London: MIND Publications.

Farahany, N. (2012) A neurological foundation for freedom. Stanford Technology Law Review, 4. Accessed on 29th November 2013 at http://stlr.stanford.edu/pdf/farahany-neurological-foundation.pdf

Faris, R.E.L. & Dunham, H.W. (1939) *Mental Disorders in Urban Areas*. Chicago: University of Chicago Press.

Faris, R.E.L. & Dunham, H.W. (1965) *Mental Disorders in Urban Areas: An ecological study of schizophrenia*. Chicago: University of Chicago Press.

Faulkner, A. & Layzell, S. (2000) *Strategies for Living: A report of user-led research into people's strategies for living with mental distress*. London: Mental Health Foundation.

FCDL (Federation for Community Development Learning) (2009) *National Occupational Standards in Community Development Work*. Accessed on 11th September 2013 at http://www.fcdl.org.uk/learning-qualifications/community-development-national-occupational-standards/

Fearon, P., Kirkbride, J., Morgan, C., Dazzan, P., Morgan, K., Lloyd, T. *et al* (2006) Incidence of schizophrenia and other psychoses in ethnic minority groups: Results from the MRC AESOP Study. *Psychological Medicine, 36*, 1541–50. doi: 10.1017/S0033291706008774.

Felitti, V., Anda, R., Nordenberg, D., Williamson, D., Spitz, A., Edwards, V. *et al* (1998) Relationship of childhood abuse and household dysfunction to many of the leading causes of death in adults: The Adverse Childhood Experiences (ACE) Study. *American Journal of Preventative Medicine, 14*, 245–58.

Fernando, S. (1991) *Mental Health, Race and Culture*. Basingstoke/London: Macmillan/MIND Publications.

Fernando, S. (2011) A 'global' mental health programme or markets for Big Pharma? *Open Mind, 168*, 22.

Fibiger, C. (2012) Psychiatry, the pharmaceutical industry, and the road to better therapeutics. *Schizophrenia Bulletin, 38*, 649–50. doi:10.1093/schbul/sbs073.

Fisher, H.L., Craig, T.K., Fearon, P., Morgan, K., Dazzan, P., Lappin, J. & Morgan, C. (2011) Reliability and comparability of psychosis patients' retrospective reports of childhood abuse. *Schizophrenia Bulletin, 37*(3), 546–53. doi: 10.1093/schbul/sbp103.

Fodor, J. (1983) *The Modularity of Mind*. Cambridge, MA: MIT Press.

Foucault, M. (1982) Afterword. In H. Dreyfus & P. Rabinow, *Michel Foucault: Beyond structuralism and hermeneutics* (pp. 208–26). New York: Harvester Wheatsheaf.

Foucault, M. (2003) *The Birth of the Clinic: An archaeology of medical perception* (Trans. A. Sheridan). Abingdon: Routledge Classics. (First published in English in 1973 by Tavistock Publications.)

Foucault, M. (1961/2006a) *History of Madness* (Preface to the 1961 ed.) (Trans. J. Murphy & J. Khalfa). Routledge: London.

Foucault, M. (2006b) *Psychiatric Power: Lectures at the Collège de France, 1973–1974*. Basingstoke: Palgrave Macmillan.

Frances, A. (2009) Whither *DSM-V*? *British Journal of Psychiatry, 195*, 391–2. doi: 10.1192/bjp.bp.109.073932.

Frank, A. (1995) *The Wounded Storyteller: Body, illness and ethics*. Chicago: University of Chicago Press.

Fraser, W.I., King, K.M., Thomas, P. & Kendell, R.E. (1986) The diagnosis of schizophrenia by language analysis. *British Journal of Psychiatry, 148*, 275–8.

Freedman, R., Lewis, D., Michel, R., Pine, D., Schultz, S. *et al* (2013) The initial field trials of *DSM-5*: New blooms and old thorns. *American Journal of Psychiatry, 170*, 1–5.

Freire, P. (1996) *Pedagogy of the Oppressed* (Trans. M. Ramos). Harmondsworth: Penguin. (Original work published 1970 by Continuum Publishing.)

Fromm-Reichmann, F. (1948) Notes on the development of treatment of schizophrenics by psychoanalytic psychotherapy. *Psychiatry, 11*, 263–73.

Fulford, K.W.M. (1989) *Moral Theory and Medical Practice*. Cambridge: Cambridge University Press.

Fulford, K.W.M. (2002) Values in psychiatric diagnosis: Executive summary of a report to the Chair of the *ICD-12/DSM-VI* Coordination Task Force (Dateline 2010). *Psychopathology, 35*, 132–8.

Fulford, K., Thornton, T. & Graham, G. (2006) *Oxford Textbook of Philosophy and Psychiatry*. Oxford: Oxford University Press.

Furnham, A. & Bower, P. (1992) A comparison of academic and lay theories of schizophrenia. *British Journal of Psychiatry, 161*, 201–10. doi: 10.1192/bjp.161.2.201.

Geddes, J. & Lawrie, S. (1995) Obstetric complications and schizophrenia: a meta-analysis. *British Journal of Psychiatry, 167*, 786–93. doi: 10.1192/bjp.167.6.786.

Geertz, C. (1975) *The Interpretation of Cultures: Selected essays*. London: Hutchinson.

Gilbert, P.L., Harris, J., McAdams, L.A. & Jeste, D.V. (1995) Neuroleptic withdrawal in schizophrenic patients: A review of the literature. *Archives of General Psychiatry, 52*, 173–88.

Gilchrist, A. (2004) *The Well-Connected Community: A networking approach to community development*. Bristol: The Policy Press.

Gillam, S., Jarman, B., White, P. *et al* (1989) Ethnic differences in consultation rates in urban general practice. *British Medical Journal, 299*, 953–7.

Gilligan, C. (1982) *In a Different Voice: Psychological theory and women's development*. Cambridge, MA: Harvard University Press.

Gillon, R. (1985) *Philosophical Medical Ethics*. Chichester: Wiley.

Goldberg, D. & Huxley, P. (1980) *Mental Illness in the Community*. London: Tavistock.

Goldman, D. (2011) Molecular etiologies of schizophrenia: Are we almost there yet? *American Journal of Psychiatry, 168*, 879–81.

Goodman, L.A., Thompson, K.M., Weinfurt, K., Corl, S., Acker, P., Mueser, K.T. & Rosenberg, S.D. (1999) Reliability of reports of violent victimization and posttraumatic stress disorder among men and women with serious mental illness. *Journal of Traumatic Stress, 12*(4), 587–99. doi: 10.1023/A:1024708916143.

Greater London Authority (2006) A Profile of Londoners by Language: An analysis of Labour Force Survey data on first language. Data Management and Analysis Group. DMAG Briefing 2006/26. London: GLA. Accessed on 17th February 2014 at http://legacy.london.gov.uk/gla/publications/factsandfigures/dmag-briefing-2006-26.pdf

Green, J., McLaughlin, K., Berglund, P., Gruber, M., Sampson, N., Zaslavsky, A. & Kessler, R. (2010) Childhood adversity and adult psychiatric disorders in the National Comorbidity Survey Replication I: Associations with first onset of *DSM-IV* disorders. *Archives of General Psychiatry, 67*, 113–23. doi: 10.1001/archgenpsychiatry.2009.186.

Greenberg, M., Szmuckler, G. & Tantam, D. (1982) Guidelines on formulating a case for the MRCPsych examination. *Psychiatric Bulletin, 6*, 160–2. doi: 10.1192/pb.6.9.160-a.

Greenhalgh, T. & Hurwitz, B. (1999) Narrative-based medicine: Why study narrative? *British Medical Journal, 318*, 48–50.

Guardian, The (2011) Stephen Lawrence murder was racially motivated, court hears. Accessed 11th December 2012 at http://www.guardian.co.uk/uk/2011/nov/15/stephen-lawrence-murder-racially-motivated-trial

Guardian, The (2012a) Disability hate crime is at its highest level since records began. Datablog accessed on 13th November 2013 at http://www.theguardian.com/news/datablog/2012/aug/14/disability-hate-crime-increase-reported-incidents-data

Guardian, The (2012b) Police officers cleared in racism trial may face misconduct hearing. Accessed on 11th December 2012 at http://www.guardian.co.uk/uk/2012/nov/30/police-cleared-racism-misconduct-hearing

Guardian, The (2012c) Kick It Out slams top clubs for 'year wasted in hypocrisy'. Accessed on 10th December 2012 at http://www.guardian.co.uk/football/2012/dec/10/kick-it-out-hypocrisy-chelsea-liverpool

Guardian, The (2012d) Young black men hit by sharp rise in unemployment. Accessed on 13th December 2012 at http://www.guardian.co.uk/business/2012/oct/17/young-black-men-unemployment-tuc

Guardian, The (2012e) Stephen Lawrence's mother criticises ministers over race discrimination. Accessed on 28th December 2012 at http://www.guardian.co.uk/uk/2012/dec/18/stephen-lawrence-mother-race-discrimination

Hague, W. (2007) *William Wilberforce: The life of the great anti-slave trade campaigner.* London: Harper Press.

Haigh, R. (2012) The philosophy of greencare: Why it matters for our mental health. *Mental Health and Social Inclusion, 16*, 127–34. doi: 10.1108/20428301211255400.

Harding, C.M., Brooks, G.W. *et al* (1987) The Vermont longitudinal study of persons with severe mental illness: I. Methodology, study sample, and overall status 32 years later. *American Journal of Psychiatry, 144*(6), 718–26.

Harland, R., Morgan, C. & Hutchinson, G. (2004) Phenomenology, science and the anthropology of the self: A new model for the aetiology of psychosis. *British Journal of Psychiatry, 185*, 361–2. doi: 10.1192/bjp.185.5.361.

Harrison, G., Owens, D., Holton, A. *et al* (1988) A prospective study of severe mental disorder in Afro-Caribbean people. *Psychological Medicine, 18*, 643–57.

Harrison, G., Cooper, J. & Gancarczyk, R. (1991) Changes in the administrative incidence of schizophrenia. *British Journal of Psychiatry, 159*, 811–16. doi: 10.1192/bjp.159.6.811.

Harrow, M. & Jobe, T. (2007) Factors involved in outcome and recovery in schizophrenia patients not on antipsychotic medications: A 15-year multifollow-up study. *Journal of Nervous and Mental Disease, 195*, 406–14.

Harrow, M. & Jobe, T. (2013) Does long-term treatment of schizophrenia with antipsychotic medications facilitate recovery? *Schizophrenia Bulletin, 39*, 962–5. doi: 10.1093/schbul/sbt034.

Harrow, M., Jobe, T. & Faull, R. (2012) Do all schizophrenic patients need antipsychotic treatment continuously throughout their lifetime? A 20-year longitudinal study. *Psychological Medicine, 42*, 2145–55. doi: 10.1017/S0033291712000220.

Hart, H. & Rubia, K. (2012) Neuroimaging of child abuse: A critical review. *Frontiers in Human Neuroscience, 6*, Article 52. doi: 10.3389/fnhum.2012.00052.

Healy, D. (1997) *The Antidepressant Era.* New York: Harvard University Press.

Healy, D. & Farquhar, G. (1998) Immediate effects of droperidol. *Human Psychopharmacology, 13*, 113–20.

Heath, I. (2001) 'A fragment of the explanation': The use and abuse of words. *Journal of Medical Ethics: Medical Humanities, 27*, 64–9.

Heidegger, M. (1962) *Being and Time* (Trans. J. Macquarrie & E. Robinson). Oxford: Basil Blackwell.

Henderson, C., Flood, C., Leese, M., Thornicroft, G., Sutherby, K. & Szmuckler, G. (2004) Effect of joint crisis plans on use of compulsory treatment in psychiatry: Single blind randomised controlled trial. *British Medical Journal, 329*, 136–38. doi: 10.1136/bmj.38155.585046.63.

Hennessy, S., Bilker, W.B., Knauss, J.S., Margolis, D.J., Kimmel, S.E., Reynolds, R.F. *et al* (2002) Cardiac arrest and ventricular arrhythmia in patients taking antipsychotic drugs: Cohort study using administrative data. *British Medical Journal, 325*, 1070.

Hickling, F. & Rodgers-Johnson, P. (1995) The incidence of first-contact schizophrenia in Jamaica. *British Journal of Psychiatry, 167*, 193–6. doi: 10.1192/bjp.167.2.193.

Ho, B.-C., Andreasen, N., Ziebell, S., Pierson, R. & Magnotta, V. (2011) Long-term antipsychotic treatment and brain volumes: A longitudinal study of first-episode schizophrenia. *Archives of General Psychiatry, 68*, 128–37.

Holmes, J. (2000) Narrative in psychiatry and psychotherapy: The evidence? *Journal of Medical Ethics: Medical Humanities, 26*, 92–6. doi: 10.1136/mh.26.2.92.

Huber, G., Gross, G. *et al* (1975) A long-term follow-up study of schizophrenia: Psychiatric course of illness and prognosis. *Acta Psychiatrica Scandinavica, 52*, 49–7.

Hunter, K. (1991) *Doctors' Stories: The narrative structure of medical knowledge.* Princeton, NJ: Princeton University Press.

Husserl, E. (1967) *The Paris Lectures.* The Hague: Martinus Nijhoff.

Hutchinson, G., Takei, N., Bhugra, D., Fahy, T., Gilvarry, C., Mallett, R. *et al* (1997) Increased rate of psychosis among African-Caribbeans in Britain is not due to an excess of pregnancy and birth complications. *British Journal of Psychiatry, 171*, 145–7.

Huxley, A. (1954) *The Doors of Perception.* London: Chatto and Windus.

Hyman, S. (2013) *Psychiatric Drug Development: Diagnosing a crisis.* Accessed on 24th February 2014 at https://www.dana.org/Cerebrum/2013/Psychiatric_Drug_Development__Diagnosing_a_Crisis/

Insel, T. (2013) *Transforming Diagnosis.* The National Institute of Mental Health (The Director's Blog, April 29th, 2013). Accessed on 11th November 2013 at http://www.nimh.nih.gov/about/director/2013/transforming-diagnosis.shtml

Ioannidis, J. (2011) Excess significance bias in the literature on brain volume abnormalities. *Archives of General Psychiatry, 68*, 773–80.

Jacobson, N.S., Dobson, K.S., Truax, P.A., Addis, M., Koerner, K., Gollan, J.K. *et al* (1996) A component analysis of cognitive-behavioural treatment for depression. *Journal of Consulting and Clinical Psychology, 64*, 295–304.

Janssen, I., Hanssen, M., Bak, R., Bijl, V., De Graaf, R., Vollebergh, W. *et al* (2003) Discrimination and delusional ideation. *British Journal of Psychiatry, 182*, 71–6.

Janssen I., Krabbendam L., Bak, R., Hanssen, M., Vollebergh, W., de Graaf, R. & van Os, J. (2004) Childhood abuse as a risk factor for psychotic experiences. *Acta Psychiatrica Scandinavica, 109*, 38–45.

Jaspers, K. (1963) *General Psychopathology* (Trans. J. Hoenig & M. Hamilton). Manchester: University of Manchester Press.

Jaynes, J. (1976) *The Origins of Consciousness in the Breakdown of the Bicameral Mind.* Boston: Houghton Mifflin.

Johnstone, L. (2000) *Users and Abusers of Psychiatry: A critical look at traditional psychiatric practice.* London: Routledge.

Jonas, S., Bebbington, P., McManus, S., Meltzer, H., Jenkins, R., Kuipers, E. *et al* (2011) Sexual abuse and psychiatric disorder in England: Results from the 2007 Adult Psychiatric Morbidity Survey. *Psychological Medicine, 41*, 709–19.

Jones, G. & Berry, M. (1986) Regional secure units: The emerging picture. In G. Edwards (Ed.) *Current Issues in Clinical Psychology IV* (pp. 111–20). London: Plenum Press.

Jones, P., Murray, R.M. & Rodgers, B. (1994) Child development preceding adult schizophrenia. *Schizophrenia Research, 11*, 97.

Joseph, J. (2003) *The Gene Illusion: Genetic research in psychiatry and psychology under the microscope.* Ross-on-Wye: PCCS Books.

Kalathil, J., Collier, B., Bhakta, R., Daniel, O., Joseph, D. & Trivedi, P. (2011) *Recovery and Resilience: African, African-Caribbean and South Asian women's narratives of recovery from mental distress.* London: Mental Health Foundation.

Kaptchuk, T., Kelley, J., Conboy, L., Davis, R., Kerr, C. *et al* (2008) Components of placebo effect: Randomised controlled trial in patients with irritable bowel syndrome. *British Medical Journal, 336*(7651), 999–1003. doi: 10.1136/bmj.39524.439618.25.

Karlsen, S. & Nazroo, J. (2002) Relation between racial discrimination, social class, and health among ethnic minority groups. *American Journal of Public Health, 92*, 624–31.

Karlsen, S., Nazroo, J., McKenzie, K., Bhui, K. & Weich, S. (2005) Racism, psychosis and common mental disorder among ethnic minority groups in England. *Psychological Medicine, 35*, 1795–803. doi: 10.1017/S0033291705005830.

Katz, M., Cole, J. & Lowery, H. (1969) Studies of the diagnostic process: The influence of symptom perception, past experience and ethnic background on diagnostic decisions. *American Journal of Psychiatry, 125*, 937–47.

Kendell, R. (1975) *The Role of Diagnosis in Psychiatry.* Oxford: Blackwell Scientific Publications.

Kendell, R. & Jablensky, A. (2003) Distinguishing between the validity and utility of psychiatric diagnoses. *American Journal of Psychiatry, 160*, 4–12.

Kendler, K. (1980) The nosological validity of paranoia (simple delusional disorder). *Archives of General Psychiatry, 37*, 699–706.

Kendler, K., Bulik, C., Silberg, J., Hettema, J., Myers, J. & Prescott, C. (2000) Childhood sexual abuse and adult psychiatric and substance use disorders in women: An epidemiological and cotwin control analysis. *Archives of General Psychiatry, 57*, 953–9. doi: 10.1001/archpsyc.57.10.953.

Khan, A., Warner, H. & Brown, W. (2000) Symptoms reduction and suicide risk in patients treated with placebo in antidepressant clinical trials. *Archives of General Psychiatry, 57*, 311–33.

Kiev, A. (1965) Psychiatric morbidity amongst West Indian immigrants in urban general practice. *British Journal of Psychiatry, 111*, 51–6.

King, M., Coker, E., Leavey, G. *et al* (1994) Incidence of psychotic illness in London: Comparison of ethnic groups. *British Medical Journal, 309*, 1115–19.

Kingdon, D. & Young, A. (2007) Research into putative biological mechanisms of mental disorders has been of no value to clinical psychiatry. *British Journal of Psychiatry, 191*, 285–90.

Kirsch, I. & Sapirstein, G. (1998) Listening to Prozac but hearing placebo: A meta-analysis of antidepressant medication. *Prevention and Treatment, 1*, Article 0002a. doi: 10.1037/1522-3736.1.1.12a.

Kirsch, I., Deacon, B.J., Huedo-Medina, T.B., Scoboria, A., Moore, T.J. & Johnson, B.T. (2008) Initial severity and antidepressant benefits: a meta-analysis of data submitted to the Food and Drug Administration. *Public Library of Science: Medicine, 5*, e45.

Kleinman, A. (1991) *Rethinking Psychiatry: From cultural category to personal experience.* New York: Free Press.

Kleinman, A. (2008) The art of medicine. Catastrophe and caregiving: The failure of medicine as an art. *Lancet, 371*, 22–3.

Knight, T. (2006) *Beyond Belief: Alternative ways of working with delusions, obsessions and unusual experiences.* Berlin/Eugene, OR/Shrewsbury: Peter Lehmann Publishing.

Koffman, J., Fulpo, N., Pashley, D. *et al* (1997) Ethnicity and use of acute psychiatric beds: One-day survey in north and south Thames regions. *British Journal of Psychiatry, 171*, 238–41.

Kohn, M. (1995) *The Race Gallery: The return of racial science.* London: Jonathan Cape.

Kraepelin, E. (1913) *Psychiatrie: ein Lehrbuch für Studierende und Aertze [Psychiatry: a textbook for students and practitioners]* (8th ed.) Vol. 3. Leipzig: Barth.

Kraepelin, E. (1919) *Dementia Praecox and Paraphrenia (from the 8th German edition of the Textbook of Psychiatry Vol. 3, Part 2)* (Trans. M. Barclay; Ed. G. Robertson). Edinburgh: Livingstone.

Kramer, M. (1961) Some problems for international research suggested by observations on differences in first admission rates to the mental hospitals of England and Wales and of the United States. *Proceedings of the Third World Congress of Psychiatry, Vol. 3* (pp. 153–60) 4–10 June, Montreal, Canada. Toronto: University of Toronto Press.

Kreitman, N. (1961) The reliability of psychiatric diagnosis. *Journal of Mental Science, 107*, 876–86.

Kua, J., Wong, K.E. *et al* (2003) A 20-year follow-up study on schizophrenia in Singapore. *Acta Psychiatrica Scandinavica, 108*(2), 118–25.

Kuhn, T. (1962) *The Structure of Scientific Revolutions* (2nd ed.). Chicago: University of Chicago Press.

Kuriansky, J., Deming, W. & Gurland, B. (1974) On trends in the diagnosis of schizophrenia. *American Journal of Psychiatry, 131*, 402–8.

Labbé, J. (2005) Ambroise Tardieu: The man and his work on child maltreatment a century before Kempe. *Child Abuse and Neglect, 29*, 311–24.

Laing, R.D. (1960) *The Divided Self: An existential study in sanity and madness.* London: Tavistock Publications.

Laing, R.D. (1967) *The Politics of Experience.* New York: Ballantine.

Laing, R.D. & Cooper, D. (1964) *Reason and Violence: A decade of Sartre's philosophy* (2nd ed.). London: Tavistock Publications.

Lataster, T., van Os, J., Drukker, M., Henquet, C., Feron, F., Gunther, N. & Myin-Germeys, I. (2006) Childhood victimisation and developmental expression of non-clinical delusional ideation and hallucinatory experiences: Victimisation and non-clinical psychotic experiences. *Social Psychiatry and Psychiatric Epidemiology, 41*, 423–8.

Laursen, T.M., Munk-Olsen, T. & Vestergaard, M. (2012) Life expectancy and cardiovascular mortality in persons with schizophrenia. *Current Opinion in Psychiatry, 25*(2), 83–8.

Lavender, H., Khondoker, A. & Jones, R. (2006) Understandings of depression: An interview study of Yoruba, Bangladeshi and White British people. *Family Practice, 23*, 651–8.

Leff, J., Kuipers, L., Berkowitz, R., Vaughn, C. & Strugeon, C. (1983) Life events, relatives' expressed emotion and maintenance neuroleptics in schizophrenic relapse. *Psychological Medicine, 13*, 799–806.

Lehtinen, V., Aaltonen, J., Koffert, T., Rakkolainen, V. & Syvalahati, E. (2000) Two-year outcome in first-episode psychosis treated according to an integrated model: Is immediate neuroleptisation always necessary? *European Psychiatry, 15*, 312–20.

Leudar, I. & Thomas, P. (2000) *Voices of Reason, Voices of Insanity.* London: Routledge.

Lewin, M. (2009) Schizophrenia 'epidemic' among African Caribbeans spurs prevention policy change. Accessed on 19th December 2012 at http://www.guardian.co.uk/society/2009/dec/09/african-caribbean-schizophrenia-policy

Lewis, B. (2011) *Narrative Psychiatry: How stories can shape clinical practice.* Baltimore, MD: Johns Hopkins University Press.

Li, P., Jones, I. & Richards, J. (1994) The collection of general practice data for psychiatric service contacts. *Journal of Public Health Medicine, 16*, 87–92.

Lieberman, J.A., Tollefson, G.D., Charles, C., Zipursky, R., Sharma, T., Kahn, R.S. *et al* (2005) Antipsychotic drug effects on brain morphology in first-episode psychosis. *Archives of General Psychiatry, 62*, 361–70.

Lloyd, K. & St Louis, L. (1996) Common mental disorders among Africans and Caribbeans. In D. Bhugra & V. Bhal (Eds.) *Ethnicity: An agenda for mental health* (pp. 60–9). London: Gaskell.

Logothetis, N. (2008) What we can do and what we cannot do with fMRI. *Nature, 453*, 869–78. doi: 10.1038/nature06976.

Longden, E. (2013) *The Voices in My Head.* Accessed on 20th September 2013 at http://www.ted.com/talks/eleanor_longden_the_voices_in_my_head.html

Longden, E., Madill, A. & Waterman, M. (2011) Dissociation, trauma, and the role of lived experience: Toward a new conceptualization of voice hearing. *Psychological Bulletin, 138*, 28–76. doi: 10.1037/a0025995.

Longmore, R.J. & Worrell, M. (2007) Do we need to challenge thoughts in cognitive behaviour therapy? *Clinical Psychology Review, 27*, 173–87.

MacIntyre, A. (1981) *After Virtue.* Notre Dame, IN: University of Notre Dame Press.

MacMillan, H., Fleming, J., Streiner, D., Lin, E., Boyle, M., Jamieson, E. *et al* (2001) Childhood abuse and lifetime psychopathology in a community sample. *American Journal of Psychiatry, 158*, 1878–83. doi: 10.1176/appi.ajp.158.11.1878.

McCabe, R. & Priebe, S. (2004) Explanatory models of illness in schizophrenia: Comparison of four ethnic groups. *British Journal of Psychiatry, 185*, 25–30. doi: 10.1192/bjp.185.1.25.

McCabe, R., Heath, C., Burns, T. & Priebe, S. (2002) Engagement of patients with psychosis in the consultation: Conversation analytic study. *British Medical Journal, 325*, 1148–51.

McCulloch, A. (2001) Social environments and health: A cross sectional survey. *British Medical Journal, 323*, 208–9.

McKenzie, K. (1999) Something borrowed from the blues? We can use Lawrence inquiry findings to help eradicate racial discrimination in the NHS. *British Medical Journal, 318*, 616–7.

McKenzie, K. (2010) Building consensus for moving forward. *Psychological Medicine, 40*, 735–6. doi: 10.1017/S0033291709005674.

McKenzie, K., Whitley, R. & Weich, S. (2002) Social capital and mental health. *British Journal of Psychiatry, 181*, 280–3.

McNicoll, A. (2013) Patients at risk as 'unsafe' mental health services reach crisis point: Community Care investigation prompts minister to pledge to end 'institutional bias against mental health' in NHS. *Community Care*, 16th October 2013. Accessed on 31st October 2013 at http://www.communitycare.co.uk/2013/10/16/patients-at-risk-as-unsafe-mental-health-services-reach-crisis-point-2/#

McQueen, D. & Smith, P. (2012) Placebo effects: A new paradigm and relevance to psychiatry. *International Psychiatry, 9*, 1–3. Maden, A., Swinton, M. & Gunn, J. (1992) The ethnic origins of women serving a prison sentence. *British Journal of Criminology, 32*, 218–21.

Malaspina, D., Goetz, R., Friedman, J., Kaufmann, C., Faraone, S., Tsuang, M. *et al* (2001) Traumatic brain injury and schizophrenia in members of schizophrenia and bipolar disorder pedigrees. *American Journal of Psychiatry, 158*, 440–6.

Mapp, Y. & Nodine, J. (1962) Psychopharmacology II: Tranquilizers and antipsychotic drugs. *Psychosomatics, 3*, 458–63.

Marcus, M., Yasamy, T., van Ommeren, M., Chishom, D. & Shekhar, S. (2012) *Depression: A global public health concern*. WHO Department of Mental Health and Substance Abuse. Accessed on 6th March 2013 at http://www.who.int/mental_health/management/depression/who_paper_depression_wfmh_2012.pdf

Marx, O. (1970) Nineteenth-century medical psychology: Theoretical problems in the work of Griesinger, Meynert, and Wernicke. *Isis, 61*, 355–70.

Masson, J. (1984) *The Assault on Truth: Freud and child sexual abuse*. New York: Farrar, Straus & Giroux.

May, P., Tuma, A., Dixon, W., Yale, C., Thiele, D. & Kraude, W. (1981) Schizophrenia: A follow-up study of five forms of treatment. *Archives of General Psychiatry, 38*, 776–84.

May, Rollo (1958) Contributions of existential psychotherapy. In R. May, E. Angel & H. Ellenberger (Eds.) *Existence: A new dimension in psychiatry and psychology* (pp. 37–91). New York: Basic Books.

May, Rollo, Angel, E. & Ellenberger, H. (Eds.) (1956) *Existence: A new dimension in psychiatry and psychology*. New York: Basic Books.

May, Rufus (2007) Reclaiming mad experience: Establishing unusual belief groups and Evolving Minds public meetings. In P. Stastny & P. Lehmann (Eds.) *Alternatives Beyond Psychiatry* (pp. 117–27). Berlin/Eugene, OR/Shrewsbury: Peter Lehmann Publishing.

May, Rufus & Longden, E. (2010) Self-help approaches to hearing voices. In F. Larøi & A. Aleman (Eds.) *Hallucinations: A practical guide to treatment* (pp. 257–79). Oxford: Oxford University Press.

Mayes, R. & Horwitz, A. (2005) *DSM-III and the revolution in the classification of mental illness. Journal of the History of the Behavioural Sciences, 41*, 249–67.

Meissner, K., Kohls, N. & Colloca, L. (Eds.) (2011) Placebo effects in medicine: mechanisms and clinical implications. *Philosophical Transactions of the Royal Society, B: Biological Sciences, 366*, 1783–9.

Menninger, K. (1963) *The Vital Balance: The life process in mental health and illness*. New York: Viking Press.

Mental Health Foundation (1997) *Knowing Our Own Minds: A survey of how people in emotional distress take control of their lives*. London: Mental Health Foundation.

Metzl, J. (2009) *The Protest Psychosis: How schizophrenia became a black disease*. Boston: Beacon Press.

Meyer, A. (1957) *Psychobiology: A science of man*. Springfield, IL: Charles C. Thomas.

Meyer, I.H., Muenzenmaier, K., Cancienne, J. & Struening, E. (1996) Reliability and validity of a measure of sexual and physical abuse histories among women with serious mental illness. *Child Abuse & Neglect, 20*(3), 213–19. doi: 10.1016/S0145-2134(95)00137-9.

MIND (2003) *Evidence to The Independent Panel of Inquiry into the Events Leading to the Death of David Bennett*. London: MIND.

Minkowitz, T. (2013) The UN asks the US to defend its use of forced psychiatric drugging. Accessed at *Mad in America* on 19th September 2013 at http://www.madinamerica.com/2013/04/un-asks-the-united-states-to-defend-its-practice-of-forced-psychiatric-drugging/

Modood, T., Berthoud, R., Lakey, J. *et al* (1998) *Ethnic Minorities in Britain: Diversity and disadvantage. The Fourth National Survey of Ethnic Minorities*. London: Policy Studies Institute.

Moerman, D. (2002) *Meaning, Medicine and the 'Placebo Effect'*. Cambridge: Cambridge University Press.

Moncrieff, J. (1997) The medicalisation of modern living. *Soundings, 6*, 63–72.

Moncrieff, J. (2003) *Is Psychiatry for Sale? An examination of the influence of the pharmaceutical industry on academic and practical psychiatry*. Maudsley Discussion Paper No. 13. London: Institute of Psychiatry. Accessed on 24th May 2012 at http://www.critpsynet.freeuk.com/pharmaceuticalindustry.htm

Moncrieff, J. (2006) Does antipsychotic withdrawal provoke psychosis? Review of the literature on rapid onset psychosis (supersensitivity psychosis) and withdrawal-related relapse. *Acta Psychiatrica Scandinavica, 114*, 3–13.

Moncrieff, J. (2007) Are antidepressants as effective as they are claimed? No, they are not effective at all. *Canadian Journal of Psychiatry, 52*, 96–7.

Moncrieff, J. (2008) *The Myth of the Chemical Cure: A critique of psychiatric drug treatment*. Basingstoke: Palgrave Macmillan.

Moncrieff, J. (2009) A critique of the dopamine theory of schizophrenia and psychosis. *Harvard Review of Psychiatry, 17*, 214–25.

Moncrieff, J. (2010) Psychiatric diagnosis as a political device. *Social Health and Theory, 8*, 370–82.

Moncrieff, J. (2013) *The Bitterest Pills: The troubling story of antipsychotic drugs*. Basingstoke: Palgrave Macmillan.

Moncrieff, J. & Kirsch, I. (2005) Efficacy of antidepressants in adults. *British Medical Journal, 331*, 155–7.

Moncrieff, J. & Leo, J. (2010) A systematic review of the effects of antipsychotic drugs on brain volume. *Psychological Medicine, 40*, 1409–22.

Moncrieff, J., Wessely, S. & Hardy, R. (1998) Meta-analysis of trials comparing antidepressants with active placebo. *British Journal of Psychiatry, 172*, 227–31.

Moodley, P. & Perkins, R. (1991) Routes to psychiatric inpatient care in an inner London borough. *Social Psychiatry and Psychiatric Epidemiology, 26*, 47–51.

Mosher, L.R. (1998) *Letter of Resignation from the American Psychiatric Association*. Accessed 7th February 2012 at http://www.moshersoteria.com/articles/resignation--from--apa/

Mosher, L.R. (1999) Soteria and other alternatives to acute psychiatric hospitalization: A personal and professional review. *Journal of Nervous and Mental Disease, 187*, 142–49.

Mosher, L.R. & Burti, L. (1994) *Community Mental Health: A practical guide*. New York & London: W.W. Norton & Company.

Mosher L.R., Vallone, R. & Menn, A. (1995) The treatment of acute psychosis without neuroleptics: Six-week psychopathology outcome data from the Soteria project. *International Journal of Social Psychiatry, 41*, 157–73.

Mosher, L.R., Hendrix, V. & Fort, D. (2004) *Soteria: Through madness to deliverance*. Bloomington, IN: XLibris.

NACRO (National Association for the Care and Resettlement of Offenders) (1989) *Race and Criminal Justice*. London: NACRO.

National Collaborating Centre for Mental Health (2010) *Schizophrenia: The NICE guidelines on core interventions in the treatment and management of schizophrenia in adults in primary and secondary care* (updated ed.). London: British Psychological Society and Royal College of Psychiatrists. Accessed on 17th April 2010 at http://www.rcpsych.ac.uk/usefulresources/publications/niceguidelines/

Nazroo, J. (1998) Genetic, cultural or socioeconomic vulnerability? Expanding ethnic inequalities in health. *Sociology of Health and Illness, 20*, 714–34.

Nelson, R., Glenny, A.M. & Song, F. (2009) Intervention review: Antimicrobial prophylaxis for colorectal surgery. *Cochrane Database of Systematic Reviews 2009, Issue 1*. Art. No: CD001181. doi: 10.1002/14651858.CD001181.pub3.

New York City Department of Health and Mental Hygiene (2013) *Program Overview*, June 4, 2013. Accessed on 7th January 2014 at http://www.nyc.gov/html/doh/html/mental/parachute.shtml

Noë, A. (2009) *Out of Our Heads: Why you are not your brain, and other lessons from the biology of consciousness*. New York: Hill and Wang.

Noë, A. (2012) *Varieties of Presence*. Cambridge, MA: Harvard University Press.

Norman, R. & Malla, A. (1993) Stressful life events and schizophrenia: I. A review of the research. *British Journal of Psychiatry, 162*, 161–6.

NSC NHS Strategic Health Authority (2003) *Independent Inquiry into the Death of David Bennett: An independent inquiry set up under HSG (94)27*. Accessed on 22nd January 2005 at http://www.irr.org.uk/pdf/bennett_inquiry.pdf

O'Hagan, M. (1996) Two Accounts of Mental Distress. In J. Read & J. Reynolds (Eds.) *Speaking Our Minds: An anthology* (pp. 44–50). London: Macmillan/Open University.

Obeyesekere, G. (1985) Depression, Buddhism, and the work of culture in Sri Lanka. In A. Kleinman & B. Good (Eds.) *Culture and Depression* (pp. 134–52). Berkeley and Los Angeles: University of California Press.

Ødegaard, O. (1932) Emigration and insanity. *Acta Psychiatrica et Neurologica Scandinavia (suppl 4)*, 1–206.

Organisation for Economic Cooperation and Development (2011) *An Overview of Growing Income Inequalities in OECD Countries: Main findings*. Accessed on 15th November 2013 at http://www.oecd.org/els/soc/49499779.pdf

Ovid (1986) *Metamorphoses: Tereus, Procne and Philomela* (Trans. A.D. Melville) (Book 6, pp. 34–42, lines 422–674). The World's Classics. Oxford: Oxford University Press.

Oyebode, F. & Humphreys, M. (2011) The future of psychiatry. *British Journal of Psychiatry, 199*, 439–40. doi: 10.1192/bjp.bp.111.092338.

Papageorgiou, A., King, M., Janmohamed, A., Davidson, O. & Dawson, J. (2002) Advance directives for patients compulsorily admitted to hospital with serious mental illness. *British Journal of Psychiatry, 181*, 513–19.

Parker, G. (1990) The parental bonding instrument. *Social Psychiatry and Psychiatric Epidemiology, 25*(6), 281–2. doi: 10.1007/BF00782881.

Pickett, K. & Wilkinson, R. (2013) Health inequality is blighting the UK. *The Independent*, 25th October. Accessed on 28th October 2013 at http://www.independent.co.uk/voices/comment/health-inequality-is-blighting-the-uk-8904398.html

Pilgrim, D. (2007) The survival of psychiatric diagnosis. *Social Science and Medicine, 65*, 536–44.

Porter, R. (1997) *The Greatest Benefit to Mankind: A medical history of humanity from antiquity to the present*. London: HarperCollins.

Prilleltensky, I. (2012) Wellness as fairness. *American Journal of Community Psychology, 49*, 1–21.

Prouty, G., Van Werde, D. & Pörtner, M. (2002) *Pre-Therapy: Reaching contact-impaired clients*. Ross-on-Wye: PCCS Books.

Putnam, H. (1982) *Reason, Truth and History*. Cambridge: Cambridge University Press.

Putnam, R.D. (1996) The strange disappearance of civic America. *The American Prospect, 7*, 1–18.

Putnam, R.D. (2000) *Bowling Alone: Collapse and revival of American community*. New York: Simon and Schuster.

Querido, A. (1966) The shaping of community mental health care. *British Journal of Psychiatry, 114*, 293–302.

Radford, L., Corral, S., Bradley, C., Fisher, H., Bassett, C., Howat, N. & Collishaw, S. (2011) *Child Abuse and Neglect in the UK Today*. London: NSPCC.

Ramesh, R. (2011) Income inequality growing faster in the UK than any other rich country, says OECD. *The Guardian*, 5th December 2011. Accessed on 31st October 2013 at http://www.theguardian.com/society/2011/dec/05/income-inequality-growing-faster-uk

Rappaport, M., Hopkins, H., Hall, K., Belleza, T. & Silverman, J. (1978) Are there schizophrenics for whom drugs may be unnecessary or contraindicated? *International Pharmacopsychiatry, 13*, 100–11.

Ray, W., Chung, C., Murray, K., Hall, K. & Stein, C. (2009) Atypical antipsychotic drugs and the risk of sudden cardiac death. *New England Journal of Medicine, 360*, 225–35.

Read, J. (1997) Child abuse and psychosis: A literature review and implications for professional practice. *Professional Psychology: Research and Practice, 28*(5), 448–56. doi: 10.1037/0735-7028.28.5.448.

Read, J. & Bentall, R.P. (2010) The effectiveness of electroconvulsive therapy: A literature review. *Epidemiologia e Psichiatria Sociale, 19*, 333–47.

Read, J. & Reynolds, J. (Eds.) (1996) *Speaking Our Minds: An anthology*. London: Macmillan/Open University.

Read, J., Perry, B.D., Moskowitz, A. & Connolly, J. (2001) The contribution of early traumatic events to schizophrenia in some patients: A traumagenic neurodevelopmental model. *Psychiatry, 64*, 319–45.

Read, J., van Os, J., Morrison, A.P. & Ross, C.A. (2005) Childhood trauma, psychosis and schizophrenia: A literature review with theoretical and clinical implications. *Acta Psychiatrica Scandinavica, 112*, 330–50. doi: 10.1111/j.1600-0447.2005.00634.x.

Read, J., Bentall, R.P. & Fosse, R. (2009) Time to abandon the bio-bio-bio model of psychosis: Exploring the epigenetic and psychological mechanisms by which adverse life events lead to psychotic symptoms. *Epidemiologia e Psichiatria Sociale, 18*(4), 299–310.

Relton, P. & Thomas, P. (2002) Acute wards: Problems and solutions. Alternatives to acute wards: Users' perspectives. *Psychiatric Bulletin, 26*, 346–7.

Rethink (2013) *Lethal Discrimination: Why people with mental illness are dying needlessly and what needs to change*. London: Rethink. Accessed on 16th January 2014 at http://www.rethink.org/media/810988/Rethink%20Mental%20Illness%20-%20Lethal%20Discrimination.pdf

Reynolds, J., Muston, R., Heller, T., Leach, J., McCormick, M., Wallcraft, J. & Walsh, M. (Eds.) (2009) *Mental Health Still Matters*. Basingstoke/Milton Keynes: Palgrave Macmillan/Open University.

Ricoeur, P. (1984) *Time and Narrative Vol. 1* (Trans. K. Mcloughlin & D. Pellauer). Chicago: University of Chicago Press.

Roberts, A. (2008) A crusade for dignity: Andrew Roberts recalls his involvement in the foundation of the Mental Patients Union. *The Guardian*, 3rd September. Accessed on 30th April 2014 at http://www.theguardian.com/society/2008/sep/03/mentalhealth.health

Robins, E. & Guze, S. (1970) Establishment of diagnostic validity in psychiatric illness: Its application to schizophrenia. *American Journal of Psychiatry, 126*, 983–7.

Rogers, A., Pilgrim, D. & Lacey, R. (1993) *Experiencing Psychiatry: Users' views of services*. London: Mind/Macmillan.

Romme, M. & Escher, S. (1993a) *Accepting Voices*. London: Mind.

Romme, M. & Escher, S. (1993b) The new approach: A Dutch experiment. In M. Romme & S. Escher (Eds.) *Accepting Voices* (pp. 11–27). London: MIND Publications.

Romme, M. & Escher, S. (2000) *Making Sense of Voices: A guide for mental health professionals working with voice hearers*. London: MIND.

Romme, M. & Escher, S. (2006) Trauma and hearing voices. In W. Larkin & A. Morrison (Eds.) *Trauma and Psychosis* (pp. 162–91). London: Routledge.

Romme, M. & Escher, S. (Eds.) (2012) *Psychosis as a Personal Crisis: An experience-based approach*. Hove: Routledge.

Romme, M., Escher, S., Dillon, J., Corstens, D. & Morris, M. (2009) *Living with Voices: 50 stories of recovery*. Ross-on-Wye: PCCS Books.

Rose, D. (2001) *Users' Voices: The perspectives of mental health service users on community and hospital care*. London: Sainsbury Centre for Mental Health.

Rose, N. (2003) Neurochemical selves. *Society, November/December*, 46–59.

Rose, S. (2001) Moving on from old dichotomies: Beyond nature–nurture towards a lifeline perspective. *British Journal of Psychiatry, 78*, s3–s7. doi: 10.1192/bjp.178.40.s3.

Rosenhan, D. (1973) On being sane in insane places. *Science, 179*, 250–8.

Rosenzweig, P., Brohier, S. & Zipfel, A. (1993) The placebo effect in healthy volunteers: Influence of experimental conditions on the adverse events profile during phase I studies. *Clinical Pharmacology and Therapeutics, 54*, 578–83.

Rushton, P. (1995) *Race, Evolution and Behaviour: A life history perspective*. New Brunswick, NJ: Transaction Publishers.

Sackett, D., Rosenberg, W., Muir Gray, J., Haynes, R. & Richardson, W. (1996) Evidence-based medicine: What it is and what it isn't. *British Medical Journal, 312*, 71–2.

Sadler, J. (2005) *Values and Psychiatric Diagnosis*. Oxford: Oxford University Press.

Salimpoor, V., van den Bosch, I., Kovacevic, N., McIntosh, A., Dagher, A. & Zatorre, R. (2013) Interactions between the nucleus accumbens and auditory cortices predict music reward value. *Science, 340*(6129), 216–19. doi: 10.1126/science.1231059.

Sanders, L. (2013) No new meds: With drug firms in retreat, the pipeline for new psychiatric medications dries up. *Science News*, 23 February 2013. Accessed on 21st October 2013 at https://www.sciencenews.org/article/no-new-meds

Sandifer, M., Pettus, C. & Quade, D. (1964) A study of psychiatric diagnosis. *Journal of Nervous and Mental Disease, 139*, 350–6.

Sargant, W. & Slater, E. (1972) *An Introduction to Physical Methods of Treatment in Psychiatry*. Edinburgh: Churchill Livingstone.

Sartre, J.-P. (1958) *Being and Nothingness*. London: Methuen.

Sashidharan, S. (1993) Afro-Caribbeans and schizophrenia: The ethnic vulnerability hypothesis re-examined. *International Review of Psychiatry, 5*, 129–44.

Sastry, J. & Ross, C. (1998) Asian ethnicity and the sense of personal control. *Social Psychology Quarterly, 61*, 10–20.

Schooler, N., Goldberg, S., Boothe, H. & Cole, J. (1967) One year after discharge: Community adjustment of schizophrenic patients. *American Journal of Psychiatry, 123*, 947–53.

Schreier, A., Wolke, D., Thomas, K., Horwood, J., Hollis, C., Gunnell, D. *et al* (2009) Prospective study of peer victimization in childhood and psychotic symptoms in a nonclinical population at age 12 years. *Archives of General Psychiatry, 66*, 527–36.

Schrödinger, E. (1992) *What is Life? With mind and matter and autobiographical sketches*. Cambridge: Cambridge University Press.

Sainsbury Centre for Mental Health (SCMH) (2002) *Breaking the Circles of Fear: A review of the relationship between mental health services and African and Caribbean communities*. London: Sainsbury Centre for Mental Health.

Searle, J. (1983) *Intentionality: An essay in the philosophy of mind*. Cambridge: Cambridge University Press.

Seebohm, P., Henderson, P., Munn-Giddings, C., Thomas, P. & Yasmeen, S. (2005) *Together We Will Change: Community development, mental health and diversity*. London: Sainsbury Centre for Mental Health.

Seebohm, P., Thomas, P. & Brown, C. (2009) Outcomes and Commissioning in Mental Health
   Services for Black and Minority Ethnic Communities: Project Report. Accessed on 18th
   September 2013 at http://mighealth.net/uk/images/5/51/Mhcomm.pdf
Seikkula, J., Alakare, B., Aaltonen, J., Holma, J., Rasinkangas, A. & Lehtinen, V. (2003) Open
   dialogue approach: Treatment principles and preliminary results of a two-year follow-up on
   first-episode schizophrenia. *Ethical Human Sciences and Services, 5,* 163–82.
Seikkula, J., Aaltonen, J., Alakare, B., Haarakangas, H., Keranen, J. & Lehtinen, K. (2006) Five-year
   experience of first-episode nonaffective psychosis in open-dialogue approach: Treatment
   principles, follow-up outcomes, and two case studies. *Psychotherapy Research, 16,* 214–28.
Sernyak, M., Leslie, D., Alarcon, R., Losonczy, M. & Rosenheck, R. (2002) Association of diabetes
   mellitus with use of atypical neuroleptics in the treatment of schizophrenia. *American Journal
   of Psychiatry, 159,* 561–6.
Shah, A.K. (1999) Difficulties experienced by a Gujarati psychiatrist in interviewing elderly
   Gujaratis in Gujarati. *International Journal of Geriatric Psychiatry, 14,* 1072–4.
Shah, P. & Mountain, D. (2007) The medical model is dead – long live the medical model. *British
   Journal of Psychiatry, 191,* 375–7.
Sharpley, M., Hutchinson, G., Murray, R. & McKenzie, K. (2001) Understanding the excess
   of psychosis among the African-Caribbean population in England: Review of current
   hypotheses. *British Journal of Psychiatry, 178:* s60–s68. doi: 10.1192/bjp.178.40.s60.
Shea, M., Elkin, I., Imber, S., Sotsky, S., Watkins, J., Collins, J. *et al* (1992) Course of depressive
   symptoms over follow-up: Findings from the National Institute of Mental Health Treatment
   of Depression Collaborative Research Program. *Archives of General Psychiatry, 49,* 782–7.
Simpson, E. & House, A. (2002) Involving users in the delivery and evaluation of mental health
   services: Systematic review. *British Medical Journal, 325,* 1265–70.
Singh, S., Greenwood, N., White, S. & Churchill, R. (2007) Ethnicity and the Mental Health Act:
   Systematic review. *British Journal of Psychiatry, 191,* 99–105. doi: 10.1192/bjp.bp.106.030346.
Slater, L. (2004) *Opening Skinner's Box: Great psychological experiments of the twentieth century.*
   London: Bloomsbury.
SOED (2007) *Shorter Oxford English Dictionary* (6th ed). Oxford: Oxford University Press.
Spandler, H. (2006) *Asylum to Action: Paddington Day Hospital, therapeutic communities and
   beyond.* London: Jessica Kingsley Publishing.
Spataro, J., Mullen, P., Burgess, P.M., Wells, D.L. & Moss, S.A. (2004) Impact of child sexual abuse
   on mental health: Prospective study in males and females. *British Journal of Psychiatry,
   184*(5), 416–21. doi: 10.1192/bjp.184.5.416.
Special Hospitals Service Authority (1993) *Report of the Committee of Inquiry into the Death in
   Broadmoor of Orville Blackwood and a Review of the Deaths of Two Other Afro-Caribbean
   Patients: 'Big, black and dangerous?'* (The Prins Report). London: Special Hospitals Service
   Authority.
Spitzer, R. & Fliess, J. (1974) A re-analysis of the reliability of psychiatric diagnosis. *British Journal
   of Psychiatry, 125,* 341–7. doi: 10.1192/bjp.125.4.341.
Stastny, P. & Lehmann, P. (2007) *Alternatives Beyond Psychiatry.* Berlin/Eugene, OR/ Shrewsbury:
   Peter Lehmann Publishing.
Steen, R.G., Mull, C., McClure, R., Hamer, R.M. & Lieberman, J.A. (2006) Brain volume in first-
   episode schizophrenia: Systematic review and meta-analysis of magnetic resonance imaging
   studies. *British Journal of Psychiatry, 188,* 510–18.
Strauss, J. & Carpenter, W. (1974a) The prediction of outcome in schizophrenia. II: Relationships
   between predictor and outcome variables. *Archives of General Psychiatry, 31,* 37–42.
Strauss, J. & Carpenter, W. (1974b) Characteristic symptoms and outcome in schizophrenia.
   Archives of General Psychiatry, 30, 429–34.
Strauss, J. & Carpenter, W. (1977) Prediction of outcome in schizophrenia. III: Five-year outcome
   and its predictors. *Archives of General Psychiatry, 34,* 159–63.

Stufflebeam, R. & Bechtel, W. (1997) PET: Exploring the myth and the method. *Philosophy of Science, 64,* Supplement. Proceedings of the 1996 biennial meetings of the Philosophy of Science Association. Part II: Symposia Papers (December 1997), S95–S106. Accessed on 2nd December 2013 at http://www.jstor.org/stable/188393

Sugarman, P. & Craufurd, D. (1994) Schizophrenia in the Afro-Caribbean community. *British Journal of Psychiatry, 164,* 474–80. doi: 10.1192/bjp.164.4.474.

Sullivan, H. (1931) The modified psychoanalytic treatment of schizophrenia. *American Journal of Psychiatry, 11,* 519–40.

Sullivan, H. (1956) *Schizophrenia as a Human Process.* New York: Norton.

Sweeney, A., Beresford, P., Faulkner, A., Nettle, M. & Rose, D. (Eds.) (2009) *This Is Survivor Research.* Ross-on-Wye: PCCS Books.

Szasz, T. (1960) The myth of mental illness. *American Psychologist, 15,* 113–18.

Szasz, T. (1972) *The Myth of Mental Illness.* London: Paladin.

Szasz, T. (1974) *The Myth of Mental Illness: Foundations of a theory of personal conduct* (rev. ed., first published 1961). New York: HarperCollins.

Szasz, T. (2007) *The Medicalization of Everyday Life.* New York: Syracuse University Press.

Tallis, R. (2011) *Aping Mankind: Neuromania, Darwinitis and the misrepresentation of humanity.* Durham: Acumen.

Tardieu, A. (1859) *Étude Médico-Légale sur les Attentats aux Moeurs.* Paris: J.B. Baillière et fils. September edition. Accessed on 2nd November 2012 at http://www.archive.org/details/tudemdicol01tard

Tardieu, A. (1860) Étude médico-légale sur les sévices et mauvais traitement exercés sur des enfants. *Annales d'Hygiène Publique et de Médecine Légale, 13,* 361–98.

Taylor, C. (1989) *Sources of the Self: The making of the modern identity.* Cambridge: Cambridge University Press.

Temerlin, M. (1968) Suggestion effects in psychiatric diagnosis. *Journal of Nervous and Mental Disease, 147,* 349–53.

Thara, R. (2004) Twenty-year course of schizophrenia: The Madras Longitudinal Study. *Canadian Journal of Psychiatry, 49*(8), 564–9.

Thomas, C., Stone, K., Osborn, M., Thomas, P. & Fisher, M. (1993) Psychiatric morbidity and compulsory admission among UK-born Europeans, Afro-Caribbeans and Asians in central Manchester. *British Journal of Psychiatry, 163,* 91–9. doi: 10.1192/bjp.163.1.91.

Thomas, P. (1997) *The Dialectics of Schizophrenia.* London: Free Association Books.

Thomas, P. (2011) Biological explanations for and responses to psychosis. In D. Pilgrim, A. Rogers & B. Pescosolido (Eds.) *The SAGE Handbook of Mental Health and Illness* (pp. 291–312). London: Sage.

Thomas, P. (2013) Soteria: Contexts, practice and philosophy. In S. Coles, S. Keenan & B. Diamond (Eds.) *Madness Contested: Power and practice* (pp 141–57). Ross-on-Wye: PCCS Books.

Thomas, P. & Bracken, P. (2011) Dualisms and the myth of mental illness. In M. Rapley, J. Moncrieff & J. Dillon (Eds.) *De-Medicalizing Misery: Psychiatry, psychology and the human condition* (pp. 10–26). Basingstoke: Palgrave Macmillan.

Thomas, P. & Cahill, A. (2004) Compulsion and psychiatry – the role of advance statements. *British Medical Journal, 329,* 122–3.

Thomas, P., Bracken, P. & Leudar, I. (2004) Hearing voices: A phenomenological-hermeneutic approach. *Cognitive Neuropsychiatry, 9,* 13–23.

Thomas, P., Bracken, P. & Timimi, S. (2012) The limits of evidence-based medicine in psychiatry. *Philosophy, Psychiatry and Psychology, 19,* 295–308.

Thomas, P., Seebohm, P., Henderson, P., Munn-Giddings, C. & Yasmeen, S. (2006) Tackling race inequalities: Community development, mental health and diversity. *Journal of Public Mental Health, 5,* 13–19.

Thomas, P. & Longden, E. (2013) Madness, childhood adversity, and narrative psychiatry: Caring and the moral imagination. *Medical Humanities, 39*, 119–25. doi: 10.1136/medhum-2012-010268.

Thomas, P., Shah, A. & Thornton, T. (2009) Language, games and interpretation: A Wittgensteinian thought experiment. *Medical Humanities, 35*, 13–18.

Thornicroft, G. (1990) Cannabis and psychosis: Is there epidemiological evidence for an association? *British Journal of Psychiatry, 157*, 25–33. doi: 10.1192/bjp.157.1.25.

Thornicroft, G. (2011) Physical health disparities and mental illness: The scandal of premature mortality. *British Journal of Psychiatry, 199*, 441–2.

Thornicroft, G., Margolius, O. & Jones, D. (1992) The TAPS project. 6: New long-stay psychiatric patients and social deprivation. *British Journal of Psychiatry, 161*, 621–4.

Tillich, P. (1952) *The Courage to Be*. New Haven, CT: Yale University Press.

Timimi, S. (2011) *No More Psychiatric Labels*. Accessed on 7th May 2012 at http://www.criticalpsychiatry.net/?p=813

TSO (The Stationery Office) (1999) *The Stephen Lawrence Inquiry: Report of an inquiry by Sir William Macpherson of Cluny*. Accessed on 14th December 2012 at http://www.archive.official-documents.co.uk/document/cm42/4262/sli-06.htm#6.34

Tyrer, P. (2012) The end of the psychopharmacological revolution. *British Journal of Psychiatry, 201*, 168. doi: 10.1192/bjp.201.2.168.

Tyrka, A., Burgers, D., Philip, N., Price, L., & Carpenter, L. (2013) The neurobiological correlates of childhood adversity and implications for treatment. *Acta Psychiatrica Scandinavica, 128*(6), 434–47. doi: 10.1111/acps.12143.

van Lutterveld, R., Diederen, K., Koops, S., Begemann, M. & Sommer, I. (2013) The influence of stimulus detection on activation patterns during auditory hallucinations. *Schizophrenia Research, 145*, 27–32. http://dx.doi.org/10.1016/j.schres.2013.01.004.

Van Orden, G. & Paap, K. (1997) Functional neuroimages fail to discover pieces of mind in the parts of the brain. *Philosophy of Science, 64*, Supplement. Proceedings of the 1996 biennial meetings of the Philosophy of Science Association. Part II: Symposia Papers (Dec, 1997), S85–S94. Accessed on 26 April 2014 at http://www.jstor.org/discover/10.2307/188392?uid=3738032&uid=2134&uid=2&uid=70&uid=4&sid=21104081691003

van Os, J., Castle, D., Takei, N. *et al* (1996) Psychotic illness in ethnic minorities: Clarification from the 1991 census. *Psychological Medicine, 26*, 203–8.

Varela, F., Thompson, E. & Rosch, E. (1991) *The Embodied Mind: Cognitive science and human experience*. Cambridge, MA: MIT Press.

Vaughn, C. & Leff, J. (1976) The influence of family life and social factors on the course of psychiatric illness: A comparison of schizophrenic and depressed neurotic patients. *British Journal of Psychiatry, 129*, 125–37.

Veiga-Martinez, C., Perez-Alvarez, M. & Garcia-Montes, J. (2008) Acceptance and commitment therapy applied to treatment of auditory hallucinations. *Clinical Case Studies, 7*, 118–35.

Viguera, A., Baldessarini, R., Hegarty, J., van Kammen, D. & Tohen, M. (1997) Clinical risk following abrupt and gradual withdrawal of maintenancy neuroleptic treatment. *Archives of Geneneral Psychiatry, 54*, 49–55.

Wallcraft, J., Read, J. & Sweeney, A. (2003) *On Our Own Terms: Users and survivors of mental health services working together for support and change*. London: Sainsbury Centre for Mental Health.

Walls, P. & Sashidharan, S. (2003) *Real Voices – Survey findings from a series of community consultation events involving black and minority ethnic groups in England*. London: Department of Health.

Wampold, B.E. (2001) *The Great Psychotherapy Debate: Models, methods, and findings*. Hillsdale, NJ: Lawrence Erlbaum.

Warner, R. (1985) *Recovery from Schizophenia: Psychiatry and political economy*. London: Routledge and Kegan Paul.

Warnock, J. (1903) Insanity from hasheesh. *Journal of Mental Science, 49*, 96–110.

Weiss, K. (2011) Albert Deutsch, 1905–1961. *American Journal of Psychiatry, 168*, 252–252. doi: 10.1176/appi.ajp.2010.10101491.

Weitzman, E.R. & Kawachi, I. (2000) Giving means receiving: The protective effect of social capital on binge drinking on college campuses. *American Journal of Public Health, 90*, 1936–9.

Wessely, S., Castle, D., Der, G. & Murray, R. (1991) Schizophrenia and Afro-Caribbeans: A case-control study. *British Journal of Psychiatry, 159*, 795–801.

Whitaker, R. (2002) *Mad in America: Bad science, bad medicine, and the enduring mistreatment of the mentally ill.* Cambridge, MA: Perseus Publishing.

Whitaker, R. (2010) *Anatomy of an Epidemic: Magic bullets, psychiatric drugs, and the astonishing rise of mental illness in America.* New York: Broadway Paperbacks.

Whitaker, R. (2013) Do antipsychotics worsen long-term schizophrenia outcomes? Martin Harrow explores the question. *Mad in America*, 26th March 2013. Accessed on 13th December 2013 at https://www.madinamerica.com/2013/03/do-antipsychotics-worsen-long-term-schizophrenia-outcomes-martin-harrow-explores-the-question/

White, M. & Epston, D. (1990) *Narrative Means to Therapeutic Ends.* New York: W.W. Norton.

WHO (1998) Sertindole application withdrawn. *WHO Pharmaceuticals Newsletter, Nos. 03 & 04.* Accessed on 14th February at http://apps.who.int/medicinedocs/en/d/Js2256e/1.12.html#Js2256e.1.12

WHO (2012a) *Depression: Fact sheet N°369.* Accessed on 6th March 2013 at http://www.who.int/mediacentre/factsheets/fs369/en/

WHO (2012b) *Depression: Evidence-based recommendations for management of depression in non-specialized health settings.* Accessed on 6th March 2012 at http://www.who.int/mental_health/mhgap/evidence/depression/en/index.html

Wildgust, H., Hodgson, R. & Beary, M. (2010) The paradox of premature mortality in schizophrenia: New research questions. *Journal of Psychopharmacology 24*, Supplement 4, 9–15.

Wilkinson, R. & Pickett, K. (2009) *The Spirit Level: Why equality is better for everyone.* London: Penguin Books.

Wilson, M. (1993) *DSM-III* and the transformation of American psychiatry: A history. *American Journal of Psychiatry, 150*, 399–410.

Winter, R. & Munn-Giddings, C. (2001) *A Handbook for Action Research in Health and Social Care.* London & New York: Routledge.

Winters, K. & Neale, J. (1983) Delusions and delusional thinking in psychotics: A review of the literature. *Clinical Psychology Review, 3*, 227–53.

Wolkowitz, O. & Pickar, D. (1991) Benzodiazepines in the treatment of schizophrenia: A review and reappraisal. *American Journal of Psychiatry, 148*, 714–26.

Wong, D.R., Wagner, H.N., Tune, L.E. *et al* (1986) Positron emission tomography reveals elevated D2 dopamine receptors in drug-naive schizophrenics. *Science, 234*, 1558–63.

Woodbridge, K. & Fulford, K.W.M. (2004) *Whose Values?* London: Sainsbury Centre for Mental Health.

World Bank (1993) *World Development Report: Investing in health research development.* Geneva: World Bank.

Wunderink, L., Nieboer, R., Wiersma, D., Sytema, S. & Nienhuis, F. (2013) Recovery in remitted first-episode psychosis at 7 years of follow-up of an early dose reduction/discontinuation or maintenance treatment strategy: Long-term follow-up of a 2-year randomized clinical trial. *JAMA Psychiatry, 70*, 913–20. doi: 10.1001/jamapsychiatry.2013.19.

Wurr, C.J. & Partridge, I.M. (1996) The prevalence of a history of childhood sexual abuse in an acute adult inpatient population. *Child Abuse & Neglect, 20*(9), 867–72. doi: 10.1016/0145-2134(96)00074-9.

Zubin J. & Spring B. (1977) Vulnerability – a new view of schizophrenia. *Journal of Abnormal Psychology, 86*, 103–26.

Index

9 781906 254728